ADVANCES IN

Surgery

Editor-in-Chief
John L. Cameron, MD

ELSEVIER

PHILADELPHIA LONDON TORONTO MONTREAL SYDNEY TOKYO

VOLUME 49

1. What Are the Indications for Resection After an Episode of Sigmoid Diverticulitis? *by Anthony A. Meyer and Timothy S. Sadiq*

2. Hospital Readmissions: Are They Preventable? *by Erin G. Brown and Richard J. Bold*

3. Recent Advances in Intestinal and Multivisceral Transplantation *by Koji Hashimoto, Guilherme Costa, Ajai Khanna, Masato Fujiki, Cristiano Quintini, and Kareem Abu-Elmagd*

4. Which Is Best for Abdominal Aortic Aneurysms Treatment with Chronic Renal Insufficiency: Endovascular Aneurysm Repair or Open Repair? *by Bao-Ngoc Nguyen and Anton N. Sidawy*

5. What Is the Optimal Treatment of Papillary Thyroid Cancer? *by Christa L. Jillard, Randall P. Scheri, and Julie Ann Sosa*

6. Does Diet Make a Difference Following Colon Surgery? *by Cheryl Lau and Edward Phillips*

7. Principles in Management of Soft Tissue Sarcoma *by Aimee M. Crago and Murray F. Brennan*

8. Hospital Accreditation and Bariatric Surgery: Is It Important? *by Juan J. Blondet, John M. Morton, and Ninh T. Nguyen*

9. Trainee Participation in Emergency Surgery: What Are the Consequences? *by George Kasotakis and Gerard Doherty*

10. Laparoscopic Pancreaticoduodenectomy: Is It an Effective Procedure for Pancreatic Ductal Adenocarcinoma? *by May C. Tee, Michael L. Kendrick, and Michael B. Farnell*

11. Bariatric Surgery versus Intensive Medical Weight Management for Type 2 Diabetes *by Monica Sethi and Manish Parikh*

12. Should Steroids Be Used During Endovascular Aortic Repair? *by Louise de la Motte, Torben V. Schroeder, and Henrik Kehlet*

13. Are Higher Hospital Venous Thromboembolism Rates an Indicator of Better Quality?: Evaluation of the Validity of a Hospital Quality Measure *by Christina A. Minami and Karl Y. Bilimoria*

14. Fluid Restriction During Pancreaticoduodenectomy: Is It Effective in Reducing Postoperative Complications? *by Timothy I. Carter, Charles J. Yeo, and Harish Lavu*

15. Is There a Relationship Between Patient Satisfaction and Favorable Surgical Outcome *by Sarah E. Tevis, Gregory D. Kennedy, and K. Craig Kent*

16. Does Volume Affect Outcome with Severe Trauma? *by Jordan A. Weinberg and Timothy C. Fabian*

17. Hyperparathyroidism: What Preoperative Imaging Is Necessary? *by Rachel R. Kelz and Douglas L. Fraker*

18. Abscess After Appendectomy: Predisposing Factors *by Daniel E. Levin and Walter Pegoli Jr*

VOLUME 48

1. Inguinal Hernia: Follow or Repair? *by Bala Ramanan, Brittney J. Maloley, and Robert J. Fitzgibbons Jr*

2. Is It Safe to Follow Side Branch IPMNs? *by Giovanni Marchegiani and Carlos Fernàndez-del Castillo*

3. Endoscopic Myotomy for Achalasia *by Christy M. Dunst, Ashwin A. Kurian, and Lee L. Swanstrom*

4. Can Interventionalists do Endovascular Aortic Aneurysm Repair As Well As Vascular Surgeons? *by Tazo Inui and Dennis F. Bandyk*

5. Does Walking Speed Predict Postoperative Morbidity? *by Nicole T. Townsend and Thomas N. Robinson*

6. Does Close Temperature Regulation Affect Surgical Site Infection Rates? *by Ira L. Leeds, Elizabeth C. Wick, and Genevieve B. Melton*

7. The Utility of the Robot in Pancreatic Resections *by Amer H. Zureikat, Melissa E. Hogg, and Herbert J. Zeh III*

8. Current Treatment for Small (<5 cm) Hepatocellular Carcinoma: Evolving Roles for Ablation and Resection *by Amudhan Pugalenthi, C. Suzanne Cutter, and Yuman Fong*

9. Screening for Pancreatic Cancer *by Katherine E. Poruk, Matthew A. Firpo, and Sean J. Mulvihill*

10. Tissue Engineering *by Ravi S. Katari, Andrea Peloso, and Giuseppe Orlando*

11. Acute Cholecystitis: Early Versus Delayed Surgery *by Werner Hartwig and Markus W. Büchler*

12. Gastrointestinal Stromal Tumors: Who Should Get Imatinib and for How Long? *by Vinod P. Balachandran and Ronald P. DeMatteo*

13. Readmission After Surgery *by Donald J. Lucas and Timothy M. Pawlik*

14. What Is Wrong with the Training of General Surgery? *by Daniel T. McKenna and Samer G. Mattar*

15. Aspirin, Clopidogrel, and the Surgeon *by Prakash A. Patel and Lee A. Fleisher*

16. Islet Autotransplantation and Total Pancreatectomy *by Piotr Witkowski, Omid Savari, and Jeffrey B. Matthews*

17. Liver Transplantation for Metastatic Neuroendocrine Tumors *by Haniee Chung and William C. Chapman*

18. Irreversible Electroporation: A Novel Therapy for Stage III Pancreatic Cancer*by Matthew J. Weiss and Christopher L. Wolfgang*

VOLUME 47

1. Repair of Giant Ventral Hernias *by Jai Bikhchandani and Robert Joseph Fitzgibbons Jr*

2. Laparoscopic Colon Resection: Is It Being Utilized? *by Sean Joseph Langenfeld, Jon S. Thompson, and Dmitry Oleynikov*

3. Safety of Surgical Resident Training *by Usama Ahmed Ali and Jon D. Vogel*

4. Current Management of the Zollinger-Ellison Syndrome *by Geoffrey W. Krampitz and Jeffrey A. Norton*

5. What Laboratory Tests Are Required for Ambulatory Surgery? *by Jaime Benarroch-Gampel and Taylor S. Riall*

6. Factors Affecting Readmission After Pancreaticoduodenectomy *by Callisia N. Clarke, Jeffrey J. Sussman, Daniel E. Abbott, and Syed A. Ahmad*

7. Should Peritoneal Lavage Be Used with Suction During Laparoscopic Appendectomy for Perforated Appendicitis? *by Shawn D. St. Peter and George W. Holcomb III*

8. Appendicitis: Changing Perspectives *by Pedro G.R. Teixeira and Demetrios Demetriades*

9. Readmission After Abdominal Aortic Aneurysm Repair: What Does it Mean? *by David Yu Greenblatt, Sara Fernandes-Taylor, and K. Craig Kent*

10. Duodenal Switch for Morbid Obesity: Is it Safe? *by Rodney J. Mason*

11. Is Propranolol of Benefit in Pediatric Burn Patients? *by Celeste C. Finnerty and David N. Herndon*

12. What Is the Optimal Means of Staging Colon Cancer? *by Elizabeth A. Arena and Anton J. Bilchik*

13. The Effect of Do-Not-Resuscitate Status on Postoperative Mortality in the Elderly Following Emergency Surgery *by John E. Scarborough and Theodore N. Pappas*

14. Incidental Gall Bladder Cancer *by Anu Behari and Vinay K. Kapoor*

15. General Surgery Residency Training Issues *by Mary E. Klingensmith and Frank R. Lewis*

16. Is the Abdominal Aortic Aneurysm Rupture Rate Decreasing? *by Andy M. Lee and Elliot L. Chaikof*

17. Stress-induced Hyperglycemia: Is It Harmful Following Trauma? *by Patrick L. Bosarge and Jeffrey D. Kerby*

18. Improvement in the Diagnosis of Appendicitis *by Frederick Thurston Drake and David Reed Flum*

VOLUME 46

1. Who Should Have or Not Have an Axillary Node Dissection with Breast Cancer? *by Richelle T. Williams, David P. Winchester, Katharine Yao, and David J. Winchester*

2. Intestinal Stomas: Indications, Management, and Complications *by Sean T. Martin and Jon D. Vogel*

3. Zero Surgical Site Infections: Is It Possible? *by C. Daniel Smith*

4. Does Simulation Training Improve Outcomes in Laparoscopic Procedures? *by Benjamin Zendejas, Roberto Hernandez-Irizarry, and David R. Farley*

5. Hypertonic Resuscitation After Severe Injury: Is it of Benefit? *by Eileen M. Bulger and David B. Hoyt*

6. What is the Prognosis After Retransplantation of the Liver? *by Ali Zarrinpar and Johnny C. Hong*

7. Screening for Abdominal Aortic Aneurysms *by Joseph L. Bobadilla and K. Craig Kent*

8. Novel Management Strategies in the Treatment of Severe *Clostridium difficile* Infection *by Ibrahim Nassour, Evie H. Carchman, Richard L. Simmons, and Brian S. Zuckerbraun*

9. The Genetic Counselor: An Important Surgical Ally in the Optimal Care of the Cancer Patient *by Erin Salo-Mullen and Jose Guillem*

10. Readmission Rates after Abdominal Surgery: Can They Be Decreased to a Minimum? *by Thomas J. Lee and Robert C.G. Martin II*

11. Superiority of Minimally Invasive Parathyroidectomy *by John W. Kunstman and Robert Udelsman*

12. Current Treatment of Papillary Thyroid Microcarcinoma *by Xiao-Min Yu, Ricardo Lloyd, and Herbert Chen*

13. Use of Computed Tomography in the Emergency Room to Evaluate Blunt Cerebrovascular Injury *by Nancy A. Parks and Martin A. Croce*

14. How Important is Glycemic Control During Coronary Artery Bypass? *by Harold L. Lazar*

15. Capillary Leak Syndrome in Trauma: What is it and What are the Consequences? *by Deborah M. Stein and Thomas M. Scalea*

16. Morbidity and Effectiveness of Laparoscopic Sleeve Gastrectomy, Adjustable Gastric Band, and Gastric Bypass for Morbid Obesity *by Timothy D. Jackson and Matthew M. Hutter*

17. Are Cancer Trials Valid and Useful for the General Surgeon and Surgical Oncologist? *by Waddah B. Al-Refaie and Selwyn M. Vickers*

18. The Current Management of Pancreatic Neuroendocrine Tumors *by Trevor A. Ellison and Barish H. Edil*

Editor: John Vassallo
Developmental Editor: Meredith Clinton

Editorial Office:
Elsevier
1600 John F. Kennedy Blvd,
Suite 1800
Philadelphia, PA 19103-2899

International Standard Serial Number: 0065-3411
International Standard Book Number: 978-0-323-44682-2

CONTRIBUTORS

ALI F. ABURAHMA, MD, Medical Director, Vascular Laboratory, Director, Vascular Surgery Fellowship and Residency Programs, Chief, Vascular & Endovascular Surgery, Co-Director, Vascular Center of Excellence; Professor, Department of Surgery, West Virginia University, Charleston, West Virginia

JOHN C. ALVERDY, MD, FACS, Sarah and Harold Lincoln Thompson Professor of Surgery, Executive Vice-Chair, Department of Surgery, The University of Chicago Medicine, University of Chicago, Chicago, Illinois

PARVIZ K. AMID, MD, Professor, Department of Surgery, David Geffen School of Medicine at University of California Los Angeles, Los Angeles, California; Lichtenstein Amid Hernia Clinic at University of California Los Angeles, Santa Monica, California

KRISTEN A. BAN, MD, Clinical Scholar in Residence, Division of Research and Optimal Patient Care, American College of Surgeons, Chicago, Illinois; Resident, Department of Surgery, Loyola University Medical Center, Maywood, Illinois

RICHARD J. BATTAFARANO, MD, PhD, Chief, Division of Thoracic Surgery, Regional Director of Thoracic Surgery for Johns Hopkins Medicine; Associate Professor of Surgery, Johns Hopkins University School of Medicine, Baltimore, Maryland

ROBERTO BERGAMASCHI, MD, PhD, FRCS, FASCRS, FACS, Division of Colon & Rectal Surgery, State University of New York at Stony Brook, Stony Brook, New York

KARL Y. BILIMORIA, MD, MS, Faculty Scholar, Division of Research and Optimal Patient Care, American College of Surgeons; Director, Surgical Outcomes and Quality Improvement Center, Department of Surgery; Member, Center for Healthcare Studies, Feinberg School of Medicine, Northwestern University, Chicago, Illinois

JAMES G. BITTNER IV, MD, FACS, Assistant Professor of Surgery; Director, Virginia Commonwealth University Minimally Invasive Surgery Center, Director, Virginia Commonwealth University Comprehensive Hernia Center; Associate Program Director, General Surgery Residency, and Co-Director, Advanced GI Minimally Invasive Surgery Fellowship, Virginia Commonwealth University, Department of Surgery, Division of Bariatric and Gastrointestinal Surgery, Medical College of Virginia, Richmond, Virginia

L. MICHAEL BRUNT, MD, Professor, Department of Surgery, Section of Minimally Invasive Surgery, Washington University School of Medicine; Team Surgeon, St. Louis Blues Hockey Club, St Louis, Missouri

DAVID C. CHEN, MD, Associate Professor, Department of Surgery, David Geffen School of Medicine at University of California Los Angeles, Los Angeles, California; Lichtenstein Amid Hernia Clinic at University of California Los Angeles, Santa Monica, California

JOANN COLEMAN, DNP, ACNP-BC, Coordinator, Sinai Center for Geriatric Surgery, Sinai Hospital, Baltimore, Maryland

CRAIG M. COOPERSMITH, MD, Professor, Department of Surgery, Emory Critical Care Center, Emory University School of Medicine, Atlanta, Georgia

RAHILA ESSANI, MD, Division of Colon & Rectal Surgery, State University of New York at Stony Brook, Stony Brook, New York

CRISTINA R. FERRONE, MD, Associate Professor, Department of Surgery, Massachusetts General Hospital, Harvard Medical School, Boston, Massachusetts

KRISTINA L. GUYTON, MD, Surgical Resident, Department of Surgery, The University of Chicago Medicine, University of Chicago, Chicago, Illinois

LYNDSAY W. HEAD, MD, Assistant Professor, Department of Anesthesiology, Emory Critical Care Center, Emory University School of Medicine, Atlanta, Georgia

NEIL H. HYMAN, MD, FACS, FASCRS, Professor, Department of Surgery, Section Chief of Colon and Rectal Surgery, The University of Chicago Medicine, University of Chicago, Chicago, Illinois

MARK R. KATLIC, MD, MMM, FACS, Chairman, Department of Surgery, Surgeon-in-Chief and Director, Sinai Center for Geriatric Surgery, Sinai Hospital, Northwest Hospital, Baltimore, Maryland

GREGORY D. KENNEDY, MD, PhD, Chief, Associate Professor, Department of Surgery, University of Wisconsin School of Medicine and Public Health, Madison, Wisconsin

CHRISTINE V. KINNIER, MD, Resident, Department of Surgery, Massachusetts General Hospital, Boston, Massachusetts

RAVI P. KIRAN, MBBS, MS, FRCS, FACS, MSc (EBM), FASCRS, Division of Colorectal Surgery, New York Presbyterian Hospital, Columbia University Medical Center; Mailman School of Public Health, Columbia University, New York, New York

ANDREW P. LOEHRER, MD, Fellow, Department of Surgery, Massachusetts General Hospital, Boston, Massachusetts

MARK A. MALANGONI, MD, Associate Executive Director, American Board of Surgery, Philadelphia, Pennsylvania

ELEFTHERIOS (TERRY) P. MAMOUNAS, MD, MPH, FACS, Medical Director, Comprehensive Breast Program, University of Florida Health Cancer Center - Orlando Health, Orlando, Florida

ALBEIR Y. MOUSA, MD, Associate Professor, Department of Surgery, West Virginia University, Charleston, West Virginia

ALICE CHARLOTTE ADELAIDE MURRAY, BSc, MBBS, MRCS, Division of Colorectal Surgery, New York Presbyterian Hospital, Columbia University Medical Center, New York, New York

DAVID K. NGUYEN, MD, Chief Resident, Department of Surgery, David Geffen School of Medicine at University of California Los Angeles, Los Angeles, California

CHRISTINA M. PAPAGEORGE, MD, General Surgery Resident, Department of Surgery, University of Wisconsin School of Medicine and Public Health, Madison, Wisconsin

DAVID W. RATTNER, MD, FACS, Chief, Division of Gastrointestinal and General Surgery, Warshaw Family Professor of Surgery, Massachusetts General Hospital, Boston, Massachusetts

THERESA ELIZABETH ROBERTSON, MD, FACS, Assistant Professor of Surgery, University of Mississippi, Jackson, Mississippi

ALEXANDRA M. ROCH, MD, MS, Department of Surgery, Indiana University School of Medicine, Indianapolis, Indiana

CHRISTIAN MAX SCHMIDT, MD, PhD, MBA, FACS, Director of IU Health Pancreatic Cyst and Cancer Early Detection Center, Department of Surgery, Indiana University School of Medicine, Indianapolis, Indiana

YULIA ZAK, MD, Assistant Professor, Department of Surgery, Mount Sinai Beth Israel, New York, New York

CONTENTS VOLUME 50 • 2016

Associate Editors xi

Contributors xiii

Management of Mixed-Type Intraductal Papillary Mucinous Neoplasm
Alexandra M. Roch and Christian Max Schmidt

Introduction 2
Definition 2
Radiographic 2
Pathologic 3
Clinicopathologic characteristics 3
Epidemiology 3
Clinical and radiographic presentation 4
Pathology 4
Classification 4
Radiographic versus pathologic classification 4
Limitation of radiographic classification 5
Heterogeneity of main-duct involvement: proposed subclassifications of mixed-type intraductal papillary mucinous neoplasm 5
Pathologic subtype in mixed-type intraductal papillary mucinous neoplasm 6
Natural history 6
Malignancy risk 6
Surveillance 7
Predictors of malignancy 8
Survival and recurrence 9
Management 10
Indications for surgery 10
Surgical decision making 10
Nonsurgical management 12
Summary 12

Minimally Invasive Esophagectomy: Is There an Advantage?
Richard J. Battafarano

Introduction 17
Historical note 18
Relationship between anastomotic leak and operative mortality 19
Comparison of the transhiatal and transthoracic esophagectomies 21

Minimally invasive esophagectomy using laparoscopic and thoracoscopic techniques 23
Is there an optimal surgical technique for performing esophagectomy? 24
Development of a maximally effective esophagectomy 26

Optimal Management of the Axilla: A Look at the Evidence
Eleftherios (Terry) P. Mamounas

Introduction 29
Development of lymphatic mapping and sentinel lymph node biopsy 30
Single-institution and multicenter studies of sentinel lymph node biopsy 30
Randomized trials of sentinel lymph node biopsy alone versus sentinel lymph node biopsy plus axillary lymph node dissection in patients with negative sentinel lymph nodes 31
Clinical significance of occult sentinel lymph node metastases 32
Randomized trials of sentinel lymph node biopsy alone versus sentinel lymph node biopsy plus axillary lymph node dissection in patients with limited sentinel lymph node involvement 32
Assessment of axillary nodal status in patients treated with neoadjuvant chemotherapy 34
Sentinel lymph node biopsy in patients treated with neoadjuvant chemotherapy 34

The Use of LINX for Gastroesophageal Reflux
Yulia Zak and David W. Rattner

History 41
Magnetic antireflux device 42
Patient selection 43
Surgical technique 44
Contraindications 45
Efficacy 46
Complications 47
Summary 47

Bowel Preparation: Are Antibiotics Necessary for Colorectal Surgery?
Alice Charlotte Adelaide Murray and Ravi P. Kiran

Introduction: background 50
Significance 50
Mechanical bowel preparation alone 51
Colonic bacteria 53
Mechanical bowel preparation plus–oral antibiotics 54
Mechanical bowel preparation plus–V antibiotics (with or without oral) 57
Current evidence 58
Rectum versus colon 61
Role of enema 62
Laparoscopic versus open 62
Present relevance and future avenues 62
Summary 62

Incarcerated/Strangulated Hernia: Open or Laparoscopic?
James G. Bittner IV

Introduction 67
Diagnosis 68
Decision-making 70
Incarcerated/strangulated inguinal hernia 70
Surgical approaches–laparoscopy 71
Laparoscopic repair for adults 71
Laparoscopic repair for children 73
Surgical approaches–open 74
Open repair for adults 74
Open repair for children 75
Summary 76

Strategies to Reduce Postoperative Urinary Tract Infections
Christina M. Papageorge and Gregory D. Kennedy

Introduction 79
Significance 80
Prevention of catheter-associated urinary tract infection 82
Sterile catheter techniques 83
Types of catheters 84
Indications for catheterization 84
Timing of catheter removal 84
Reducing postoperative urinary retention 85
Prophylactic antibiotics 87
Screening for asymptomatic bacteriuria 87
Summary 88

The Aging Surgeon
Mark R. Katlic and JoAnn Coleman

Introduction 93
Case report 94
Is the aging surgeon still a problem? 94
Are surgeons human? 95
Is a mandatory retirement age the answer? 97
But does the surgical profession police itself? 98
The aging surgeon program 99
Summary 102

Maintenance of Certification
Mark A. Malangoni

Background 105
Recertification established 107
Introduction of maintenance of certification 107
Requirements for the American Board of Surgery maintenance of certification program 109
Relevance of American Board of Surgery maintenance of certification 111

Treatment of Locally Advanced Pancreatic Ductal Adenocarcinoma

Andrew P. Loehrer, Christine V. Kinnier, and Cristina R. Ferrone

Introduction 115
Significance of resectability 116
Neoadjuvant chemotherapy 117
FOLFIRINOX 117
Neoadjuvant chemoradiation 119
Surgical resection and intraoperative therapy 120
Intraoperative radiotherapy 121
Intraoperative electroporation 122
Adjuvant therapy 122
Future Directions 123
Summary 124

Prevention of Perioperative Anastomotic Healing Complications: Anastomotic Stricture and Anastomotic Leak

Kristina L. Guyton, Neil H. Hyman, and John C. Alverdy

Anastomotic complications: a spectrum of clinical presentations 129
Beyond tension and ischemia: physics is important, but biology is a major factor in anastomotic healing 130
Current understanding: we have probabilistic measurements and we now need deterministic analyses 131
Anastomotic stricture 131
Anastomotic leak 131
The challenge of defining anastomotic healing complications 132
Anastomotic stricture 132
Anastomotic leak 133
Specific interventions to prevent anastomotic healing complications 133
Anastomotic stricture 133
Anastomotic leak: hand sewn versus stapling, intraoperative evaluation, and diverting ileostomy 134
The biology of anastomotic healing 135
Microbes: the common denominator of anastomotic complications? 136
Preparing the bowel for anastomotic surgery: how we got it right, why we still have it wrong 137
Summary: how do we move forward in the prevention of anastomotic healing complications? 138

Is Health Services Research Important for Surgeons?

Kristen A. Ban and Karl Y. Bilimoria

Introduction 143
Significance of health services research for surgeons 144
Defining health services research 144

A framework for health sciences research: structure, process, and outcomes 144
Structure 144
Process 146
Outcomes 147
Disciplines within health services research and research modalities 148
Patient/disease-management level 148
Hospital level 151
Health policy level 154
Summary 154

Robotic Colorectal Surgery: Advance or Expense?
Rahila Essani and Roberto Bergamaschi

Introduction 157
Operating in confines of narrow bony pelvis 158
Impact of coning on circumferential resection margin in rectal cancer 159
Suturing and knot-tying 162
Hand-sewn ileocolic anastomoses 163
Rectopexy 165
Transanal minimally invasive surgery 165
Transanal total mesorectal excision 166
Summary 167

Ventilator Management: A Systematic Approach to Choosing and Using New Modes
Theresa Elizabeth Robertson

Introduction 173
Significance 174
Initial approach 175
Hypoxia 175
High pressures 180
Dyssynchrony and comfort 182
Ventilator liberation 183
Present relevance and future avenues 184
Summary 184

Hernia Management in the Athlete
L. Michael Brunt

Background and epidemiology of groin injuries 188
Differential diagnosis 189
Clinical evaluation 191
Diagnostic evaluation and imaging 192
Pathophysiology of athletic pubalgia 193
Surgical indications and operative approaches 194
Inguinal hernia 194
Athletic pubalgia 195
Role of adductor tenotomy 199

Postoperative management and return to sport 200
Summary 200

Groin Pain After Inguinal Hernia Repair
David K. Nguyen, Parviz K. Amid, and David C. Chen

Introduction 203
Significance 204
Definition 204
Etiology 204
Risk factors 207
Symptomatology and diagnosis 208
History 208
Physical examination 208
Diagnostic imaging and tests 210
Treatment 211
Nonsurgical management 211
Surgical management 213
Future directions 215

Evolution of Sepsis Management: From Early Goal-Directed Therapy to Personalized Care
Lyndsay W. Head and Craig M. Coopersmith

Definition of sepsis 222
Pathobiology of sepsis 223
Therapy for sepsis 225
Early goal-directed therapy 225
Efficacy of early goal-directed therapy 227
Why did early goal-directed therapy fail? 228
Changes in sepsis management over time 228
Efficacy of individual elements of early goal-directed therapy 229
Personalized care: today 230
Personalized care: the future 232
Summary 232

Current Status of Carotid Stenting Versus Endarterectomy
Ali F. AbuRahma and Albeir Y. Mousa

Review of randomized controlled carotid trials (carotid artery stenting vs carotid endarterectomy) 236
The Carotid and Vertebral Artery Transluminal Angioplasty Study 236
The Stenting and Angioplasty with Protection in Patients at High Risk for Endarterectomy Trial 236
The Endarterectomy Versus Angioplasty in Patients with Symptomatic Severe Carotid Stenosis Trial 237
The Stent-supported Percutaneous Angioplasty of the Carotid Artery Versus Endarterectomy Trial 237
The Carotid and Vertebral Artery Transluminal Angioplasty Study 2 (also called International Carotid Stenting Study) 238

Carotid Revascularization Endarterectomy Versus Stenting Trial 238
Metaanalysis of Clinical Trials: Carotid Artery Stenting Versus Carotid Endarterectomy 240
Carotid artery stenting results in the real world 243
Outcomes After Carotid Artery Stenting in Medicare Beneficiaries, 2005 to 2009 (Carotid Artery Stenting Linked to High Real-world Mortality) 244
Comparison of Trends and Outcomes of Carotid Artery Stenting and Carotid Endarterectomy in the United States (2001–2010) 244
Comparative Effectiveness of Carotid Revascularization Treatment: Evidence from a National Hospital Discharge Database 246
Systematic Review and Metaanalysis of Carotid Artery Stenting Versus Endarterectomy for Carotid Stenosis: a Chronologic and Worldwide Study 247
Repeat Carotid Endarterectomy Versus Carotid Artery Stenting for Patients with Restenosis After Carotid Endarterectomy: Systematic Review and Metaanalysis 247
Society for Vascular Surgery Carotid Vascular Registry: Carotid Artery Stenting Versus Carotid Endarterectomy Outcome Comparison 248
Other Negative Predictors for Carotid Artery Stenting 248
Effect of Age on Carotid Artery Stenting Results 248
Effect of Gender on Carotid Artery Stenting Results 249
Carotid Artery Stenting Is More Costly than Carotid Endarterectomy 249
Should the United States Centers for Medicare and Medicaid Services Extend Reimbursement Indications for Carotid Artery Stenting? 249
Guidelines of Various Specialties in Treating Carotid Artery Stenosis and the Differences in Their Recommendations for the Role of Carotid Artery Stenting 250
For Symptomatic Carotid Artery Stenosis 251
For Asymptomatic Carotid Artery Stenosis 251
Recent Carotid Artery Stenting Data: Using the Enroute Transcarotid System (Investigation of Transcarotid CAS With Dynamic Flow Reversal in Subjects With Significant Extracranial Carotid Stenosis [ROADSTER Trial]) 252
Final Recommendation for the Role of Carotid Artery Stenting Versus Carotid Endarterecomy 252
Summary 253

Advances in Surgery 50 (2016) 1–15

ADVANCES IN SURGERY

Management of Mixed-Type Intraductal Papillary Mucinous Neoplasm

Alexandra M. Roch, MD, MS[a],
Christian Max Schmidt, MD, PhD, MBA[b,*]

[a]Department of Surgery, Indiana University School of Medicine, 980 W Walnut Street R3-C541, Indianapolis, IN 46202, USA; [b]IU Health Pancreatic Cyst and Cancer Early Detection Center, Department of Surgery, Indiana University School of Medicine, 545 Barnhill Drive, EH 129, Indianapolis, IN 46202, USA

Keywords

• Intraductal papillary mucinous neoplasm • Main-duct-involved IPMN • Mixed-type IPMN • Pancreatic mucinous cystic lesion • Pancreatic cyst

Key points

- Radiologic diagnosis of mixed-type IPMN is inaccurate overestimating main pancreatic duct involvement in 20% of patients.
- Radiologic diagnosis of branch-duct IPMN is inaccurate underestimating main pancreatic duct involvement in up to 30% of patients.
- Multiple pathologic definitions of mixed-type IPMN exist.
- Classification of mixed-type IPMN as a subcategory of main-duct IPMN may be an oversimplification.
- Mixed type-IPMN are a heterogeneous group of lesions with various phenotypes and thus their management should be tailored according to the patient and biology of the lesion.

Disclosure Statement: Dr C.M. Schmidt is founder of B9, Inc. B9 seeks to identify diagnostic biomarkers for benign conditions. He also consults for Redpath Integrated Pathology, Asuragen, and Mauna Kea Technologies, all of which have technologies that aid in the management of patients with pancreatic cysts. Dr A.M. Roch has nothing to disclose.

*Corresponding author. 980 West Walnut Street C522, Indianapolis, IN 46202. *E-mail address*: maxschmi@iupui.edu

0065-3411/16/$ – see front matter
http://dx.doi.org/10.1016/j.yasu.2016.03.001

INTRODUCTION

In 1982, Ohashi and colleagues [1] described four cases of a rare pancreatic entity they called "mucin-producing cancer." It affected the main pancreatic duct and produced excessive quantities of mucus, which filled and distended the pancreatic ductal system. This type of pancreatic tumor, later in 1996 named intraductal papillary mucinous neoplasm (IPMN) [2], is believed to account today for up to 70% of all cystic neoplasms of the pancreas. Reasons for the IPMN epidemic are unknown, but likely result from increased awareness, recognition, and detection with improved imaging resolution. IPMN are classified into branch-duct (BD-IPMN), main-duct (MD-IPMN), and mixed (MT-IPMN) types according to the radiographic topography of ductal involvement [3,4]. Patients who undergo surgical resection are definitively classified according to the pathologic topography of ductal involvement. It is well established that all IPMN types harbor a real but variable risk of malignant transformation following a stepwise progression pattern similar to that of adenomatous polyps in colonic cancer [5,6]. Over the last 30 years, more than 2000 articles on IPMN have been indexed in the PubMed/Medline database. Few papers, however, specifically focus on MT-IPMN, which account for 28% to 41% of all IPMN in surgical series [7–9]. Historically, the management of MT-IPMN has been lumped into the management of MD-IPMN because of the presence of main pancreatic duct involvement and a presumed similar risk of malignant progression [10,11]. MT-IPMN is unable to be accurately established preoperatively in up to 30% of cases when compared with the gold standard, surgical pathology. Even in pathologically proven MT-IPMN, main-duct involvement represents a spectrum from minimal to extensive, which positively correlates with the incidence of higher grades of IPMN dysplasia. Thus, the classification and optimal management of these lesions is evolving [12].

DEFINITION

MT-IPMN is characterized by IPMN involvement of both the main pancreatic duct and the branch ducts of the pancreas. Criteria used to differentiate MT-IPMN from isolated MD-IPMN and BD-IPMN are not uniform in the literature. Most studies use the results of imaging studies alone [10,11]. Following surgery, patients are definitively classified as MT-IPMN only if there is pathologic involvement of both main and branch ducts.

Radiographic

MT-IPMN is diagnosed with a reasonable degree of certainty based on cross-sectional (multidetector computed tomography [CT], magnetic resonance cholangiopancreatography [MRCP]) and/or endoscopic (endoscopic ultrasound, endoscopic retrograde cholangiopancreatography, pancreatic ductoscopy) imaging. It is radiographically defined, according to the 2012 revised International Consensus Guidelines, as the association of segmental or diffuse main pancreatic duct dilation of greater than or equal to 5 mm (without any non-IPMN cause of obstruction) and single/cluster or multiple pancreatic "cysts" greater than or equal to 5 mm communicating with the main pancreatic duct (branch ducts) (Fig. 1) [11].

Pathologic

MT-IPMN can also be defined histologically in a surgical specimen. Histology confirms MT-IPMN if it shows a neoplasm with tall, columnar, mucin-producing epithelium, with or without papillary proliferations, arising within the epithelial lining of both the main pancreatic duct and branch ducts in the absence of ovarian-type stroma [6,10,11]. In the absence of significant ductal dilation (≥5 mm or ≥10 mm cutoffs), some pathologists classify these same histopathologic features as main-duct or branch-duct pancreatic intraepithelial neoplasia instead of IPMN [3,5].

CLINICOPATHOLOGIC CHARACTERISTICS

MT-IPMN has overlapping similarities with MD-IPMN in regards to clinicopathologic and epidemiologic characteristics [9,13].

Epidemiology

MD-IPMN and MT-IPMN occur more frequently in men (55% of MD-IPMN and 56% of MT-IPMN), whereas BD-IPMN occur more frequently in women (57%) (gender ratio MT-IPMN vs BD-IPMN; $P = .01$) [9,13]. The median age at diagnosis is similar among the three IPMN types. Patients with invasive MD-IPMN and MT-IPMN are significantly older than those with noninvasive lesions [9,14].

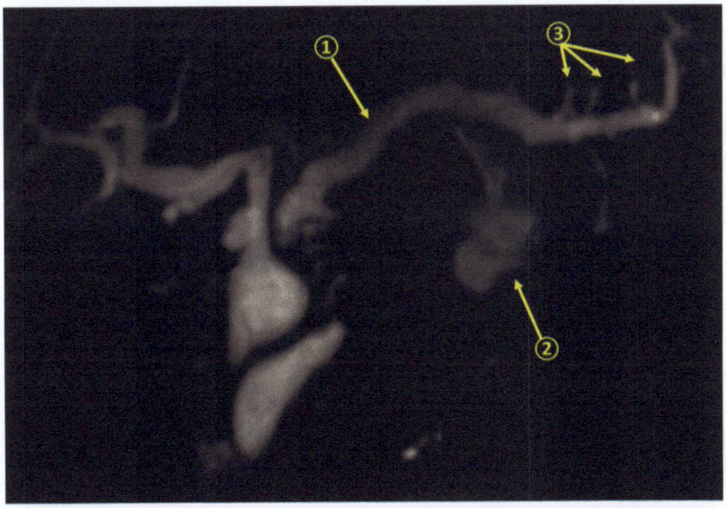

Fig. 1. Magnetic resonance cholangiopancreatography showing multifocal mixed-type intraductal papillary mucinous neoplasm with diffuse dilation of the main pancreatic duct and multifocal branch-duct dilation. (*1*) Main pancreatic duct dilation. (*2*) Large branch-duct dilation. (*3*) Multifocal branch-duct dilation.

Clinical and radiographic presentation

Incidental diagnosis of IPMN is significantly more common in BD-IPMN (34% of asymptomatic lesions) compared with MD-IPMN (13%) and MT-IPMN (19%). Objective signs/symptoms (ie, jaundice, weight loss) are more frequent in MD-IPMN and MT-IPMN. Radiographically diffuse (as opposed to segmental) IPMN are found in 10% of MT-IPMN [9,13].

Pathology

Based on mostly surgical series, the prevalence of low-grade dysplasia in MD-IPMN and MT-IPMN is significantly lower (11% and 8%, respectively, vs 44% in BD-IPMN). Conversely, invasive cancer rate is significantly higher in MD-IPMN (48%) and MT-IPMN (42%) compared with BD-IPMN (11%). The rate of malignancy (high-grade dysplasia or invasive) in MT-IPMN averages 54%, and the risk of invasive lesion is 38% to 40% (Table 1) [11,14–25]. Because the incidence of invasive IPMN is higher in MD-IPMN and it increases with age, this suggests MD-IPMN and MT-IPMN have an aggressive biology characterized by progression with time to invasive cancer.

CLASSIFICATION

Radiographic versus pathologic classification

The classification of MT-IPMN based on imaging findings has substantial value in preoperative management algorithms, as shown in the 2006 Sendai and revised 2012 International Consensus Guidelines [10,11]. An accurate distinction of main-duct involvement versus not is likely the single most reliable

Table 1
Rates of malignancy (HGD and invasive carcinoma) in MT-IPMN

Authors, y	Type of study	Number	Malignant, n (%)	HGD, n (%)	Invasive, n (%)
Sohn et al, [15] 2004	Surgical/retrospective	33	>13 (>40)	NA	13 (40)
Suzuki et al, [16] 2004	Surgical/retrospective	228	>148 (>65)	NA	148 (65)
Lee et al, [17] 2005	Surgical/retrospective	5	2 (40)	0 (0)	2 (40)
Schnelldorfer et al, [7] 2008	Surgical/retrospective	48	18 (38)	NA	NA
Nagai et al, [18] 2008	Surgical/retrospective	8	4 (50)	2 (25)	2 (25)
Ohno et al, [19] 2009	Surgical/retrospective	25	14 (56)	8 (32)	6 (24)
Nara et al, [8] 2009	Surgical/retrospective	38	30 (79)	4 (11)	26 (68)
Bournet et al, [20] 2009	Surgical/retrospective	52	18 (35)	8 (15)	10 (19)
Hwang et al, [21] 2012	Surgical/retrospective	41	19 (46)	7 (17)	12 (29)
Crippa et al, [9] 2010	Surgical/retrospective	149	92 (62)	30 (20)	62 (42)
Masuda et al, [22] 2013	Surgical/retrospective	45	25 (56)	11 (24)	14 (31)
Sahora et al, [23] 2014	Surgical/retrospective	209	123 (59)	66 (32)	57 (27)
Roch et al, [24] 2014	Surveillance/ prospective	70	>9 (>13)	NA	9 (13)
Total		951	>515 (54)	—	361–379 (38–40)

Abbreviations: HGD, high-grade dysplasia; NA, non available.

predictor of malignant potential in a patient with IPMN. Radiographic classification of IPMN type, however, is not always reliable.

Limitation of radiographic classification

The main-duct dilation in IPMN is thought to be caused by an inherent change in the ductal wall elasticity and ductal hypertension from obstruction caused by mucin hypersecretion and increased mucin viscosity [10,11]. The main pancreatic duct may dilate because of several other factors including senescence, pancreatitis, ductal obstruction, and pancreatic resection. Histopathologic examination not uncommonly reveals involvement of the main duct with IPMN when none was suspected radiographically or vice versa. A recent study showed that in 21% of patients with a preoperative radiologic diagnosis of isolated BD-IPMN, final pathology demonstrated main pancreatic duct involvement. Conversely, 30% of patients with main pancreatic duct dilation greater than or equal to 5 mm on cross-sectional imaging did not reveal main pancreatic duct involvement on surgical pathology [26]. Overall, preoperative cross-sectional imaging studies (CT, MRI-MRCP) demonstrate low sensitivity (78%) and specificity of (72%) for the diagnosis of main pancreatic duct involvement (accuracy, 75%). Once pathology confirms main-duct involvement, there is no consensus on the extent of pathologic involvement of the main duct necessary to qualify the lesion as sufficient to meet criteria for MD-IPMN or MT-IPMN. Essentially, any degree of involvement qualifies. In light of these data, preoperatively, patients with IPMN and main-duct dilation are more accurately classified as having suspected main-duct involvement.

Heterogeneity of main-duct involvement: proposed subclassifications of mixed-type intraductal papillary mucinous neoplasm

Because the epidemiologic and clinicopathologic characteristics of MD-IPMN and MT-IPMN are similar based on outcomes in surgical series [9,13,14], both types are commonly grouped together. It is unclear whether MT-IPMN are an extension of MD-IPMN into the branch ducts, an extension of BD-IPMN into the main duct, either, or neither (ie, a distinct disease entity). Pathologic MT-IPMN with radiographic main duct less than or equal to 4 mm (below the International Consensus Guidelines accepted radiographic cutoff for main-duct involvement) are sometimes called early main-duct-involved IPMN. These often have less aggressive biology [26]. In examining pathology in these patients, there is often minimal IPMN involvement of the main duct. Minimal involvement of the main duct may also occur when radiographic main-duct dilation is greater than 4 mm, but this is less common. In a recent study from Massachusetts General Hospital [23], the authors identified pathologic heterogeneity in MT-IPMN. Based on pathologic evaluation, they defined two types of MT-IPMN based on extensive or minimal involvement of the main duct. Minimal involvement was defined as noncircumferential microscopic involvement of the main pancreatic duct (limited to one or a few histologic sections), in the absence of gross main pancreatic duct abnormality (except for main pancreatic duct dilation). The minimal involvement MT-IPMN is difficult to differentiate preoperatively from BD-IPMN and represents approximately 22% of all cases of pathologic MT-IPMN. As others have suggested, this group indicates minimal involvement MT-IPMN has a less aggressive biology.

In minimal involvement MT-IPMN, the lesions are more likely to be identified incidentally compared with extensive involvement MT-IPMN (70% vs 29%; $P<.0001$). Conversely, patients with extensive involvement MT-IPMN present more frequently with symptoms of weight loss (30% vs 11%; $P = .009$) and jaundice (14% vs 0%; $P = .007$), similar to MD-IPMN.

Mean main pancreatic duct diameter was significantly larger in extensive involvement MT-IPMN (9 mm [2–140] vs minimal involvement MT-IPMN 2 mm [2–12]; $P<.0001$). Patients with minimal involvement MT-IPMN were more likely to have an observation period before operation (41% vs 10%; $P<.0001$), and an increase in cyst size was the leading indication for resection in this group. Conversely, most patients with extensive involvement MT-IPMN underwent operation because of a suspicious nodule or mass (18% vs 4.3%; $P = .019$). One-third of minimal involvement MT-IPMN demonstrates segmental (as opposed to diffuse) dilation of the main pancreatic duct on imaging studies.

Pathologic subtype in mixed-type intraductal papillary mucinous neoplasm

According to recent studies, IPMN type is associated with pathologic subtype (gastric, intestinal, pancreatobiliary). Branch-duct IPMN is associated with predominantly gastric subtype, MD-IPMN with intestinal subtype, and MT-IPMN is split [27]. In comparing MT-IPMN with minimal versus extensive pathologic main-duct involvement, 89% of minimal involvement MT-IPMN is gastric subtype (comparable with BD-IPMN 81%). Even when the branch-duct component exhibits another epithelium subtype (intestinal or pancreatobiliary), the main-duct component of minimal involvement MT-IPMN is exclusively gastric subtype. Conversely, nearly half of extensive involvement MT-IPMN and 80% of MD-IPMN exhibits intestinal type epithelium. All invasive carcinomas arising in minimal involvement MT-IPMN and most of those arising in BD-IPMN are of the tubular type, whereas 26% of those arising in extensive involvement MT-IPMN and 45% of those arising in MD-IPMN are of the colloid type.

NATURAL HISTORY

The Sendai criteria and the 2012 revised International Consensus Guidelines recommend surgical resection of all main-duct-involved IPMN (MD-IPMN and MT-IPMN) in fit patients, because of their malignant potential [10,11]. Because these guidelines are largely accepted and followed among surgeons, it is uncommon that patients with MT-IPMN undergo primary surveillance. Thus, their natural history remains unclear.

Malignancy risk

There is little question that the existence of main pancreatic duct involvement is associated with a more aggressive behavior in IPMN. This seems to be true whether or not the main pancreatic duct involvement by IPMN is accompanied by BD-IPMN involvement. For example, in a large multi-institutional (University of Verona and Massachusetts General Hospital) study by Crippa and colleagues [9], the frequency of invasive carcinoma in MT-IPMN (42%) was comparable with MD-IPMN (48%), but distinctly different from isolated BD-IPMN (11%). These findings, based almost exclusively on surgical series, have been corroborated in numerous studies (see Table 1) [15–24].

According to Barron and colleagues [26], radiographic BD-IPMN with main pancreatic duct involvement on final pathology are more often malignant (ie, high-grade dysplasia, invasive carcinoma) or invasive compared with pathologic isolated BD-IPMN (29.4% vs 11.5%, $P = .015$ or 20.6% vs 6.9%, $P = .025$, respectively). Conversely, radiographic main-duct involvement without main pancreatic duct involvement on final pathology is less malignant or invasive compared with pathologic main-duct involvement (24% vs 57.5%, $P = .0001$ and 4% vs 36.7%, $P = .0001$, respectively). Similarly, Salvia and colleagues [28] reported that the final pathologic diagnosis matched the preoperative diagnosis for main pancreatic duct involvement in only 78% of cases, and that the risk of harboring malignancy was significantly higher in MT-IPMN that were preoperatively misclassified as BD-IPMN on imaging. Fritz and colleagues [29] also found malignancy in 8% of histologically proven BD-IPMN (8 out of 100) versus 30% (20 out of 67) of misclassified BD-IPMN with involvement of the main pancreatic duct on pathology ($P < .001$). In Massachusetts General Hospital experience, MT-IPMN (n = 209) and MD-IPMN (n = 20) harbored a 41% rate of malignant lesions. However, high-grade dysplasia and invasive carcinoma were observed less frequently in minimal involvement MT-IPMN than in extensive involvement MT-IPMN (11% and 6% vs 37% and 33%, respectively; $P = .001$ and $P < .0001$). The rates of high-grade dysplasia and invasive carcinoma in minimal involvement MT-IPMN in this study were actually comparable with BD-IPMN [23].

Surveillance

Indiana University recently published a series of 70 patients with MT-IPMN who underwent primary surveillance for a median of 4.5 years [24]. Surgery was contraindicated in 42% because of major comorbidities (American Association of Anesthesiologists score $\geq$3), in 51% because the patient refused surgery after being appropriately informed of the invasive potential of their disease and the indication for surgical management, and in 7% because of borderline radiographic criteria for MT-IPMN (main pancreatic duct dilation range, 5–6 mm). Nine patients (12.9%) progressed to an invasive carcinoma during follow-up, at a median of 2.7 years. There was a stepwise increase in the incidence of invasive carcinoma with duration of surveillance, resulting in 3- and 5-year invasive progression risks of 7.1% and 10%, respectively. The rate of patients with MT-IPMN who developed invasive carcinoma was lower than that reported in previous surgical series. This finding may be caused in part by a selection bias, because surgical patients are more likely to present with criteria suspicious for malignant progression. Furthermore, most surgical series report pathologic main-duct involvement, a finding only confirmed after surgery. This series, despite cytopathologic confirmation of IPMN, may include patients with isolated BD-IPMN despite radiographic main-duct dilation meeting criteria for main-duct involvement.

Forty-four percent of patients who progressed in the Indiana University study did so in a range of 3.8 to 9 years. Although there is no specific data on MT-IPMN, these results are not consistent with previous small case studies on primarily surveillance of main-duct-involved IPMN (MD-IPMN and MT-IPMN) that suggested that malignancy developed over a shorter time period. Obara and colleagues [30] reported malignant progression in three out of three main-duct-involved IPMNs over a 26-month period, two invasive and one high-grade dysplasia on final surgical pathology. Similarly, Kobayashi and colleagues [31] described progression of three out of four main-duct-involved IPMNs during 29 months, one invasive and two high-grade dysplasia on final surgical pathology. In Takuma and colleagues [32] study, 20% of main-duct-involved IPMN developed invasive carcinomas in a range of 17 to 65 months. Conversely, 35% did not progress over a 12- to 156-month follow-up. One possible explanation for the development of invasive carcinoma in shorter periods may be the failure to detect high-risk lesions at the beginning of surveillance. In most of these small case studies, no baseline endoscopic ultrasound with fine-needle aspiration (and cytopathology) was performed before surveillance.

Predictors of malignancy

Several articles have studied the risk factors for malignancy in IPMN, with controversial results [10,11,33–35]. Most studies, however, have focused on BD-IPMN, and few have specifically analyzed predictors of malignancy in MT-IPMN.

In the Indiana University study [24], univariate analysis yielded weight loss, diffuse main-duct dilation, absence of intra-abdominal extrapancreatic cysts, increase of main-duct diameter, shorter time from isolated branch-ducts to main pancreatic duct involvement, elevated serum CA19-9 level (defined as >37 units/mL), and elevated serum alkaline phosphatase level (defined as >125 ng/mL) as potential predictors of invasive progression. Rather than the maximal diameter of the main pancreatic duct, the percentage change or differential change in millimeters may be more predictive of invasive progression in MT-IPMN. Regarding the branch-duct component of MT-IPMN, neither the size nor fluctuations in size were predictive of invasive carcinoma. Usual predictors of invasiveness used in the Sendai criteria and in the 2012 revised International Consensus Guidelines [10,11] (mural nodule, maximum main-duct diameter, maximal branch-duct size, main-duct diameter >10 mm, and branch-duct size >30 mm) were not significant in univariate analysis. In logistic regression, diffuse main-duct dilation, elevated serum CA19-9 level, elevated serum alkaline phosphatase level, and absence of intra-abdominal extrapancreatic cysts were independent predictors of invasive progression with odds ratios of 7.4, 10, 6.9, and 12.3, respectively. The receiver operating characteristics curve indicated that the combination of these four predictors achieved a sensitivity of 78% and a specificity of 98% in predicting invasive MT-IPMN (accuracy, 98%) in this select group of patients undergoing primary surveillance for MT-IPMN. Of the 12 patients in this population who had two predictive factors, 25% showed an invasive progression. Of the five patients with three predictors, 80% developed an invasive lesion during follow-up. In this model, a surgical intervention for patients with MT-IPMN and two predictive factors or less would result in potential overtreatment of 60 out of 63 (95%) patients with noninvasive lesions. Conversely, nonsurgical management of patients with three or four predictors would result in undertreatment of six out of seven (86%) patients with invasive carcinoma. There was a median time frame of almost 2 years before invasive carcinoma develops when the second predictor is diagnosed, which could potentially represent a window of opportunity for surgical management even in patient who are less fit.

In a recent Japanese study of 45 MT-IPMN, immunohistochemical reactivity against anti–mucin 2 (MUC2) was a predictive factor of malignancy [22]. The prevalence of high-grade dysplasia and invasive carcinoma in MUC2-positive MT-IPMN was significantly higher than that in MUC2-negative MT-IPMN (high-grade dysplasia and invasive carcinoma 88% vs 38%, $P = .0017$; invasive carcinoma 50% vs 21%, $P = .042$). Univariate analysis and multivariate analysis yielded MUC2 expression on surgical pathology specimen as an independent predictive factor of high-grade dysplasia and invasive carcinoma in MT-IPMN (odds ratio, 14.6).

Survival and recurrence

From one of the largest surgical series on MT-IPMN [9], 5-year survival was 77%. The 5-year disease-specific survival was 100% and 64% for noninvasive and invasive MT-IPMN, respectively. Twenty-seven patients developed tumor recurrence after a mean of 18.5 months. Of these, 25 originally had invasive MT-IPMN, accounting for a recurrence rate of 40% in this subgroup of patients during this same timeframe.

In Roch and colleagues [24] surveillance study, in the subgroup of patients who did not progress (n = 61), 1-year survival and 3-year survival rates were 98.3% and 72.1%, respectively. Median survival from diagnosis of MT-IPMN in the nine patients with invasive progression was 4.2 years, but median survival from the diagnosis of invasive IPMN was only 0.8 years.

Preliminary analysis of Indiana University experience with 71 invasive IPMN (39 MT-IPMN, 17 MD-IPMN, and 15 BD-IPMN) suggests that median overall survival of invasive MT-IPMN was significantly longer than that of invasive MD-IPMN, but comparable with that of invasive BD-IPMN. In patients with invasive main-duct-involved IPMN (MD-IPMN and MT-IPMN), Cox regression disclosed MT-IPMN as an independent predictor of longer overall. These results corroborate a recent study from Massachusetts General Hospital on the heterogeneity of all (not just invasive) MT-IPMN [23]. Minimal involvement MT-IPMN has similar outcomes as BD-IPMN (disease-specific 5- and 10-year survival rates of 97% and 97%, respectively), compared with extensive involvement MT-IPMN whose poorer prognosis was similar to that of MD-IPMN (disease-specific 5- and 10-year survival rates of 83% and 83%, respectively).

MANAGEMENT

Indications for surgery

The specific surgical indications of MT-IPMN are not clearly defined in the 2006 or the 2012 revised International Consensus Guidelines [10,11]. Because of the clinicopathologic similarities with MD-IPMN, and comparable risk of malignant/invasive lesions, the International Consensus Guidelines recommend the same management strategy for MD-IPMN and MT-IPMN. Surgical resection is recommended when the main pancreatic duct dilation reaches 10 mm or greater, in all fit patients. In cases of moderate main pancreatic dilation (5–9 mm), further evaluation (endoscopic ultrasound or endoscopic retrograde cholangiopancreatography) is considered to improve diagnostic accuracy before surgical resection [11]. There is no consensus on predictors of malignancy in MT-IPMN (especially diameter of main pancreatic duct, size of index cyst, mural nodule, or presence of symptoms) [11,24,33–35]. Close surveillance (as stated in the 2012 revised International Consensus Guidelines) may be complicated and of limited benefit. Thereby, when a diagnosis of MT-IPMN is confirmed (classic radiographic appearance and/or a combination of historic, demographic, radiographic, cytopathologic, and biochemical evidence), resection should be offered in fit patients.

Surgical decision making

Because the risk of malignant/invasive component in MT-IPMN is significant, segmental pancreatectomy with regional lymphadenectomy according to the site and extent of the IPMN should be considered the gold standard and preferred to parenchyma-sparing procedures. Segmental involvement of the main duct in the head or body/tail of pancreas should be treated with pancreaticoduodenectomy or distal pancreatectomy, respectively. In patients undergoing distal pancreatectomy, splenectomy is selectively performed. Splenectomy may improve staging, so is recommended if based on preoperative and intraoperative assessments an invasive IPMN is present or highly likely to be present. Dilation of the main pancreatic duct and its involvement with IPMN are not always correlated. Patients with diffuse MT-IPMN (nonsegmental) on imaging without an obvious target in the body/tail (eg, solid mass in the tail of pancreas) should undergo pancreaticoduodenectomy to ensure removal of any obstructive process in the head of pancreas causing diffuse dilation of the main pancreatic duct. At operation, an intraoperative frozen section of the pancreatic neck should be performed to determine if additional resection is indicated based on the degree of dysplasia present. An intraoperative frozen section margin with high-grade dysplasia or invasive IPMN would necessitate extension of the resection and possibly a total pancreatectomy if margin clearance is not possible. Total pancreatectomy is indicated in few patients with MT-IPMN involving the entire gland, and should be avoided if possible because of its significant risk of morbidity and mortality [36–38].

Several clinical and molecular studies have suggested that the presence of IPMN in the pancreas increases the risk of malignant/invasive transformation of not only ductal epithelial cells within the IPMN but also within the entire pancreatic gland. Clinically, this field defect may manifest as skip lesions (6%–21%) [39–42], with invasive carcinoma identified in an area of the pancreas distinct from the index IPMN lesion undergoing surveillance [31,43–45], or a new lesion in the remnant pancreas after surgical resection with well-documented negative margins [46,47]. Patients with MT-IPMN and MD-IPMN have skip lesions slightly more frequently than those without main pancreatic duct involvement [41]. These skip lesions may be heterogeneous and clonally distinct from each other [48].

To minimize recurrence, some have advocated resection to margins negative for IPMN. If frozen-section biopsy reveals low-grade or moderate-grade dysplasia at the margin, further resection to obtain a negative margin remains controversial and debated. Main pancreatic duct margin status of "negative for IPMN" versus "low/moderate-grade IPMN dysplasia" during partial pancreatectomy does not convincingly affect the remnant pancreas recurrence rate or patient prognosis [40,47]. Indeed, patients may recur with negative transection margins (3%–15% of main pancreatic duct involved–IPMN) [49,50]. Thus, the resection margin status guides the extent of resection, but does not guarantee the absence of IPMN in the remnant.

Okada's team has introduced the notion of "distance of tumor spread in the main pancreatic duct of IPMN" [51]. They found that the mean main pancreatic duct spread in MD-IPMN (66 $\pm$ 33 mm) was longer than that of MT-IPMN (38 $\pm$ 28 mm), although it did not reach statistical significance ($P = .09$). They conclude that the distance of tumor spread in the main pancreatic duct may offer important insights about the most appropriate resection line.

Cytology and pancreatoscopy have been used to better assess the extent of MT-IPMN, and thus optimize the resection line. According to Eguchi and colleagues [41] technique, a single-lumen catheter is inserted across the cut surface in the main pancreatic duct of the cranial pancreas and a triple-lumen catheter is inserted into the caudal pancreas to obtain the pancreatic juice separately from each portion of the pancreatic head, body, and tail. In the pilot study, they described eight skip IPMN lesions (19%) proven on final pathology, five of them detected by intraoperative cytology only. Peroral pancreatoscopy has been used to examine the main pancreatic duct preoperatively. Thorough observation of the entire main pancreatic duct has proved difficult technically because of the acute angle formed by the junction of the ducts of Wirsung and Santorini. Intraoperative pancreatoscopy (wirsungoscopy) overcomes this difficulty and allows serial staged biopsies to detect skip IPMN lesions in the main pancreatic duct. Kaneko and colleagues [52] evaluated the performance characteristics of intraoperative pancreatoscopy in a small series of 24 patients. Intraoperative pancreatoscopy detected 10 skip IPMN lesions that could not be detected by endoscopic ultrasound or endoscopic retrograde cholangiopancreatography, 3 out of 10 requiring additional resection. For diagnosis of mucinous papillary lesions, the sensitivity, specificity, and accuracy of intraoperative pancreatoscopy were all 100%. Some teams have optimized the use of intraoperative pancreatoscopy by adding narrow band imaging to allow for a better identification of the vascular pattern of the lesion [53]. Aside from time and expense, the main limitation of intraoperative pancreatoscopy is that it is only technically feasible if the main pancreatic duct is dilated. In patients with apparent isolated BD-IPMN, nearly 30% have IPMN involvement of the main duct despite the absence of main pancreatic duct dilation.

Nonsurgical management

In a select and older population, where the mortality/morbidity associated with pancreatectomy may outweigh the risk of malignant transformation, primary surveillance may be an option. From the Indiana University study on surveillance of MT-IPMN [24], four multivariate predictors of invasive progression were discovered. These were elevated serum CA19-9, elevated serum alkaline phosphatase, diffuse main pancreatic duct dilation, and the absence of non-pancreatic intra-abdominal cysts. Tracking these with blood tests and CT in select patients may be less injurious and more economical than other treatment (resection) and detection (serial MRI-MRCP and endoscopic ultrasound) strategies. Univariate predictors (weight loss, increase in size of the main pancreatic duct, and time from involvement of the branch duct to the involvement of the main pancreatic duct) should also be followed prospectively to aid in patient management. We speculate that informed surveillance of select patients unfit for surgical resection may offer a better strategy, and in some (in particular the "surgery averse") a potential window of opportunity if multivariate risk factors develop for secondary surgical resection before invasive IPMN develops.

A parallel or alternative strategy has been promulgated by two teams (United States and Japan) [22,23]. Each demonstrated that MT-IPMN consist of heterogeneous lesions with differential prognosis according to their morphologic subtype (MUC2-negative vs MUC2-positive; gastric type vs intestinal type; minimal involvement MT-IPMN vs extensive involvement MT-IPMN). They suggest that management should be tailored to the subtype of MT-IPMN. Specifically, MUC2-negative, gastric type, or minimal involvement MT-IPMN share histopathologic characteristics and less aggressive biology akin to BD-IPMN, and should therefore be offered primary surveillance. MUC2-positive, intestinal type, or extensive involvement MT-IPMN are associated with high invasive rate and poor prognosis, and thus should undergo surgical resection.

SUMMARY

No consensus exists regarding definition, classification, or even management of MT-IPMN. Since their description, because of a higher risk of malignant/

invasive lesions than BD-IPMN, they have usually been classified as MD-IPMN and resected. Because the 2006 Sendai criteria and the 2012 revised International Consensus Guidelines recommend resection for all main pancreatic duct involved IPMN [10,11], very little is known about the natural history of these lesions. The rate of malignancy from surgical series averages 54%, justifying as a general rule, compliance with the guidelines. The actual rate, however, of clinically relevant malignancy may be much lower in the short term, as suggested in primary surveillance series (13%) [24]. Several recent studies question the conventional classification of MT-IPMN and promulgate individualized management of MT-IPMN, because this IPMN type may be more complex than previously appreciated, displaying multiple and varied phenotypes [22,23]. Thus, the management of MT-IPMN continues to evolve.

References

[1] Ohashi K, Murakami Y, Maruyama M, et al. Four cases of mucous secreting pancreatic cancer. Prog Dig Endosc 1982;20:348–51.

[2] Kloppel G, Solcia E, Longnecker DS, et al. Histological typing of tumors of the exocrine pancreas. In: World Health Organization, editor. International classification of tumors. 2nd edition. Berlin: Springer; 1996. p. 11–20.

[3] Hruban RH, Takaori K, Klimstra DH, et al. An illustrated consensus on the classification of pancreatic intraepithelial neoplasia and intraductal papillary mucinous neoplasms. Am J Surg Pathol 2004;28:977–87.

[4] Adsay NV, Fukushima N, Furukawa T, et al. Intraductal neoplasm of the pancreas. In: Bosman FT, Carneiro F, Hruban RH, et al, editors. WHO classification of tumors of the digestive system. Lyon (France): WHO press; 2010. p. P304–13.

[5] Maitra A, Fukushima N, Takaori K, et al. Precursors to invasive pancreatic cancer. Adv Anat Pathol 2005;12(2):81–91.

[6] Shi C, Hruban RH. Intraductal papillary mucinous neoplasm. Hum Pathol 2012;43:1–16.

[7] Schnelldorfer T, Sarr MG, Nagorney DM, et al. Experience with 208 resections for intraductal papillary mucinous neoplasm of the pancreas. Arch Surg 2008;143:639–46.

[8] Nara S, Onaya H, Hiraoka N, et al. Preoperative evaluation of invasive and non-invasive intraductal papillary mucinous neoplasms of the pancreas: clinical, radiological and pathological analysis of 123 cases. Pancreas 2009;38:8–16.

[9] Crippa S, Fernandez-del Castillo C, Salvia R, et al. Mucin-producing neoplasms of the pancreas: an analysis of distinguishing clinical and epidemiologic characteristics. Clin Gastroenterol Hepatol 2010;8:213–9.

[10] Tanaka M, Chari S, Adsay V, et al. International consensus guidelines for management of intraductal papillary mucinous neoplasms and mucinous cystic neoplasms of the pancreas. Pancreatology 2006;6:17–32.

[11] Tanaka M, Fernandez del Castillo C, Adsay V, et al. International consensus guidelines 2012 for the management of IPMN and MCN of the pancreas. Pancreatology 2012;12(3):183–97.

[12] Tanaka M. Controversies in the management of pancreatic IPMN. Nat Rev Gastroenterol Hepatol 2011;8:56–60.

[13] Salvia R, Crippa S, Partelli S, et al. Differences between main-duct and branch-duct intraductal papillary mucinous neoplasms of the pancreas. World J Gastrointest Surg 2010;2(10): 342–6.

[14] Schmidt CM, White PB, Waters JA, et al. Intraductal papillary mucinous neoplasms: predictors of malignant and invasive pathology. Ann Surg 2007;246:644–51.

[15] Sohn TA, Yeo CJ, Cameron JL, et al. Intraductal papillary mucinous neoplasms of the pancreas: an updated experience. Ann Surg 2004;239:788–97.

[16] Suzuki Y, Atom Y, Sugiyama M, et al. Cystic neoplasm of the pancreas: a Japanese multi institutional study of intraductal papillary mucinous tumor and mucinous cystic tumor. Pancreas 2004;28:241–6.
[17] Lee SY, Lee KT, Lee JK, et al. Long-term follow-up results of intraductal papillary mucinous tumors of the pancreas. J Gastroenterol Hepatol 2005;20:1379–84.
[18] Nagai K, Doi R, Kida A, et al. Intraductal papillary mucinous neoplasms of the pancreas: clinicopathologic characteristics and long-term follow-up after resection. World J Surg 2008;32:271–8.
[19] Ohno E, Hirooka Y, Itoh A, et al. Intraductal papillary mucinous neoplasms of the pancreas: differentiation of malignant and benign tumors by endoscopic ultrasonography findings of mural nodules. Ann Surg 2009;249:628–34.
[20] Bournet B, Kirzin S, Carrere N, et al. Clinical fate of branch duct and mixed forms of intraductal papillary mucinous neoplasia of the pancreas. J Gastroenterol Hepatol 2009;24: 1211–7.
[21] Hwang DW, Jang JY, Lee SE, et al. Clinicopathologic analysis of surgically proven intraductal papillary mucinous neoplasms of the pancreas in SNUH: a 15-year experience at a single academic institution. Langenbecks Arch Surg 2012;397:93–102.
[22] Masuda A, Arisaka Y, Hara S, et al. MUC2 expression and prevalence of high grade dysplasia and invasive carcinoma in MT-intraductal papillary mucinous neoplasm of the pancreas. Pancreatology 2013;13:583–8.
[23] Sahora K, Fernandez-del Castillo C, Dong F, et al. Not all MT-intraductal papillary mucinous neoplasms behave like main-duct lesions: implications of minimal involvement of the main pancreatic duct. Surgery 2014;156:611–21.
[24] Roch AM, Ceppa EP, Al-Haddad MA, et al. The natural history of main duct-involved, MT-intraductal papillary mucinous neoplasm. Parameters predictive of progression. Ann Surg 2004;260:680–90.
[25] Correa-Gallego C, Ferrone CR, Thayer SP, et al. Incidental pancreatic cysts: do we really know what we are watching? Pancreatology 2010;10:144–50.
[26] Barron MR, Roch AM, Waters JA, et al. Does preoperative imaging accurately predict main duct involvement in intraductal papillary mucinous neoplasm? J Gastrointest Surg 2014;18(3):447–56.
[27] Furukawa T, Hatori T, Fujita I, et al. Prognostic relevance of morphological types of intraductal papillary mucinous neoplasms of the pancreas. Gut 2011;60:509–16.
[28] Salvia R, Malleo G, Marchegiani G, et al. Pancreatic resections for cystic neoplasms: from the surgeon's presumption to the pathologist's reality. Surgery 2012;152:135–42.
[29] Fritz S, Klauss M, Bergmann F, et al. Pancreatic main duct involvement in branch duct IPMNs. An underestimated risk. Ann Surg 2014;260:848–56.
[30] Obara T, Maguchi H, Saitoh Y, et al. Mucin-producing tumor of the pancreas: Natural history and serial pancreatogram changes. Am J Gastroenterol 1993;88:564–9.
[31] Kobayashi G, Fujita N, Noda Y, et al. Mode of progression of intraductal papillary mucinous tumor of the pancreas: Analysis of patients with follow-up EUS. J Gastroenterol 2005;40:744–51.
[32] Takuma K, Kamisawa T, Anjiki H, et al. Predictors of malignancy and natural history of main duct intraductal papillary mucinous neoplasm of the pancreas. Pancreas 2011;40(3): 371–5.
[33] Salvia R, Fernandez del Castillo C, Bassi C, et al. Main-duct intraductal papillary mucinous neoplasms of the pancreas: clinical predictors of malignancy and long-term survival following resection. Ann Surg 2004;239:678–85.
[34] Sugiyama M, Izumisato Y, Abe N, et al. Predictive factors for malignancy in intraductal papillary mucinous tumors of the pancreas. Br J Surg 2003;90:1244–9.
[35] Ogura T, Masuda D, Kurisu Y, et al. Potential predictors of disease progression for main duct intraductal papillary mucinous neoplasms of the pancreas. J Gastroenterol Hepatol 2013;28:1782–6.

[36] Muller MW, Friess H, Kleeff J, et al. Is there still a role for total pancreatectomy? Ann Surg 2007;246:966–74.
[37] Murphy MM, Knauss WJ, Ng SC, et al. Total pancreatectomy: a national study. HPB (Oxford) 2009;11:476–82.
[38] Ihse I, Anderson H, Andren S. Total pancreatectomy for cancer of the pancreas: Is it appropriate? World J Surg 1996;20:288–93.
[39] Raut CP, Cleary KR, Staerkel GA, et al. Intraductal papillary mucinous neoplasms of the pancreas: effect of invasion and pancreatic margin status on recurrence and survival. Ann Surg Oncol 2006;13:582–94.
[40] D'Angelica M, Brennan MF, Suriawinata AA, et al. Intraductal papillary mucinous neoplasms of the pancreas: an analysis of clinicopathologic features and outcomes. Ann Surg 2004;239:400–8.
[41] Eguchi H, Ishikawa O, Ohigashi H, et al. Role of intraoperative cytology combined with histology in detecting continuous and skip type intraductal cancer existence for intraductal papillary mucinous carcinoma of the pancreas. Cancer 2006;107:2567–75.
[42] Sauvanet A, Couvelard A, Belghiti J. Role of frozen section assessment for intraductal papillary mucinous tumor of the pancreas. World J Gastrointest Surg 2010;2:352–8.
[43] Ingkakul T, Sadakari Y, Ienaga J, et al. Predictors of the presence of concomittant invasive ductal carcinoma in intraductal papillary mucinous neoplasm of the pancreas. Ann Surg 2010;251:70–5.
[44] Tanno S, Nakano Y, Sugiyama Y, et al. Incidence of synchronous and metachronous pancreatic carcinoma in 168 patients with branch duct intraductal papillary mucinous neoplasm. Pancreatology 2010;10:173–8.
[45] Uehara H, Nakaizumi A, Ishikawa O, et al. Development of ductal carcinoma of the pancreas during follow-up of branch duct intraductal papillary mucinous neoplasm of the pancreas. Gut 2008;57:1561–5.
[46] Miller JR, Meyer JE, Waters JA, et al. Outcomes of the pancreatic remnant following segmental pancreatectomy for non-invasive intraductal papillary mucinous neoplasm. HPB 2011;13:759–66.
[47] Tamura K, Ohtsuka T, Ideno N, et al. Treatment strategy for main duct intraductal papillary mucinous neoplasms of the pancreas based on the assessment of recurrence in the remnant pancreas after resection. Ann Surg 2014;259:36–8.
[48] Matthaei H, Norris AL, Tsiatis AC. Clinicopathological characteristics and molecular analyses of multifocal intraductal papillary mucinous neoplasms of the pancreas. Ann Surg 2012;255:326–33.
[49] White R, D'Angelica M, Katabi N, et al. Fate of the remnant pancreas after resection of non-invasive intraductal papillary mucinous neoplasm. J Am Coll Surg 2007;204:987–93.
[50] Chari ST, Yadouv D, Smyrk TC, et al. Study of recurrence after surgical resection of intraductal papillary mucinous neoplasm of the pancreas. Gastroenterology 2002;123:1500–7.
[51] Okada K, Imaizumi T, Hirabayashi K, et al. The distance of tumor spread in the main pancreatic duct of an intraductal papillary mucinous neoplasm: where to resect and how to predict it. J Hepatobiliary Pancreat Sci 2010;17:516–22.
[52] Kaneko T, Nakao A, Nomoto S, et al. Intraoperative pancreatoscopy with the ultrathin pancreatoscope for mucin producing tumors of the pancreas. Arch Surg 1998;133:263–7.
[53] Yelamali A, Mansard HJ, Dama R, et al. Intraoperative pancreatoscopy with narrow band imaging: a novel method for assessment of resection margins in case of intraductal papillary mucinous neoplasm. Surg Endosc 2012;26:3682–5.

Advances in Surgery 50 (2016) 17–28

ADVANCES IN SURGERY

Minimally Invasive Esophagectomy

Is There an Advantage?

Richard J. Battafarano, MD, PhD

Division of Thoracic Surgery, Johns Hopkins University School of Medicine, 600 North Wolfe Street, Blalock 240, Baltimore, MD 21287, USA

Keywords

• Minimally invasive esophagectomy • Transhiatal esophagectomy • Transthoracic esophagectomy • Anastomotic complications of esophagectomy • Morbidity and mortality associated with esophagectomy

Key points

- The operative morbidity and mortality associated with esophagectomy for esophageal cancer remain significant.
- There has been an evolution of surgical procedures used to treat this disease beginning with the transthoracic esophagectomy and the transhiatal esophagectomy.
- More recently, advanced laparoscopic and thoracoscopic techniques have been applied to esophageal resection and reconstruction, and this procedure is now described as a minimally invasive esophagectomy.
- Surgeons and hospitals caring for patients with esophageal cancer must remain focused on performing esophagectomies with a low incidence of anastomotic complications and a low mortality regardless of which operative procedure is performed.

INTRODUCTION

The American Cancer Society estimates that 18,170 men and women (14,660 men and 3510 women) will be diagnosed with esophageal cancer in 2014, and the per-capita incidence of this lethal disease continues to increase. Although squamous cell carcinoma is the most common esophageal malignancy

The author has nothing to disclose.

E-mail address: rbattaf1@jhmi.edu

0065-3411/16/$ – see front matter
http://dx.doi.org/10.1016/j.yasu.2016.03.002

diagnosed worldwide, the incidence of adenocarcinoma in the United States has increased dramatically and now accounts for approximately 70% of newly diagnosed esophageal cancers. Importantly, esophageal cancer is now the seventh leading cause of cancer death in American men and will be responsible for more than 15,000 cancer deaths this year [1].

For those patients with esophageal cancer without distant metastatic disease, every effort is made to offer esophageal resection to these patients as part of the overall care of this disease. Despite improvements in anesthesia, surgical technique, and postoperative care, the morbidity and potential mortality associated with esophagectomy remain significant. Advances in laparoscopic and thoracoscopic techniques have been applied to esophageal resection and reconstruction, and this procedure is now described as a minimally invasive esophagectomy (MIE). Analysis of how this procedure might contribute to the overall care of patients with esophageal cancer is the focus of this review.

HISTORICAL NOTE

The first resection of the intrathoracic esophagus followed by esophagogastric reconstruction was reported by Ohsawa [2] in Japan in 1933. This approach was adopted in the United States after Adams and Phemister [3] reported their experience in 1939. However, transthoracic resection of the esophagus via laparotomy and right thoracotomy as treatment for esophageal cancer was not routinely performed until it was popularized by the English surgeon Ivor Lewis [4] in 1946; this operation continues to bear his name. McKeown [5] introduced the 3-incision procedure in order to improve proximal margins by first mobilizing the intrathoracic esophagus via a right thoracotomy followed by completion of the resection and reconstruction via laparotomy and neck incisions. Other variations of the transthoracic approach include the wide en-bloc esophagogastectomy popularized by Skinner [6], DeMeester, and Altorki and colleagues [7]. The left thoracoabdominal approach allows excellent visualization of both the intrathoracic esophagus and stomach in one operative field [8,9].

In an effort to decrease the morbidity and mortality of transthoracic resection of the esophagus, Orringer and colleagues [10,11] at the University of Michigan popularized the transhiatal esophagectomy (THE) performed via a laparotomy and left neck incision. By eliminating the thoracotomy incision, they hoped to limit the respiratory complications associated with the transthoracic procedure. In addition, they hoped to avoid the creation of intrathoracic anastomoses that historically were associated with high mortality by creating the anastomosis in the neck. Luketich and colleagues [12,13] at the University of Pittsburgh popularized the MIE using laparoscopic and thoracoscopic techniques. They initially performed a laparoscopic/thoracoscopic 3-incision procedure (McKeown), but more recently have converted to a laparoscopic/thoracoscopic operation with placement of the esophagogastric anastomosis in the right thorax.

The controversy associated with determining which operation is "best" in the management of patients with esophageal cancer continues until the present time. The core of this debate centers on optimizing the oncologic benefits of esophageal resection while minimizing the morbidity and mortality of this procedure. Comparing the results of previously published series using these different operative techniques as a rationale for choosing which operation to use at this time is difficult for several reasons: (1) esophageal cancer has changed from primarily being a disease of mid-esophageal squamous cancers to a disease of distal esophageal adenocarcinomas; (2) the routine use of neoadjuvant chemoradiation therapy for most esophageal cancers has resulted in the utilization of a gastric conduit that has been irradiated; (3) improvement in postoperative analgesia via patient-controlled epidural catheters has limited the morbidity associated with the thoracic incision. Despite these limitations, there is value in reviewing the recent literature examining transthoracic esophagectomy (TTE), THE, and MIEs in regard to operative morbidity and mortality and oncologic outcomes.

RELATIONSHIP BETWEEN ANASTOMOTIC LEAK AND OPERATIVE MORTALITY

The oncologic benefits of esophageal resection can only be realized if esophagectomy can be performed with limited morbidity and mortality. The importance of the relationship between surgical complications and survival was reported by Rizk and his colleagues [14] at Memorial Sloan Kettering Cancer Center. Of the 510 patients studied, 138 (27%) had complications directly attributable to surgical technique, such as an anastomotic leak, a paralyzed vocal cord, or chylothorax. Technical complications were associated with increased length of stay (median 23 days vs 11 days, $P<.001$), increased in-hospital mortality (12.3% vs 3.8%, $P<.001$), and a higher rate of medical complications (77.5% vs 47.3%, $P<.001$). Importantly, only 43 of 138 patients (31%) with technical complications were alive at 3 years, whereas 179 of 372 patients (48%) without technical complications were alive. After controlling for age, medical comorbidities, use of induction therapy, tumor stage, histology, location, and completeness of resection, the presence of a technical complication remained highly predictive of worse overall survival (hazard ratio = 1.41, $P = .008$). Anastomotic leak was the most common complication in this series and was the primary determinate of in-hospital mortality.

Because the severity of anastomotic leaks can vary from radiologic leaks in asymptomatic patients to conduit necrosis and septic shock, a standard classification system for esophagogastric anastomotic leaks has been adopted and is based on work by the Surgical Infection Study Group [15], a systematic review by Urschel [16], and a thoracic surgical working group led by Lerut [17]. This system categorizes leaks into 4 groups according to their clinical presentation and subsequent outcome. Radiological leaks are made up of clinically silent leaks that are found incidentally during routine postoperative contrast studies in patients with no systemic signs of infection. The leak identified is contained by surrounding structures and often drains back into the lumen through the anastomotic defect. These leaks require no change in the clinical management of the patient and will resolve with time.

Group 2 consists of clinically minor leaks. Patients with cervical anastomoses often develop wound erythema associated with fever and an elevated white blood cell count. Initial management requires reopening the wound at the bedside. In most patients, the leak will be contained in the neck by the surrounding tissues, and opening the wound and performing frequent dressing changes are all that is required. Management of contained intrathoracic leaks is dictated by their location and the patient's clinical course. Most respond to treatment with antibiotics and delaying oral intake. However, contained leaks close to the aorta and the trachea should be considered for drainage because of the risk of developing fistulas to these vital structures [18–20].

Group 3 includes clinically major leaks. These leaks are often identified by the development of a pneumothorax or pleural effusion associated with septic deterioration and demonstrate significant disruption of the anastomosis at the time of endoscopy. This complication can be associated with both intrathoracic and cervical anastomoses and requires an aggressive management approach. The 3 critical principles in the management of this problem are (1) complete drainage of the pleural space; (2) adequate control of the esophagogastric fistula; and (3) re-expansion of the lung. Small anastomotic leaks will often heal if the lung is completely expanded because the visceral pleura functions to buttress the leak. Chest tube drainage alone, thoracoscopic drainage and repair, and reoperative thoracotomy with direct repair and muscle flap reinforcement of the leak all can be successfully used to treat this complication as long as adherence to the above principles is followed. Because the mortality associated with anastomotic dehiscence ranges from 20% to 60%, an aggressive approach to this problem is required [21,22].

Group 4 constitutes early fulminant leaks that often present within the first 48 hours and are usually caused by gastric necrosis. These patients present with septic shock and require immediate operative intervention. Resection of nonviable portions of the stomach, creation of a cervical end esophagostomy, and placement of a drainage abdominal gastrostomy are required. This complication occurs infrequently but is often fatal without prompt aggressive treatment.

Because a significant number of esophageal surgeons obtain contrast esophagrams only in patients manifesting clinical signs of an anastomotic leak, anastomotic leak rates reported in the literature primarily reflect clinically significant leaks. Specific attention to the relationship between anastomotic leak and operative mortality has been demonstrated in the Society of Thoracic Surgeons Thoracic Surgery Database [23]. In a review of 7595 esophagectomies entered into the database from 2001 to 2011, the overall anastomotic leak rate was 10.6% (12.3% in the neck, 9.3% in the chest) and the 30-day operative mortality for the entire cohort was 3.6%. However, the mortality was 7.2% for patients with anastomotic leak and 3.1% without an anastomotic leak. Importantly, anastomotic leak was not only associated with an increase in mortality but also significantly associated with postoperative atrial arrhythmia, ventricular arrhythmia, deep vein thrombosis, pneumonia and acute respiratory distress syndrome, reintubation, empyema, sepsis, and renal failure [24].

Other single-institutional series have also demonstrated significant anastomotic leak rates and their subsequent negative effects on postoperative outcomes. Sepesi and his colleagues [25] from the MD Anderson Cancer Center reported their experience with 607 patients who underwent esophagectomy with thoracic anastomosis between January 2001 and August 2011. Anastomotic leak occurred in 51 of 607 patients (8.4%), and 30-day operative mortality was 2.6%. Because patients treated with omentum reinforcement of the anastomosis had a significantly lower anastomotic leak rate (4.7%) compared with patients without omentum (10.5%), they recommended routine use of omentum as a method for reducing anastomotic leaks.

Price and colleagues [26] from the Mayo Clinic reported their experience with 432 consecutive esophagectomies performed via a variety of surgical techniques using both intrathoracic and cervical esophagogastric anastomoses at their institution from July 2004 through December 2008. The anastomotic leak rate was 11% with the anastomotic leak rate being higher in cervical anastomoses (21%) compared with intrathoracic anastomoses (5.9%). The operative mortality was 3.7%. In this series, 17 (3.9%) patients required reoperation for anastomotic leaks, including anastomotic revision in 12 patients, esophageal exclusion in 3 patients, and drainage in 2 patients.

All of the reports described were primarily based on esophagectomies performed since 2000 and reflect the modern anastomotic leak rates and operative mortalities in North America. Moreover, these results clearly demonstrated that anastomotic complications result in significant morbidity and mortality. Attempts to reduce operative morbidity and mortality and to improve outcomes in this disease will have to focus on reducing the incidence and severity of anastomotic complications.

COMPARISON OF THE TRANSHIATAL AND TRANSTHORACIC ESOPHAGECTOMIES

Because Orringer and his colleagues at the University of Michigan introduced the THE in an effort to decrease the morbidity of esophageal resection, many consider the THE to be the first "minimally invasive esophagectomy." The introduction of the THE was initially associated with a significant amount of controversy. Proponents of the transthoracic approach argued that this approach allows for a complete lymphadenectomy together with esophageal resection following the standard oncologic principles for cancer resections. Proponents of the THE argued that decreasing the operative morbidity and mortality is the most important goal in choosing the surgical approach for esophagectomy. Two relatively recent analyses (a large meta-analysis of published reports and a prospective randomized trial) in the literature have attempted to answer this question.

Hulscher and his colleagues [27] identified 50 articles in the literature from 1990 to 1999, including 6 prospective comparative studies of which 3 were randomized. The overall in-hospital mortality in both groups taken together was 7.5%. However, the in-hospital mortality was significantly higher after transthoracic resections (9.2% vs 5.7%, relative risk [RR] 1.60, 95% confidence interval [CI] 1.42–1.89). Transthoracic resections also had a higher risk of pulmonary complications (18.7% vs 12.7%, RR 1.47, 95% CI 1.29–1.68), chylous leakage (2.4% vs 1.4%, RR 1.70, 95% CI 1.05–2.72), and wound infection (7.7% vs 4.3%, RR 1.76, 95% CI 1.37–2.27). Anastomotic leakage (7.2% vs 13.6%, RR 0.53, 95% CI 0.45–.063) and vocal cord paralysis (3.5% vs 9.5%, RR 0.36, 95% CI 0.27–0.47) were more frequent after transhiatal resections. However, overall survival at 3 years (26.7 vs 25.0) and at 5 years (23.0 vs 21.7) was not significantly different.

Because the investigators observed that data from the prospective studies included in their meta-analysis suggested an advantage to the transthoracic approach, they conducted a prospective randomized trial comparing TTE to THE. In this study, 220 patients with adenocarcinoma of the distal esophagus or esophagogastric junction were randomized to THE (106) or TTE (114) with extended en-bloc lymphadenectomy. The technique for the TTE used a 3-incision approach (McKeown) with creation of the anastomosis in the neck. No patients in this study received neoadjuvant therapy [28].

Examination of the postoperative course revealed that the overall in-hospital mortality for the entire group of patients was 3.2% and was not statistically different between THE and TTE (1.9% vs 4.4%, $P = .45$). However, there was a lower incidence of pulmonary complications in patients undergoing THE compared with TTE (27% vs 57%, $P < .001$) that translated into statistical differences in the need for mechanical ventilation, time in the intensive care unit, and length of hospital stay. As one might expect, anastomotic leak rates were similar (14% vs 16%, $P = .85$) because all anastomoses were created in the neck.

The primary endpoints of the study were overall survival and disease-free survival. Importantly, there was no difference between the 2 groups in cancer histology, TNM stage, or adequacy of resection as measured by the residual tumor classification system (R0-R2). The investigators had included, as a secondary endpoint, the total number of lymph nodes resected as a surrogate marker for the adequacy of the lymphadenectomy. In this regard, the total number of lymph nodes resected was lower in patients undergoing THE compared with those that underwent TTE (16 ± 9 vs 31 ± 14, $P < .001$). However, there was no difference in overall survival between patients that underwent THE and TTE (1.8 years vs 2.0 years, $P = .38$) or in disease-free survival (1.4 y vs 1.7 years, $P = .15$).

Analysis of this comparison of the TTE and THE suggests that avoidance of the thoracotomy incision reduces postoperative pulmonary complications and may even decrease early postoperative mortality. However, esophagogastric anastomoses created in the cervical position have higher rates of anastomotic leak rate and recurrent laryngeal nerve injury. Because all of these complications appear to negatively affect long-term survival, attempts to improve outcomes in the care of patients with esophageal cancer will need to focus on reducing both pulmonary and anastomotic complications in the perioperative period.

MINIMALLY INVASIVE ESOPHAGECTOMY USING LAPAROSCOPIC AND THORACOSCOPIC TECHNIQUES

The technique of MIE using a right thoracoscopic approach was initially described by Cushieri in 1992 [29,30], and the technique of laparoscopic THE was introduced in 1995 [31]. Since that time, several surgeons have adopted a minimally invasive approach to this procedure. In order to attempt to determine if there was an advantage of MIE versus the traditional TTE, Biere and his European colleagues [32] performed a multicenter, open-label, randomized controlled trial across 5 study centers between 2009 and 2011. Patients with resectable cancer of the esophagus or esophagogastric junction were randomly assigned via a computer-generated randomization sequence to receive either open transthoracic or minimally invasive TTE. The primary outcome was pulmonary infection within the first 2 weeks after surgery and during the whole stay in hospital.

In this study, 56 patients were randomized to TTE and 59 patients were randomized to MIE. The esophagogastric anastomosis was created in the neck in 65% of all patients, and this did not differ between the TTE and MIE groups. The combined 30-day and in-hospital mortality for the entire cohort of 115 patients was 2.6% and did not differ between the groups. Similarly, the overall anastomotic leak rate was 9.6% and did not differ between TTE and MIE (7% vs 12%, $P = .39$). However, there were significantly more pulmonary infections in the TTE group compared with the MIE group (34% vs 12%; $P = .005$) validating their hypothesis that MIE would reduce pulmonary complications.

The largest series of MIE was reported by Luketich and his colleagues [13] from the University of Pittsburgh in 2012. A total of 1011 consecutive patients underwent MIE with either a cervical anastomosis (481) or intrathoracic anastomosis (530) from 1996 to 2011. Initially, they used a laparoscopic/thoracoscopic 3-incision (McKeown) procedure with creation of the esophagogastric anastomosis in the neck. The investigators then converted to a laparoscopic/thoracoscopic (Ivor-Lewis) procedure with creation of the anastomosis in the right thorax.

In this series, the combined 30-day and in-house mortality for the entire group was 2.8%. Although the 30-day mortality did not differ significantly between the MIE-Ivor-Lewis and the MIE-McKeown groups (0.9% vs 2.5%, $P = .83$), there was a difference in the combined 30-day and in-house mortality between the groups that did achieve significance (1.7% vs 3.95%, $P = .035$). The overall incidence of postoperative adverse events did not differ between the MIE-Ivor-Lewis and the MIE-McKeown group. However, injury to the recurrent laryngeal nerve was more common in patients undergoing the MIE-McKeown procedure (8% vs 1%, $P < .001$) as was the development of acute respiratory distress syndrome (4% vs 2%, $P = .03$).

This series demonstrated that the MIE can be performed with acceptable mortality and low morbidity. Moreover, it suggests that the MIE-Ivor-Lewis approach appears to be better tolerated by patients than the MIE-McKeown technique. Because the investigators did not routinely obtain contrast esophagrams in all patients, an anastomotic leak rate was not reported. However, 5% of the patients in the series developed an anastomotic leak requiring operative intervention, and this did not differ between the 2 different MIE techniques.

IS THERE AN OPTIMAL SURGICAL TECHNIQUE FOR PERFORMING ESOPHAGECTOMY?

In reviewing the modern reports describing the outcomes associated with esophagectomy in the management of patients with esophageal cancer, there has been a steady decline in the operative mortality from approximately 5% to 6% in the 1990s to the current rate of approximately 2% to 4%. However, overall anastomotic leak rates have remained relatively high (8%–14%), and a significant number of patients undergoing esophagectomy require operative intervention for anastomotic leaks (4%–5%). Importantly, anastomotic complications significantly contribute to the morbidity and mortality associated with esophagectomy and potentially mitigate the oncologic benefits of this procedure.

In an effort to decrease anastomotic complications and their negative impact on survival, several changes were made in the surgical management of patients with esophageal cancer undergoing esophagectomy. Because the literature clearly has demonstrated that esophagogastric anastomoses created in the neck have a higher leak rate, the creation of neck anastomoses were avoided unless absolutely necessary to achieve a negative proximal margin. All procedures used an upper midline laparotomy and a right posterolateral thoracomy. A left neck incision was added in those patients that required a cervical anastomosis in order to achieve a negative proximal margin. The esophagogastric anastomoses were created on the greater curvature of the stomach just distal to the gastroepiploic arterial arcade that had a strong pulse. If there was a diminution in the pulse over the last few arcades of the gastroepiploic artery, the anastomosis was created more proximally on the greater curvature to ensure an adequate blood flow for anastomotic healing. Importantly, all of the esophagogastric anastomoses performed in the thorax (Ivor-Lewis) were created using a circular stapler no smaller than 28 mm in diameter after liberally mobilizing the esophagus to allow creation of a tension-free esophagogastric anastomosis. All patients had patient-controlled epidural catheters as their primary mode of perioperative analgesia. All patients began receiving enteral nutrition via a feeding jejunostomy tube by the third postoperative day and continued with enteral nutrition for at least 30 days following surgery. All patients underwent a contrast esophagram to determine the adequacy of the anastomosis and to assure gastric emptying.

Eighty-one consecutive patients underwent esophagectomy following neoadjuvant chemoradiation therapy using this operative strategy. There was a preponderance of male patients with esophageal adenocarcinomas, and most patients underwent an Ivor-Lewis esophagogastrectomy via a laparotomy and right thoracotomy. However, 3 patients with squamous cell carcinoma of the midesophagus required a 3-incision (McKeown) esophagectomy with creation of a neck anastomosis in order to achieve a negative proximal margin (Table 1).

Three (3.7%) patients developed an anastomotic leak following surgery. Two of these leaks occurred in patients whose anastomoses were created in the neck. One of these patients developed necrosis of the fundus of the gastric conduit requiring reoperation. This patient ultimately died of multisystem organ failure and was the only mortality (1.2%) in this group. Of the 78 patients that underwent an Ivor-Lewis esophagectomy and creation of the esophagogastric anastomosis in the upper thorax using a circular stapler, there was 1 anastomotic leak and no operative deaths. This leak was radiographically noted, but not clinically apparent, and this leak did not require operative intervention.

One patient developed a late (postoperative day 43) fistula between the esophagus and the right main stem bronchus that was not present on the postoperative contrast esophagram performed on day 8. This fistula was successfully repaired with a second operation. Respiratory failure requiring reintubation occurred in 9 (11.1%) patients, and an additional 14 (17.2%) patients were treated for pneumonia. New-onset atrial fibrillation was the single most frequent complication following esophagectomy and occurred in 21 (25.9%) patients.

The data from this series suggest that adopting a systematic approach to the surgical management of patients with esophageal cancer following neoadjuvant chemoradiation therapy can result in a low anastomotic leak rate and a low

Table 1
Characteristics of 81 consecutive patients that underwent esophagectomy following neoadjuvant chemoradiation therapy

Gender	
Male	65
Female	16
Histology	
Adenocarcinoma	73
Squamous cell carcinoma	8
Procedure	
McKeown	3
Ivor-Lewis	78
Anastomotic technique	
Hand-sewn	2
Linear stapler	1
Circular stapler (28 mm)	78

mortality. The results of this series compare very favorably with the results of Mathisen and colleagues [33] in which there were no intrathoracic anastomotic leaks and a 2.3% operative mortality in 104 esophagectomy patients. However, none of these patients received neoadjuvant chemoradiation therapy. Cerfolio and colleagues [34] reported a series of 90 patients that underwent Ivor-Lewis esophagogastrectomy, of which 52 (58%) patients received neoadjuvant therapy. No patient was noted to have an anastomotic leak on contrast esophagram. However, 4 (4.4%) patients died in the postoperative period, and all of these received neoadjuvant chemoradiation therapy. The investigators also observed that patients treated with neoadjuvant therapy had a higher overall complication rate (Table 2).

DEVELOPMENT OF A MAXIMALLY EFFECTIVE ESOPHAGECTOMY

Over the last 40 years, there have been many advances in the operative management of patients with locally advanced esophageal cancer that have resulted in an overall decrease in the operative mortality of esophagectomy. However, additional work remains to decrease the operative morbidity associated with this procedure, especially in those patients treated with neoadjuvant chemoradiation therapy. During this period, THE and MIE have been added to the TTE in an effort to decrease the pulmonary complications associated with this procedure. Moving forward, however, it will be critical that all institutions involved in the care of patients with esophageal cancer be able to demonstrate a marked diminution in the rate of anastomotic complications in order to decrease the morbidity and mortality following esophagectomy. Whether surgeons perform a THE, an MIE, or a TTE, the goal should be for anastomotic complication rates of less than 5% and operative mortalities of less that 2%. The question for all those involved in the care of patients with esophageal cancer is not whether MIE is "better" than THE or TTE, but rather, which operative strategy at each institution is associated with the lowest anastomotic

Table 2
Complications associated with esophagectomy following neoadjuvant therapy (N = 81)

Complication	N	%
Anastomotic leak	3	3.7
Operative mortality	1	1.2
Tracheoesophageal fistula	1	1.2
Respiratory failure	9	11.1
Pneumonia	14	17.2
Chyle leak	5	6.2
New-onset atrial fibrillation	21	25.9
Myocardial infarction	1	1.2
Recurrent laryngeal nerve injury	4	4.9
Pulmonary embolus	1	1.2
Deep vein thrombosis	3	3.7

complication rate and lowest operative mortality. There is no doubt that in the future there will be an increasing number of esophagectomies performed using laparoscopic, thoracoscopic, and even robotic techniques. However, the focus at each institution must remain on performing a maximally effective esophagectomy associated with low anastomotic complication and low mortalities.

References

[1] Siegel R, Ma J, Zou Z, et al. Cancer statistics. CA Cancer J Clin 2014;2014(64):9–29.
[2] Ohsawa T. The surgery of the esophagus. Arch Jpn Chir 1933;10:605–8.
[3] Adams W, Phemister D. Carcinoma of the lower thoracic esophagus: report of a successful resection and esophagogastrectomy. J Thorac Cardiovasc Surg 1939;7:621–8.
[4] Lewis I. The surgical treatment of carcinoma of the oesophagus; with special reference to a new operation for growths of the middle third. Br J Surg 1946;34:18–31.
[5] McKeown KC. The surgical treatment of carcinoma of the oesophagus. J R Soc Med 1974;67:389–95.
[6] Skinner DB. En bloc resection for neoplasms of the esophagus and cardia. J Thorac Cardiovasc Surg 1983;85:59–71.
[7] Altorki NK, Girardi L, Skinner DB. En bloc esophagectomy improves survival for stage III esophageal cancer. J Thorac Cardiovasc Surg 1997;114:948–55.
[8] Sweet RH. Transthoracic resection of the esophagus and stomach for carcinoma: analysis of the postoperative complications, causes of death, and late results of operation. Ann Surg 1945;121:272–84.
[9] Ma J, Zhan C, Wang L, et al. The sweet approach is still worthwhile in modern esophagectomy. Ann Thorac Surg 2014;97:1728–33.
[10] Orringer MB, Sloan H. Esophagectomy without thoracotomy. J Thorac Cardiovasc Surg 1978;76:643–54.
[11] Orringer MB, Marshall B, Iannettoni MD. Transhiatal esophagectomy: clinical experience and refinements. Ann Surg 1999;230:392–400.
[12] Luketich JD, Fernando HC, Christie NA, et al. Outcomes after minimally invasive esophagomyotomy. Ann Thorac Surg 2001;72:1909–12.
[13] Luketich JD, Pennathur A, Awais O, et al. Outcomes after minimally invasive esophagectomy: review of over 1000 patients. Ann Surg 2012;256:95–103.
[14] Rizk NP, Bach PB, Schrag D, et al. The impact of complications on outcomes after resection for esophageal and gastroesophageal junction carcinoma. J Am Coll Surg 2004;198:42–50.
[15] Peel AL, Taylor EW. Proposed definitions for the audit of postoperative infection: a discussion paper. Surgical Infection Study Group. Ann R Coll Surg Engl 1991;73:385–8.
[16] Urschel JD. Esophagogastrostomy anastomotic leaks complicating esophagectomy: a review. Am J Surg 1995;169:634–40.
[17] Lerut T, Coosemans W, Decker G, et al. Anastomotic complications after esophagectomy. Dig Surg 2002;19:92–8.
[18] Marty-Ane CH, Prudhome M, Fabre JM, et al. Tracheoesophagogastric anastomosis fistula: a rare complication of esophagectomy. Ann Thorac Surg 1995;60:690–3.
[19] Bartels HE, Stein HJ, Siewert JR. Tracheobronchial lesions following oesophagectomy: prevalence, predisposing factors and outcome. Br J Surg 1998;85:403–6.
[20] Matory YL, Burt M. Esophagogastrectomy: reoperation for complications. J Surg Oncol 1993;54:29–33.
[21] Patil PK, Patel SG, Mistry RC, et al. Cancer of the esophagus: esophagogastric anastomotic leak–a retrospective study of predisposing factors. J Surg Oncol 1992;49:163–7.
[22] Tam PC, Fok M, Wong J. Reexploration for complications after esophagectomy for cancer. J Thorac Cardiovasc Surg 1989;98:1122–7.
[23] Wright CD, Kucharczuk JC, O'Brien SM, et al. Predictors of major morbidity and mortality after esophagectomy for esophageal cancer: a Society of Thoracic Surgeons General

Thoracic Surgery Database risk adjustment model. J Thorac Cardiovasc Surg 2009;137: 587–95.
[24] Kassis ES, Kosinski AS, Ross P Jr, et al. Predictors of anastomotic leak after esophagectomy: an analysis of the Society of Thoracic Surgeons general thoracic database. Ann Thorac Surg 2013;96:1919–26.
[25] Sepesi B, Swisher SG, Walsh GL, et al. Omental reinforcement of the thoracic esophagogastric anastomosis: an analysis of leak and reintervention rates in patients undergoing planned and salvage esophagectomy. J Thorac Cardiovasc Surg 2012;144:1146–50.
[26] Price TN, Nichols FC, Harmsen WS, et al. A comprehensive review of anastomotic technique in 432 esophagectomies. Ann Thorac Surg 2013;95:1154–60.
[27] Hulscher JB, Tijssen JG, Obertop H, et al. Transthoracic versus transhiatal resection for carcinoma of the esophagus: a meta-analysis. Ann Thorac Surg 2001;72:306–13.
[28] Hulscher JB, van Sandick JW, de Boer AG, et al. Extended transthoracic resection compared with limited transhiatal resection for adenocarcinoma of the esophagus. N Engl J Med 2002;347:1662–9.
[29] Cuschieri A. Endoscopic subtotal oesophagectomy for cancer using the right thoracoscopic approach. Surg Oncol 1993;2(Suppl 1):3–11.
[30] Cuschieri A. Thoracoscopic subtotal oesophagectomy. Endosc Surg Allied Technol 1994;2: 21–5.
[31] DePaula AL, Hashiba K, Ferreira EA, et al. Laparoscopic transhiatal esophagectomy with esophagogastroplasty. Surg Laparosc Endosc 1995;5:1–5.
[32] Biere SS, van Berge Henegouwen MI, Maas KW, et al. Minimally invasive versus open oesophagectomy for patients with oesophageal cancer: a multicentre, open-label, randomised controlled trial. Lancet 2012;379:1887–92.
[33] Mathisen DJ, Grillo HC, Wilkins EW Jr, et al. Transthoracic esophagectomy: a safe approach to carcinoma of the esophagus. Ann Thorac Surg 1988;45:137–43.
[34] Cerfolio RJ, Bryant AS, Bass CS, et al. Fast tracking after Ivor Lewis esophagogastrectomy. Chest 2004;126:1187–94.

Advances in Surgery 50 (2016) 29–40

ADVANCES IN SURGERY

Optimal Management of the Axilla: A Look at the Evidence

Eleftherios (Terry) P. Mamounas, MD, MPH

Comprehensive Breast Program, University of Florida Health Cancer Center - Orlando Health, 1400 South Orange Avenue, MP 700, Orlando, FL 32806, USA

Keywords

• Breast cancer • Axillary staging • Sentinel lymph node biopsy • Axillary dissection

Key points

- The development and validation of sentinel lymph node biopsy (SLNB) for early-stage breast cancer has challenged the primacy of axillary lymph node dissection (ALND) for staging the axilla.
- Randomized clinical trials established the role of SLNB alone as the standard of care for patients with negative SLN(s).
- Additional clinical trials have evaluated the use of SLNB alone in patients with limited SLN involvement and in those treated with neoadjuvant chemotherapy.
- These trials have helped to expand the role of SLNB (either alone or with axillary radiotherapy) for the majority of patients with early-stage breast cancer.

INTRODUCTION

The surgical management of the axilla in patients with operable breast cancer has undergone significant evolution during the past 30 years. Axillary lymph node dissection (ALND) was established as the undisputed standard of care at the end of the nineteenth century as part of the Halsted radical mastectomy and remained so for the better part of the twentieth century until its therapeutic role was challenged by a randomized clinical trial (National Surgical Adjuvant Breast and Bowel Project [NSABP] B-04) [1,2]. That trial showed that elective ALND or axillary radiotherapy did not improve long-term outcomes for patients with clinically negative axilla. However, even following publication of the results of the B-04 trial in the late 1970s, the procedure still remained the

Disclosure: The author has nothing to disclose.

E-mail address: terry.mamounas@orlandohealth.com

0065-3411/16/$ – see front matter
http://dx.doi.org/10.1016/j.yasu.2016.03.003

standard of care for axillary staging because of the need to obtain the prognostic information of pathologic nodal status and the need to identify candidates for adjuvant chemotherapy. In addition, ALND in patients with pathologically positive axillary nodes provided excellent control of the disease in the axilla [2].

Over the ensuing years, elective ALND remained the gold standard for staging the axilla because no imaging modality was shown to be as accurate as pathologic examination of the axillary nodes in predicting axillary nodal status. However, by the late 1980s, widespread use of screening mammography resulted in an increasing proportion of patients presenting without axillary involvement at the time of ALND. Such patients do not derive any therapeutic benefit from ALND but are at risk for its sequelae. The need to avoid the morbidity of ALND in these histologically node-negative patients without losing prognostic information led to the development of lymphatic mapping and sentinel lymph node biopsy (SLNB) [3,4].

DEVELOPMENT OF LYMPHATIC MAPPING AND SENTINEL LYMPH NODE BIOPSY

The sentinel lymph node (SLN) concept dictates that lymphatic drainage from the breast to the regional nodes follows an orderly pattern to a primary node or SLN and from there to secondary nodes or non-SLNs. Although it was initially thought that different parts of the breast may drain to different SLNs, recent data support the principle that different parts of the breast drain to the same SLNs [5,6].

Single-institution and multicenter studies of sentinel lymph node biopsy

Multiple single-institution series have evaluated SLNB plus ALND [7]. Most used a combination of blue dye and radiocolloid for lymphatic mapping. In general, the identification rates (IRs) were higher when radiocolloid was used either alone or combined with blue dye rather than when dye alone was used. The false-negative rate (FNR) varied widely (0%–19%) and tended to be higher when radiocolloid was not included in the mapping.

Several multicenter studies evaluated SLNB plus ALND in the mid to late 1990s [8–12]. Altogether, these studies included more than 3300 patients. Lymphatic mapping included blue dye, radiocolloid, or the combination of both. SLN IR ranged between 74% and 94% and FNR ranged between 4% and 13%. These studies provided information on the ability to successfully perform lymphatic mapping and SLNB in various clinical settings and by surgeons with different levels of experience with the procedure.

A meta-analysis [13] of 69 studies and more than 10,000 patients undergoing SLNB plus ALND showed a greater than or equal to 90% IR in about half of the studies and an overall FNR of 8.4%. Based on the information discussed earlier, the American College of Surgeons Oncology Group (ACOSOG) eventually conducted a multicenter study (ACOSOG Z-0010) that prospectively evaluated SLNB without completion ALND in patients with negative SLNs showing low rates of axillary recurrence [14].

Randomized trials of sentinel lymph node biopsy alone versus sentinel lymph node biopsy plus axillary lymph node dissection in patients with negative sentinel lymph nodes

Several randomized trials have compared SLNB alone with SLNB plus ALND in patients with negative SLNs (Milan, NSABP B-32, Axillary Lymphatic Mapping Against Nodal Axillary Clearance [ALMANAC]) [15–20]. The aims of these trials were to compare the 2 procedures in terms of disease-free survival (DFS) and overall survival (OS), axillary recurrence, morbidity, and quality of life (QOL).

The first randomized trial to report results was the Milan trial [15], in which 516 patients with tumors less than or equal to 2 cm were randomized to SLNB plus ALND or to SLNB alone with ALND only in case of SLN involvement. SLNB alone resulted in less pain and better arm mobility. In the ALND group, 32% had positive SLNs. The FNR was 4.6%. With 46 months' median follow-up, there were no differences in axillary recurrence between the two groups. Updated results, with 79 months' median follow-up, showed no significant OS differences between the two groups (96.4% with ALND and 98.4% with SLN; log-rank $P = .1$) [16]. Only 1 overt axillary metastasis occurred in the group that did not receive ALND. Because of its small sample size, the trial does not have the statistical power to detect small DFS and OS differences between the two groups.

The ALMANAC trial [20] compared arm/shoulder morbidity and QOL outcomes in 1031 patients with clinically node-negative invasive breast cancer who were randomized to SLNB versus ALND. Intention-to-treat analyses at 1, 3, 6, and 12 months after surgery were conducted. The relative risks of any lymphedema and sensory loss for SLNB versus ALND at 12 months were 0.37 (absolute rates: 5% vs 13%) and 0.37 (absolute rates: 11% vs 31%), respectively. Drain usage, length of hospital stay, and time to resumption of normal day-to-day activities after surgery were statistically significantly lower with SLNB versus ALND (all $P < .001$). Overall patient-recorded QOL and arm functioning scores were significantly better with SLNB throughout (all $P \leq .003$), whereas no increase in anxiety levels was noted with SLNB only ($P > .05$).

The largest randomized trial to date (NSABP B-32) randomized 5611 patients with operable breast cancer and clinically negative axillary nodes to SLNB alone versus SLNB plus ALND. Patients in the SLNB-alone group with positive SLNs also underwent full ALND. The technical outcomes of the trial showed an IR of 97.2% and an FNR of 9.8% [18]. Tumor location, type of biopsy, and number of removed SLNs significantly affected the FNR (FNR was 17.7% with 1 SLN, 10.0% with 2 SLNs, 6.9% with 3 SLNs, 5.5% with 4 SLNs, and 1% with 5 or more SLNs). Significant improvement in 3-year postsurgical morbidity levels was noted with SLNB alone versus SLNB plus ALND in terms of relative shoulder abduction deficits, relative arm volume differences, arm numbness, and arm tingling [17]. Long-term outcome results of the trial were reported in 2010 [19] with a mean time on study for SLN-negative patients of 95.6 months. There were no significant differences in DFS or OS between the two groups (8-year DFS, 82.4% vs 81.5%; hazard ratio [HR], 1.05; *P* = .54. OS, 91.8% vs 90.3%; HR, 1.20; *P* = .12 with SLNB plus ALND vs SLNB alone). There were 8 regional node recurrences as first events in the SLNB plus ALND group and 14 in the SLNB-alone group (*P* = .22). These results indicate that when SLNB is negative, SLNB alone is an appropriate, safe, and effective therapy for patients with operable breast cancer and clinically negative axilla.

Clinical significance of occult sentinel lymph node metastases

Retrospective and observational analyses suggest that presence of occult lymph node metastases is an important prognostic factor of outcome in early-stage breast cancer. However, prospective data from randomized trials according to SLN involvement have been lacking. Thus, an additional objective of the B-32 trial was to examine the prognostic significance of immunohistochemistry (IHC)-detected tumor cells in SLNs when routine hematoxylin and eosin (H&E) stain was negative [21]. Paraffin-embedded tissue blocks of SLNs from patients with pathologically negative SLNs were centrally evaluated for occult metastases. Both routine staining and IHC staining for cytokeratin were used at 2 widely spaced additional tissue levels. Treating physicians were unaware of the findings. Occult metastases were detected in 15.9% of 3887 patients (about two-thirds were isolated tumor cells and one-third micrometastases). Patients with occult metastases versus those without had significantly worse DFS (HR, 1.40; *P* = .02), distant disease-free interval (HR, 1.31; *P* = .04) and OS (HR, 1.30; *P* = .03). However, absolute differences in outcomes were small (5-year OS with occult metastases vs without were 94.6% and 95.8%, respectively). These results support that occult metastases in the SLNs are independent prognostic predictors of outcome but, because the magnitude of the outcome differences is small, there is little clinical benefit of additional evaluation of negative SLNs, including IHC analysis. This recommendation has also been included in the current American Society of Clinical Oncology guidelines [22].

The results of the randomized trials discussed earlier, along with the collective experience from single-institution and multicenter trials of SLNB plus ALND, helped establish SLNB alone as the gold standard for staging the axilla when the SLNs are negative. More importantly, they paved the way for the conduct of a series of clinical trials evaluating the role of SLNB alone (or with axillary radiotherapy) in patients with positive SLNs.

Randomized trials of sentinel lymph node biopsy alone versus sentinel lymph node biopsy plus axillary lymph node dissection in patients with limited sentinel lymph node involvement

The most influential trial evaluating SLNB alone in patients with positive SLNs was the ACOSOG Z0011 trial [23], a phase 3, noninferiority trial designed to determine the effects of completion ALND on survival of patients with SLN metastasis. Eligible patients had clinical T1 to T2 invasive breast cancer, no palpable adenopathy, and 1 to 2 positive SLNs identified by frozen section, touch preparation, or H&E staining on permanent section. Target enrollment was 1900 women with final analysis after 500 deaths, but the trial closed early (46.9% of the preplanned accrual, 94 deaths) because of slow accrual and lower-than-expected mortality. All patients underwent lumpectomy and whole-breast irradiation, although high breast tangents were frequently used and approximately 19% of patients also received regional node irradiation [24]. Patients with 1 to 2 positive SLNs were randomized to ALND (n = 445) or not (n = 446). With median follow-up of 6.3 years, the 5-year OS was 91.8% with SLNB plus ALND and 92.5% with SLNB alone (not inferior). The 5-year DFS was 82.2% with SLNB plus ALND and 83.9% with SLNB alone. Ipsilateral axillary recurrences were rare in both groups (0.5% with SLNB plus ALND and 0.9% with SLNB alone). Based on these findings, the investigators concluded that, in patients with limited SLN involvement treated with breast-conserving surgery, breast radiotherapy and adjuvant systemic therapy, use of SLNB alone compared with SLNB plus ALND did not result in inferior survival.

The findings from the ACOSOG Z0011 trial were further corroborated by the findings of another randomized clinical trial (IBCSG 23–01) designed to evaluate whether no ALND was noninferior to ALND in patients with 1 or more SLNs with micrometastases ($\leq$2 mm) and primary tumor of less than or equal to 5 cm [25]. The primary end point was DFS and noninferiority was defined as an HR of less than 1.25 for no ALND versus ALND by intention to treat. Patients treated with mastectomy were eligible. Although target accrual was 1960 patients (analysis after 558 events), slow accrual led to early termination of accrual with 934 patients (98 events). With median follow-up of 5.0 years, the 5-year DFS was 87.8% without ALND and 84.4% with ALND (log-rank $P = .16$; HR for no ALND vs ALND, 0.78; non-inferiority $P = .0042$). Long-term surgical events such as sensory neuropathy, lymphedema, and motor neuropathy were mainly seen in the group that underwent ALND. Based on these findings, the investigators concluded that ALND could be avoided in patients with early breast cancer and limited SLN involvement, thus minimizing complications of axillary surgery.

A third randomized trial that has informed axillary management in patients with positive SLNs was the AMAROS (After Mapping of the Axilla: Radiotherapy or Surgery) trial [26]. This open-label, randomized, noninferiority trial was designed to assess whether axillary radiotherapy provides comparable regional control with fewer side-effects compared with ALND. Eligible patients with T1 to T2 primary breast cancer and no palpable lymphadenopathy who were found to have positive SLNs at surgery were randomly assigned to ALND or axillary radiotherapy. Extracapsular nodal extension was not an exclusion criterion and 18% of patients were treated with mastectomy. The primary end point was noninferiority of 5-year axillary recurrence, considered to be not more than 4% with axillary radiotherapy versus an expected 2% with

ALND. Of the 1425 patients with positive SLNs, 744 were randomized to ALND and 681 to axillary radiotherapy. With median follow-up of 6.1 years, 5-year axillary recurrence was 0.43% after ALND versus 1.19% after axillary radiotherapy. Because of the low number of events, the planned noninferiority test was underpowered. Ipsilateral arm lymphedema was noted significantly more often after ALND than after axillary radiotherapy (at 1, 3, and 5 years). Based on the findings, the investigators concluded that after a positive SLNB, ALND and axillary radiotherapy provide excellent and comparable axillary control but axillary radiotherapy results in significantly less morbidity.

The results of the ACOSOG Z0011 and the IBCSG 23-01 have been rapidly adopted in clinical practice [27,28]. One large study based on information from the National Cancer Data Base examined use of SLNB alone in patients who did and did not fulfill Z0011 eligibility criteria from 1998 to 2011 [28]. The proportion of lumpectomy patients receiving SLNB increased from 6.1% in 1998 to 23.0% in 2009 to 56.0% in 2011 ($P<.001$). However, patients outside of Z0011 criteria also underwent SLNB alone: 54% of patients with tumors greater than 5 cm, 52.5% who received no radiation therapy or accelerated partial breast irradiation, 35.9% with clinically positive nodes, 22.3% who underwent mastectomy, and 12.9% who had greater than 3 tumor-positive nodes. These results underscore the need for careful patient selection when attempting to apply the results of randomized clinical trials to everyday practice.

Assessment of axillary nodal status in patients treated with neoadjuvant chemotherapy

In patients who are considered for NC, absence of information on pathologic axillary nodal status at presentation is often of concern. Thus, assessing axillary nodal status with noninvasive/minimally invasive techniques is essential. Axillary ultrasonography with fine-needle aspiration (FNA) or core needle biopsy of abnormal lymph nodes is a simple, minimally invasive study that can help establish axillary lymph node involvement and provide direct evidence of chemosensitivity of axillary metastases to NC [29]. SLNB is another option for assessing axillary nodal status before NC and its feasibility and accuracy in typical candidates for NC has previously been shown in small series [30,31] and as part of multicenter and randomized trials [9–11,15]. However, as discussed later, the use of SLNB before NC is controversial.

Sentinel lymph node biopsy in patients treated with neoadjuvant chemotherapy

NC downstages involved axillary lymph nodes in a considerable proportion of patients [32–35]. With SLNB becoming the standard of care for staging the axilla in early-stage breast cancer, patients who present with either overt or subclinical involvement of the axilla could potentially be spared from ALND if, following NC, the SLN is found to be negative. This approach is naturally predicated on the demonstration of the feasibility and accuracy of SLNB after NC, which has been assessed in single-institution series, multicenter series, and meta-analyses.

Single-institution studies of sentinel lymph node biopsy after neoadjuvant chemotherapy
Single-institution studies have shown great variability in IR and FNR of SLNB. When early single-institution studies (2000–2004) are examined collectively, the average IR is around 89% and the average FNR is around 11% [36]. Although the IR is lower than that with up-front SLNB, the FNR seems to be comparable between the two approaches [3,4,9,10]. When more recent, single-institution studies (2005–2009) are examined collectively [36], the IR is around 86% (still lower than with up-front SLNB) and the FNR is around 10% (comparable with that with up-front SLNB) [3,4,9,10]. The largest single-institution experience with SLNB after NC comes from MD Anderson Cancer Center [37]. The study also compared the accuracy of SLNB after NC (n = 575) with that of up-front SLNB (n = 3171). SLN IR was 97.4% in the NC group and 98.7% in the surgery-first group (P = .017). FNRs were similar between the two groups: 5.9% with NC vs 4.1% in the surgery-first group (P = .39).

Multicenter studies of sentinel node biopsy after neoadjuvant chemotherapy
A retrospective analysis from the NSABP B-27 trial [38] included 428 patients treated with NC who underwent SLNB plus ALND. The IR was 85% and the FNR was 11%. FNR was numerically lower when radiocolloid was used for lymphatic mapping (8%) versus when lymphazurin alone was used (14%). The FNR was not significantly different in patients who presented with clinically negative versus clinically positive axillary nodes (12.4% vs 7.0% respectively; P = .51). The prospective, multicenter study from France (GANEA [Ganglion Sentinelle et Chimiotherapie Neoadjuvante]) [39] evaluated 195 patients with $T_{0\text{-}3}N_{0\text{-}1}$ breast cancer who underwent dual-agent lymphatic mapping. The IR was 90% and the FNR was 11.5%. Patients with clinical N_0 before NC had a higher IR versus those with clinical N_1 but there were no significant differences in FNR between the two groups. When these two multicenter studies are examined together, the overall IR is 86.5% (lower than with up-front SLNB) but the overall FNR is 10.9%, (comparable with that with up-front SLNB) [36].

Meta-analysis of studies evaluating sentinel lymph node biopsy after neoadjuvant chemotherapy
The first reported meta-analysis of SLNB plus ALND before NC [40] included 21 studies and 1273 patients. The pooled estimate of IR was 90% and the pooled estimate of the FNR was 12%. A second meta-analysis [41] included 24 studies and 1799 patients. The summary of successful IR was 89.6% and the summary FNR was 8.4%, both with no significant heterogeneity. Both meta-analyses concluded that SLNB is a reliable tool for planning treatment in patients treated with NC as an alternative to completion ALND.

Sentinel lymph node biopsy after neoadjuvant chemotherapy in patients with known axillary involvement at diagnosis
Based on the evidence presented earlier, most surgeons have now adopted SLNB after NC for patients who present with clinically N_0 disease. However,

there is still concern over the feasibility and accuracy of SLNB in patients who present with documented involvement of the axilla. Initial small, single-institution, retrospective studies produced conflicting results [42–44]. One study that included patients with locally advanced features (clinical T_4N_2) showed significantly higher FNR compared with up-front SLNB [42], whereas 2 others showed comparable FNRs between the two approaches [43,44].

Three prospective studies were recently reported that provide additional important information on the subject [45–47]. The ACOSOG Z0171 was a single-arm trial of SLNB plus ALND in 756 patients with $T_{0\text{-}4}N_{1\text{-}2}$ breast cancer and biopsy-proven axillary lymph node involvement [45]. The primary end point was FNR in women with cN_1 disease greater than or equal to 2 SLNs removed. The SLN IR was 92.9%. Positive SLNs had metastases greater than 0.2 mm on H&E only. For patients with cN_1 disease and greater than or equal to 2 SLNs identified, the FNR was 12.6%. FNR was 10.8% with dual-agent mapping and 9.1% when greater than or equal to 3 sentinel nodes (SNs) were removed. Because the observed FNR was higher than the prespecified study end point of 10%, the investigators suggested further analyses of factors associated with FNR before widespread use of SLN in these patients. Additional analyses of Z1071 from the 2014 San Antonio Breast Cancer Symposium [48], based on 470 patients with cN_1 disease and greater than or equal to 2 SLNs, for which pathologic evaluation with IHC was available, showed an FNR of 8.7%. A resulting increase in unnecessary ALND occurred in only 2.1% of the patients (positive SLN with isolated tumor cells and no non-SLNs with metastases >0.2 mm). An unplanned subgroup analysis of Z1071 also examined patients who had a clip placed in the positive node at time of biopsy (32% of the total). When the clip was identified in the removed SLNs the FNR was 6.8%. If the clip was not identified in the SLNs, the FNR was much higher (39%).

The second prospective study (SENTINA trial [SENTinel NeoAdjuvant]) [46] was a 4-arm prospective multicenter cohort study designed to evaluate a specific algorithm for the timing of a standardized SLNB procedure after NC. As part of the trial, patients with clinical nodal involvement before NC (biopsy proof was not mandatory) who converted to clinically node negative after NC underwent SLNB plus ALND. The SLNB detection rate was 80.1% and the FNR was 14.2%. In the multivariate regression analysis, the number of removed SLNs was a significant predictor of FNR (odds ratio for >1 vs 1 SLN removed, .505; $P = .008$). The FNR was 24.3% with 1 SLN removed versus 9.6% with 2 or more SLNs removed. In addition, the FNR was 16% when radiocolloid alone was used versus 8.6% when radiocolloid plus blue dye was used for lymphatic mapping.

The third prospective trial (SN FNAC [Sentinel Node Following NeoAdjuvant Chemotherapy]) evaluated SLNB plus ALND after NC in 153 T0-3, $N_{1\text{-}2}$ patients with biopsy-proven, node-positive breast cancer [47]. In this study, use of IHC was mandatory and eligible patients had any size SLN metastases (ypN_0(i+), ypN_1mi, or ypN_1). The SLN IR was 87.6%. The FNR was

9.6%. Use of dual mapping was associated with numerically lower FNR compared with the use of radiocolloid alone (5.2% vs 16.0%). FNR was 8.4% when only patients with central review were included and 4.9% when greater than or equal to 2 SLNs were removed. Using the ACOSOG Z1071 definition of positive SNs (metastases >0.2 mm), the FNR in patients with greater than or equal to 2 SNs in the SN FNAC trial was 11.5% (comparable with the FNR of 12.4% in Z1071) [45].

The findings from these three trials support that SLNB after NC in patients with documented axillary lymph node involvement before NC is feasible but, in order to optimize its performance characteristics, several steps need to be taken: (1) appropriate patient selection for SLNB ($T_{1\text{-}3}N_1$); (2) dual-agent lymphatic mapping (isotope plus blue dye); (3) identification and removal of greater than 2 SNs; (4) clip placement in the positive node with clip localization and retrieval at SLNB; and (5) consideration of performing IHC staining in the SLN with completion ALND even with N_0i+ disease.

For patients who present with documented axillary lymph node involvement and are found to have a positive SLNs after NC, the currently ongoing ALLIANCE 11202 trial (https://clinicaltrials.gov/ct2/show/NCT01901094) randomizes patients to completion ALND versus not (assuming that regional nodal radiotherapy will be used). This clinical trial has the potential to further decrease the need for ALND in patients with early-stage breast cancer.

Sentinel lymph node biopsy before neoadjuvant chemotherapy: advantages and limitations

In patients with clinically negative axillae who are considered for NC, the timing of SLNB (before or after NC) has been the subject of controversy. However, after a decade of fierce debate, it seems that performing SLNB after NC has become the arguable standard for patients with operable breast cancer. This approach capitalizes on the downstaging effect of NC on subclinically involved axillary nodes. The main advantage of SLNB before NC is that it provides information on axillary nodal status without the confounding effects of NC, which can be helpful if the SLN is negative. However, the main limitation of this approach is that, if the SLN proves to be positive, the potential for axillary nodal downstaging with NC is lost and such patients generally require an axillary node dissection either before or after NC [36]. In addition, SLNB before NC eventually requires a second surgical procedure for definitive management whether the SLN is negative or positive. More importantly, the prognostic significance of negative axillary nodes after NC and prior positive SLNB is questionable because pathologically negative axillary nodes in this situation may reflect axillary nodal downstaging from NC or just prior removal of all positive nodes by SLNB [36]. One of the strongest arguments for SLNB before NC may be that pathologic nodal status before NC can help identify optimal candidates for postoperative locoregional radiotherapy (XRT). Although limited information exists on rates and patterns of loco-regional recurrence (LRR) after NC, independent predictors of LRR in patients treated with NC include clinical factors at presentation as well as pathologic tumor response to NC [49]. By using these independent predictors, groups at low, intermediate, and high risk of LRR could be identified and this, in turn, could help in the decision-making process regarding adjuvant locoregional XRT without need for SLNB before NC. A prospective, randomized phase III clinical trial led by NSABP and RTOG (NSABP B-51/RTOG 1304) is currently evaluating the benefit from LRR in patients who present with documented involvement of axillary nodes before NC (by FNA or core needle biopsy) but who are found to have histologically negative nodes after NC.

References

[1] Fisher B, Montague E, Redmond C, et al. Comparison of radical mastectomy with alternative treatments for primary breast cancer. A first report of results from a prospective randomized clinical trial. Cancer 1977;39:2827–39.
[2] Fisher B, Redmond C, Fisher ER, et al. Ten-year results of a randomized clinical trial comparing radical mastectomy and total mastectomy with or without radiation. N Engl J Med 1985;312:674–81.
[3] Krag DN, Weaver DL, Alex JC, et al. Surgical resection and radiolocalization of the sentinel lymph node in breast cancer using a gamma probe. Surg Oncol 1993;2:335–9 [discussion: 340].
[4] Giuliano AE, Kirgan DM, Guenther JM, et al. Lymphatic mapping and sentinel lymphadenectomy for breast cancer. Ann Surg 1994;220:391–8 [discussion 398–401].
[5] Linehan DC, Hill AD, Akhurst T, et al. Intradermal radiocolloid and intraparenchymal blue dye injection optimize sentinel node identification in breast cancer patients. Ann Surg Oncol 1999;6:450–4.
[6] Klimberg VS, Rubio IT, Henry R, et al. Subareolar versus peritumoral injection for location of the sentinel lymph node. Ann Surg 1999;229:860–4 [discussion 864–5].
[7] Mamounas EP. Breast cancer surgical management. Textbook of breast cancer: a clinical guide to therapy. 3rd edition. Boca Raton, FL: CRC Press; 2005. p. 115–61.
[8] Noguchi M, Motomura K, Imoto S, et al. A multicenter validation study of sentinel lymph node biopsy by the Japanese Breast Cancer Society. Breast Cancer Res Treat 2000;63:31–40.
[9] Krag D, Weaver D, Ashikaga T, et al. The sentinel node in breast cancer–a multicenter validation study. N Engl J Med 1998;339:941–6.
[10] McMasters KM, Tuttle TM, Carlson DJ, et al. Sentinel lymph node biopsy for breast cancer: a suitable alternative to routine axillary dissection in multi-institutional practice when optimal technique is used. J Clin Oncol 2000;18:2560–6.
[11] Tafra L, Lannin DR, Swanson MS, et al. Multicenter trial of sentinel node biopsy for breast cancer using both technetium sulfur colloid and isosulfan blue dye. Ann Surg 2001;233:51–9.
[12] Shivers S, Cox C, Leight G, et al. Final results of the Department of Defense multicenter breast lymphatic mapping trial. Ann Surg Oncol 2002;9:248–55.
[13] Kim T, Giuliano AE, Lyman GH. Lymphatic mapping and sentinel lymph node biopsy in early-stage breast carcinoma: a metaanalysis. Cancer 2006;106:4–16.
[14] Hunt KK, Ballman KV, McCall LM, et al. Factors associated with local-regional recurrence after a negative sentinel node dissection: results of the ACOSOG Z0010 trial. Ann Surg 2012;256:428–36.
[15] Veronesi U, Paganelli G, Viale G, et al. A randomized comparison of sentinel-node biopsy with routine axillary dissection in breast cancer. N Engl J Med 2003;349:546–53.
[16] Veronesi U, Paganelli G, Viale G, et al. Sentinel-lymph-node biopsy as a staging procedure in breast cancer: update of a randomised controlled study. Lancet Oncol 2006;7:983–90.

[17] Ashikaga T, Krag DN, Land SR, et al. Morbidity results from the NSABP B-32 trial comparing sentinel lymph node dissection versus axillary dissection. J Surg Oncol 2010;102:111–8.
[18] Krag DN, Anderson SJ, Julian TB, et al. Technical outcomes of sentinel-lymph-node resection and conventional axillary-lymph-node dissection in patients with clinically node-negative breast cancer: results from the NSABP B-32 randomised phase III trial. Lancet Oncol 2007;8:881–8.
[19] Krag DN, Anderson SJ, Julian TB, et al. Sentinel-lymph-node resection compared with conventional axillary-lymph-node dissection in clinically node-negative patients with breast cancer: overall survival findings from the NSABP B-32 randomised phase 3 trial. Lancet Oncol 2010;11:927–33.
[20] Mansel RE, Fallowfield L, Kissin M, et al. Randomized multicenter trial of sentinel node biopsy versus standard axillary treatment in operable breast cancer: the ALMANAC Trial. J Natl Cancer Inst 2006;98:599–609.
[21] Weaver DL, Ashikaga T, Krag DN, et al. Effect of occult metastases on survival in node-negative breast cancer. N Engl J Med 2011;364:412–21.
[22] Lyman GH, Temin S, Edge SB, et al. Sentinel lymph node biopsy for patients with early-stage breast cancer: American Society of Clinical Oncology clinical practice guideline update. J Clin Oncol 2014;32:1365–83.
[23] Giuliano AE, Hunt KK, Ballman KV, et al. Axillary dissection vs no axillary dissection in women with invasive breast cancer and sentinel node metastasis: a randomized clinical trial. JAMA 2011;305:569–75.
[24] Jagsi R, Chadha M, Moni J, et al. Radiation field design in the ACOSOG Z0011 (Alliance) Trial. J Clin Oncol 2014;32:3600–6.
[25] Galimberti V, Cole BF, Zurrida S, et al. Axillary dissection versus no axillary dissection in patients with sentinel-node micrometastases (IBCSG 23-01): a phase 3 randomised controlled trial. Lancet Oncol 2013;14:297–305.
[26] Donker M, van Tienhoven G, Straver ME, et al. Radiotherapy or surgery of the axilla after a positive sentinel node in breast cancer (EORTC 10981-22023 AMAROS): a randomised, multicentre, open-label, phase 3 non-inferiority trial. Lancet Oncol 2014;15: 1303–10.
[27] Wright GP, Mater ME, Sobel HL, et al. Measuring the impact of the American College of Surgeons Oncology Group Z0011 trial on breast cancer surgery in a community health system. Am J Surg 2015;209:240–5.
[28] Yao K, Liederbach E, Pesce C, et al. Impact of the American College of Surgeons Oncology Group Z0011 randomized trial on the number of axillary nodes removed for patients with early stage breast cancer. J Am Coll Surg 2015;221:71–81.
[29] Krishnamurthy S, Sneige N, Bedi DG, et al. Role of ultrasound-guided fine-needle aspiration of indeterminate and suspicious axillary lymph nodes in the initial staging of breast carcinoma. Cancer 2002;95:982–8.
[30] Bedrosian I, Reynolds C, Mick R, et al. Accuracy of sentinel lymph node biopsy in patients with large primary breast tumors. Cancer 2000;88:2540–5.
[31] Chung MH, Ye W, Giuliano AE. Role for sentinel lymph node dissection in the management of large (> or = 5 cm) invasive breast cancer. Ann Surg Oncol 2001;8:688–92.
[32] Fisher B, Brown A, Mamounas E, et al. Effect of preoperative chemotherapy on local-regional disease in women with operable breast cancer: findings from National Surgical Adjuvant Breast and Bowel Project B-18. J Clin Oncol 1997;15:2483–93.
[33] Bear HD, Anderson S, Brown A, et al. The effect on tumor response of adding sequential preoperative docetaxel to preoperative doxorubicin and cyclophosphamide: preliminary results from National Surgical Adjuvant Breast and Bowel Project Protocol B-27. J Clin Oncol 2003;21:4165–74.
[34] Gianni L, Pienkowski T, Im YH, et al. Efficacy and safety of neoadjuvant pertuzumab and trastuzumab in women with locally advanced, inflammatory, or early HER2-positive breast

cancer (NeoSphere): a randomised multicentre, open-label, phase 2 trial. Lancet Oncol 2012;13:25–32.
[35] Gianni L, Eiermann W, Semiglazov V, et al. Neoadjuvant chemotherapy with trastuzumab followed by adjuvant trastuzumab versus neoadjuvant chemotherapy alone, in patients with HER2-positive locally advanced breast cancer (the NOAH trial): a randomised controlled superiority trial with a parallel HER2-negative cohort. Lancet 2010;375:377–84.
[36] Mamounas EP. Impact of neoadjuvant chemotherapy on locoregional surgical treatment of breast cancer. Ann Surg Oncol 2015;22:1425–33.
[37] Hunt KK, Yi M, Mittendorf EA, et al. Sentinel lymph node surgery after neoadjuvant chemotherapy is accurate and reduces the need for axillary dissection in breast cancer patients. Ann Surg 2009;250:558–66.
[38] Mamounas EP, Brown A, Anderson S, et al. Sentinel node biopsy after neoadjuvant chemotherapy in breast cancer: results from National Surgical Adjuvant Breast and Bowel Project Protocol B-27. J Clin Oncol 2005;23:2694–702.
[39] Classe JM, Bordes V, Campion L, et al. Sentinel lymph node biopsy after neoadjuvant chemotherapy for advanced breast cancer: results of Ganglion Sentinelle et Chimiotherapie Neoadjuvante, a French prospective multicentric study. J Clin Oncol 2009;27:726–32.
[40] Xing Y, Foy M, Cox DD, et al. Meta-analysis of sentinel lymph node biopsy after preoperative chemotherapy in patients with breast cancer. Br J Surg 2006;93:539–46.
[41] Kelly AM, Dwamena B, Cronin P, et al. Breast cancer sentinel node identification and classification after neoadjuvant chemotherapy-systematic review and meta analysis. Acad Radiol 2009;16:551–63.
[42] Shen J, Gilcrease MZ, Babiera GV, et al. Feasibility and accuracy of sentinel lymph node biopsy after preoperative chemotherapy in breast cancer patients with documented axillary metastases. Cancer 2007;109:1255–63.
[43] Lee S, Kim EY, Kang SH, et al. Sentinel node identification rate, but not accuracy, is significantly decreased after pre-operative chemotherapy in axillary node-positive breast cancer patients. Breast Cancer Res Treat 2007;102:283–8.
[44] Newman EA, Sabel MS, Nees AV, et al. Sentinel lymph node biopsy performed after neoadjuvant chemotherapy is accurate in patients with documented node-positive breast cancer at presentation. Ann Surg Oncol 2007;14:2946–52.
[45] Boughey JC, Suman VJ, Mittendorf EA, et al. Sentinel lymph node surgery after neoadjuvant chemotherapy in patients with node-positive breast cancer: the ACOSOG Z1071 (Alliance) clinical trial. JAMA 2013;310:1455–61.
[46] Kuehn T, Bauerfeind I, Fehm T, et al. Sentinel-lymph-node biopsy in patients with breast cancer before and after neoadjuvant chemotherapy (SENTINA): a prospective, multicentre cohort study. Lancet Oncol 2013;14:609–18.
[47] Boileau JF, Poirier B, Basik M, et al. Sentinel node biopsy after neoadjuvant chemotherapy in biopsy-proven node-positive breast cancer: the SN FNAC study. J Clin Oncol 2015;33(3): 258–64.
[48] Boughey JC, Ballman K, Symmans WF, et al. Methods impacting the false negative rate of sentinel lymph node surgery in patients presenting with node positive breast cancer (T0-T4,N1-2) who receive neoadjuvant chemotherapy – Results from a prospective trial – ACOSOG Z1071 (Alliance). Cancer Res 2015;75(9 Suppl) [abstract: P2-01-02].
[49] Mamounas EP, Anderson SJ, Dignam JJ, et al. Predictors of locoregional recurrence after neoadjuvant chemotherapy: results from combined analysis of National Surgical Adjuvant Breast and Bowel Project B-18 and B-27. J Clin Oncol 2012;30:3960–6.

Advances in Surgery 50 (2016) 41–48

ADVANCES IN SURGERY

The Use of LINX for Gastroesophageal Reflux

Yulia Zak, MD[a,*], David W. Rattner, MD[b]

[a]Mount Sinai Beth Israel, First Avenue at 16th Street, New York, NY 10003, USA;
[b]Massachusetts General Hospital, 55 Fruit Street, Boston, MA 02114, USA

Keywords

• Magnetic sphincter augmentation • LINX • Gastroesophageal reflux

Key points

- For a variety of reasons, the number of antireflux operations has been decreasing, creating a demand for alternatives to the laparoscopic Nissen procedure.
- The LINX device is an expandable chain of magnetic titanium beads that augments the abnormal lower esophageal sphincter and prevents its inappropriate relaxation.
- It is placed laparoscopically, and has been shown to be safe and effective in initial studies.
- There is a need for long-term outcomes and safety data with regard to this device compared with laparoscopic fundoplication.

HISTORY

Laparoscopic Nissen fundoplication (lap Nissen) was first reported in 1991 by Dr Bernard Dallemagne of Liege, Belgium. The introduction of a laparoscopic approach to treat gastroesophageal reflux led to a marked increase in antireflux surgery, particularly once laparoscopic suturing aids entered the marketplace. Lap Nissen was certainly less painful than open antireflux surgery and provided a much more rapid return to work than the existing alternative operations. For a variety of reasons, however, the volume of antireflux operations has decreased in the past decade. A major contributing factor was a relatively high rate of technically unsuccessful operations that left a population of patients suffering from significant side effects that were difficult to manage with medications. Not surprisingly, gastroenterologists became reluctant to refer their

The authors have nothing to disclose.

*Corresponding author. *E-mail address:* yulia.zak@gmail.com

0065-3411/16/$ – see front matter
http://dx.doi.org/10.1016/j.yasu.2016.03.004

patients for surgery and generally managed refractory complaints with increasing doses and types of medications. Patients, however, were not always satisfied and continued to seek out a definitive solution to their complaints. This dynamic has created a demand for both endoscopic and laparoscopic alternatives to the Nissen fundoplication. This article discusses only magnetic sphincter augmentation, or the LINX procedure.

The efforts to develop these alternatives are really driven by both the long-term failure rate of lap Nissen and side effects (bloating, flatulence, dysphagia) that many patients undergoing this procedure experience [1–3]. Among the alternatives developed are implantable devices aimed at recreation or augmentation of a functional lower esophageal sphincter (LES). The first such invention was the Angelchik prosthetic ring, first described in 1979. This doughnut-shaped prosthesis was made of an elastomer shell filled with a silicone gel, and was placed around the gastroesophageal junction. Although it was easy to insert and was shown to be effective, the device fell out of favor because of instances of device migration with esophageal erosion and fairly high rates of dysphagia resulting in a 15% reoperation rate [4]. After the withdrawal of the Angelchik device from the market, almost 3 decades elapsed before a new prosthesis was introduced.

The recent development of the LINX Reflux Management System (Torax Medical, St. Paul, MN, USA) has allowed for the restoration of the competency of the LES without significantly altering esophagogastric anatomy. This device is placed using a minimally invasive approach and aims to address a patient population whose reflux disease is not well-controlled on medical therapy yet still has relatively preserved anatomy and esophageal motility.

MAGNETIC ANTIREFLUX DEVICE

The LINX device was approved for use by the US Food and Drug Administration in 2012. It consists of a chain of titanium beads with hermetically sealed magnetic cores that are linked together by sliding titanium wires into a flexible ring (Fig. 1).

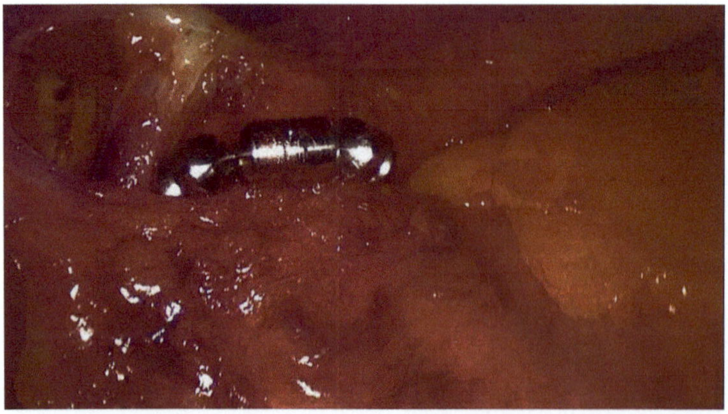

Fig. 1. LINX device implanted at the gastroesophageal junction.

Each bead can move independently but cannot fully separate from the others. At rest, there is minimal compression on the gastroesophageal junction, because the beads are in contact with each other. At the same time, the expandable ring augments the natural resistance of the LES to opening and prevents its abnormal opening [5]. The ring is designed to require a force of more than 27 mm Hg to overcome the magnetic field to open and allow food to pass. Because the average amplitude of peristaltic contraction in the esophagus is between 40 and 100 mm Hg, the LINX device allows passage of food and liquids with swallowing. The ring can expand to more than twice its diameter before returning to its original conformation after the food bolus has passed. Conversely, it is unusual in the normal course of digestion or at rest for the stomach to generate pressures high enough to open the ring, and hence the device augments the resting pressure in the LES and probably also prevents inappropriate transient relaxation of the LES. An advantage of the LINX is that vomiting generates enough force to overcome the pressure in the device so that emesis can occur. This feature is the biggest attraction to patients seeking a LINX procedure because many patients have read horror stories of others' inability to vomit after Nissen fundoplication.

PATIENT SELECTION

Because symptoms are not always a reliable indicator of gastroesophageal reflux, it is essential to prove that a patient's complaints are in fact caused by pathologic acid reflux. Some patients who are not satisfied with proton pump inhibitor (PPI) therapy and cannot get referred to a surgeon by their gastroenterologist will learn of LINX on the Internet and present to a surgeon's office requesting an operation. Failure of symptoms to respond to PPIs should be a red flag and raise concerns that the patient may have an element of visceral hypersensitivity, a motility disorder, or another cause for their complaints. Given that LINX is really targeted at symptom relief, it is essentially mandatory that patients undergo 24-hour pH probe testing (or endoscopy with Bravo capsule) to establish a cause and effect relationship between pathologic acid reflux and reported symptoms. This study should be performed off medications because suppression of acid prevents one from making the necessary correlations. Likewise, the surgeon and patient must appreciate that adequate peristalsis generating pressures of greater than 40 mm Hg is necessary for food to pass through the device. Therefore, esophageal motility testing is also a prerequisite to deciding whether a patient is a suitable candidate for a LINX procedure. As with any other antireflux procedure, upper gastrointestinal endoscopy must be performed preoperatively to exclude a neoplasm, identify if a hiatal hernia is present, and detect Barrett's esophagus. Patients with hiatal hernias greater than 3 cm and patients with Barrett's esophagus are not currently felt to be good candidates for LINX. Because patients often experience dysphagia in the early postoperative period, it is important to be certain that patients will be able to carefully follow dietary instructions during this phase of recovery. Patients with a history of noncompliance or those who seem unable to tolerate a setback in their recovery may have difficulty as they progress through the middle phase of their recovery.

SURGICAL TECHNIQUE

The procedure is performed under general anesthesia, and patients need to be intubated using techniques that minimize the risk of aspiration. The patient is positioned supine and secured to allow for a steep reverse Trendelenburg position. After establishing pneumoperitoneum, a 5- or 12-mm camera port is inserted several centimeters superior and to the left of the umbilicus. The rest of the laparoscopic ports are placed under direct vision in a configuration similar to a fundoplication procedure, with the exception of the right subcostal 5 mm working port (used for instruments in the left hand). This port should be placed well lateral to the midclavicular line to allow for better alignment when creating the retroesophageal window and placing the LINX esophagus sizing tool. The second 12-mm working port is placed along the left midclavicular line subcostally, and a 5-mm assistant port is added subcostally along the anterior axillary line on the left. An additional liver retractor port is positioned according to the type of the retractor used.

We start the procedure by carefully dissecting the fat pad in the angle of His away from the gastroesophageal junction on the left, and opening the phrenoesophageal ligament along the anterior border of the left crus. Once we can see the plane between the esophagus and the left crus, we move to the right side of the hiatus. The gastrohepatic ligament is incised and the hepatic branch of the vagus nerve coursing through it is preserved. The gastroesophageal junction is identified in the area between this vagal branch and the inferior leaf of the phrenoesophageal ligament [5]. The peritoneum is opened along the anterior border of the right crus just cephalad to the crural decussation, and the posterior vagus is identified. A retroesophageal window is created with 2 blunt instruments between the posterior vagus nerve and the wall of the esophagus (Fig. 2). This retroesophageal tunnel is then connected to the original dissection along the left crus. A vessel loop is passed through the window to assist in the

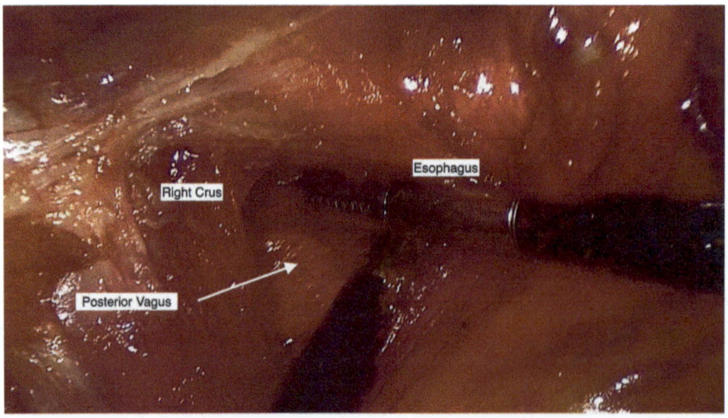

Fig. 2. Creation of the retroesophageal tunnel before placing LINX device. The magnetic ring will eventually pass between the posterior vagus nerve and the posterior wall of the esophagus.

manipulation of the esophagus during device positioning. Only the minimum dissection required to accommodate the LINX device without disrupting the existing anatomic antireflux mechanism of the phrenoesophageal ligaments should be performed. The proprietary esophagus sizing tool is then inserted using the left hand working port, and its soft tip is advanced through the retroesophageal tunnel. The tip is then curled around the esophagus at the level of the LES (Fig. 3). The sizer must be oriented perpendicular to the esophagus and should fit snugly but without any indentation or compression of the esophagus. The esophagus should not be under stretch from the vessel loop when measurements are obtained. The circumference is measured several times for selection of the implant of the correct size (from 10 to 18 beads). The LINX is then inserted through the 12-mm left subcostal port (right hand working port), and passed through the retroesophageal window to encircle the esophagus. The 2 magnetic ends of the device are brought together anteriorly and snapped into place, using the preattached green and white traction sutures.

Postoperatively, the patients are kept on a soft diet for 24 hours and antiemetics are provided as needed. They are then discharged home on a soft diet without any acid-suppressing medications. Soft, frequent meals are recommended to keep the reflux ring active and minimize scar tissue formation. Some surgeons recommend having patients eat small amounts of food or yogurt on an hourly basis for the first 3 to 4 weeks to help keep the beads of the LINX moving. Patients who cannot comply with this type of intense dietary manipulation are not good candidates for LINX implantation.

CONTRAINDICATIONS

There are minimal data on procedural outcomes in patients with large hiatal hernias, because most published studies exclude patients with hernias 3 cm or larger. The current consensus is that such patients should undergo a formal

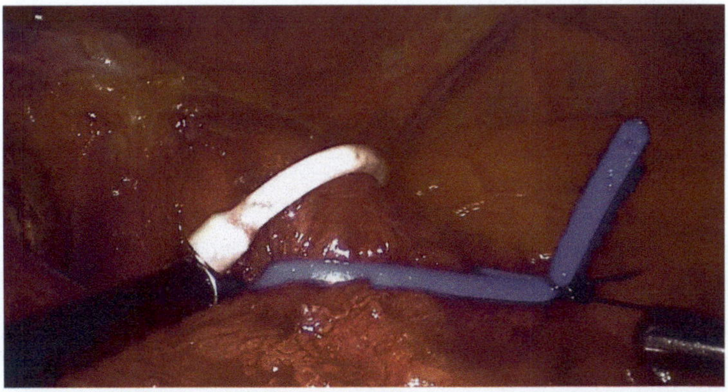

Fig. 3. The sizing device is used to determine the appropriate size LINX prosthesis. The vessel loop holds the retroesophageal tunnel open but should not place the esophagus on stretch during the sizing maneuver.

hiatal hernia repair with a fundoplication procedure. If an unexpected hiatal hernia is found during the dissection for LINX placement, however, it should be repaired before device implantation.

Patients with advanced esophagitis or esophageal dysmotility are not appropriate candidates for LINX placement. These patients are recommended to undergo laparoscopic fundoplication instead. Other patient factors that may preclude device placement include allergy to titanium, stainless steel, nickel, or ferrous materials. Even though the current version of the LINX implant is considered "MRI conditional" for MRI systems up to 1.5 T, caution should be exercised in those who may require long-term MRI surveillance (Box 1).

EFFICACY

The longest term outcomes to date were published by Lipham and colleagues on a prospective multiinstitutional case series of 100 patients with an 85% 3-year follow-up. Sixty-four percent of the subjects achieved a 50% or greater reduction in esophageal acid exposure on follow-up pH monitoring, and 58% had normalization of exposure. There was a corresponding 50% or greater improvement in gastroesophageal reflux disease health-related quality of life score in 92% of the patients. Ninety-three percent of the patients were able to reduce their daily PPI dose by at least 50% [6]. Comparative studies between LINX and lap Nissen have found that both procedures were similarly effective in resolving gastroesophageal reflux disease when assessed by symptoms control, with some showing lower postoperative PPI use after LINX placement

Box 1: Patient selection for LINX procedure

Favorable

Symptoms responsive to proton pump inhibitors
Normal esophageal peristalsis
Hypotensive lower esophageal sphincter
No hiatal hernia
Minimal or no esophagitis on endoscopy
No prior hiatal or foregut surgery

Unfavorable

Symptoms poorly or nonresponsive to proton pump inhibitors
Barrett's esophagus
Hiatal hernia greater than 2 cm
Abnormal esophageal peristalsis
Need for MRI
Morbid Obesity
Inability to comply with postoperative instructions

[7,8]. The LINX patients, as expected, have a greater ability to vomit and belch, and have less bloating complaints than those undergoing a fundoplication [7–9]. In assessing the currently available literature, it is important to note that there may be selection bias in the populations of patients that are being compared and hence a prospective randomized trial will ultimately be required to establish a truly valid comparison between LINX and lap Nissen.

COMPLICATIONS

Overall, LINX has an excellent safety profile in short- and medium-term studies [10,11]. The most common side effect is temporary or persistent dysphagia. Over time, the beads of the device become encapsulated in scar tissue, which is thought to limit the ability of the device to expand and allow passage of a food bolus. In contrast with fundoplications, dysphagia does not occur in the immediate postoperative period, rather developing 10 to 21 days after implantation. Usually patients can be coached through this phase of recovery, but in some instances esophageal dilation is necessary to relieve symptoms. Current US experience shows a 3.4% nonemergent device removal rate after median implant duration of 94 days, most commonly owing to dysphagia (2.2% of the patients) [10]. Six cases of endoluminal perforation have been described to date. Most of these were managed with a combination of endoscopic and laparoscopic removal of the ring, with 1 successful completely endoscopic removal [10,12]. To remove the device, the overlying ring of scar tissue around the gastroesophageal junction often must be opened sharply to allow access to the magnetic chain. The wire between the magnets can then be cut with laparoscopic scissors (or the DC Clip Cutter made for removal of the OTSC-clip [Ovesco Endoscopy AG, Tübingen, Germany], if accessing endoscopically). Because the connecting wires are dumbbell shaped, the ring must be cut in 2 places to remove beads individually. Once the chain is disrupted, the device can be removed. Conversion to a conventional fundoplication can be undertaken at the same time or at a later date.

SUMMARY

Treatment of gastroesophageal reflux disease has evolved over the past several years, and magnetic LES augmentation with the LINX device has been shown to provide a safe and efficacious alternative for patients who are hesitant to undergo laparoscopic fundoplication. It is a technically straightforward and reversible procedure that does not preclude future fundoplication, although long-term outcomes data are still pending. At present, fundoplication remains the gold standard surgical treatment for patients with large hiatal hernias or erosive esophagitis.

References

[1] Richter JE. Gastroesophageal reflux disease treatment: side effects and complications of fundoplication. Clin Gastroenterol Hepatol 2013;11(5):465–71 [quiz: e39].

[2] Hunter JG, Smith CD, Branum GD, et al. Laparoscopic fundoplication failures: patterns of failure and response to fundoplication revision. Ann Surg 1999;230(4):595–604 [discussion: 604–6].
[3] Niebisch S, Fleming FJ, Galey KM, et al. Perioperative risk of laparoscopic fundoplication: safer than previously reported-analysis of the American College of Surgeons National Surgical Quality Improvement Program 2005 to 2009. J Am Coll Surg 2012;215(1): 61–8 [discussion: 68–9].
[4] Varshney S, Kelly JJ, Branagan G, et al. Angelchik prosthesis revisited. World J Surg 2002;26(1):129–33.
[5] Bonavina L, Saino G, Lipham JC, et al. LINX((R)) Reflux Management System in chronic gastroesophageal reflux: a novel effective technology for restoring the natural barrier to reflux. Therap Adv Gastroenterol 2013;6(4):261–8.
[6] Ganz RA, Peters JH, Horgan S. Esophageal sphincter device for gastroesophageal reflux disease. N Engl J Med 2013;368(8):719–27.
[7] Sheu EG, Nau P, Nath B, et al. A comparative trial of laparoscopic magnetic sphincter augmentation and Nissen fundoplication. Surg Endosc 2015;29(3):505–9.
[8] Warren HF, Reynolds JL, Lipham JC, et al. Multi-institutional outcomes using magnetic sphincter augmentation versus Nissen fundoplication for chronic gastroesophageal reflux disease. Surg Endosc 2015. [Epub ahead of print].
[9] Reynolds JL, Zehetner J, Nieh A, et al. Charges, outcomes, and complications: a comparison of magnetic sphincter augmentation versus laparoscopic Nissen fundoplication for the treatment of GERD. Surg Endosc 2015. [Epub ahead of print].
[10] Lipham JC, Taiganides PA, Louie BE, et al. Safety analysis of first 1000 patients treated with magnetic sphincter augmentation for gastroesophageal reflux disease. Dis Esophagus 2015;28(4):305–11.
[11] Loh Y, McGlone ER, Reddy M, et al. Is the LINX reflux management system an effective treatment for gastro-oesophageal reflux disease? Int J Surg 2014;12(9):994–7.
[12] Bauer M, Meining A, Kranzfelder M, et al. Endoluminal perforation of a magnetic antireflux device. Surg Endosc 2015;29(12):3806–10.

Advances in Surgery 50 (2016) 49–66

ADVANCES IN SURGERY

Bowel Preparation

Are Antibiotics Necessary for Colorectal Surgery?

Alice Charlotte Adelaide Murray, BSc, MBBS, MRCS[a], Ravi P. Kiran, MBBS, MS, FRCS, MSc (EBM)[a,b,*]

[a]Division of Colorectal Surgery, New York Presbyterian Hospital, Columbia University Medical Center, Herbert Irving Pavilion, 161 Fort Washington Avenue, Floor: 8, New York, NY 10032, USA; [b]Mailman School of Public Health, Columbia University, 722 W 168th Street, New York, NY 10032, USA

Keywords

• Mechanical bowel preparation • Antibiotics • Colorectal surgery • Surgical site infection • Anastomotic leak • Outcomes • Complications • Quality

Key points

- The goal of bowel preparation is to facilitate safe surgery and reduce postoperative complications.
- The use of antibiotic prophylaxis in colorectal surgery is essential, not controversial.
- Historical evidence supports the use of oral antibiotics in combination with mechanical cleansing for the reduction of infectious complications.
- Prophylactic intravenous antibiotic administration at induction in clean-contaminated surgery is now both routine and mandatory.
- Oral and intravenous antibiotics with mechanical bowel preparation show improved colectomy-specific outcomes compared with no preparation or mechanical bowel preparation plus intravenous antibiotics alone.

The authors have nothing to disclose.

*Corresponding author. Division of Colorectal Surgery, New York Presbyterian Hospital, Columbia University Medical Center, Herbert Irving Pavilion, 161 Fort Washington Avenue, Floor: 8, New York, NY 10032. *E-mail address*: rpk2118@columbia.edu

0065-3411/16/$ – see front matter
http://dx.doi.org/10.1016/j.yasu.2016.03.005

INTRODUCTION: BACKGROUND

The aim of bowel preparation is to prime the colon for surgery, reduce septic complications and facilitate safe surgery. Evidence for the benefits of antibiotic preparation in colorectal surgery has existed for more than 50 years. The argument concerning combined use of antibiotics and mechanical bowel preparation (MBP), as well as any of the individual components, has continued to evolve. Recent recommendations suggest dispensing with bowel preparation be altogether. However, the pendulum is swinging back towards maximal preparation with MBP and oral antibiotics.

In 1938, Garlock and Seley [1] first published results demonstrating improved outcomes following antimicrobial use as an aid to colon surgery. The use of MBP in combination with oral antibiotics became routine practice in the 1970s with the preparation proposed by Nichols and Condon [2] emerging as the standard preoperative regimen. A significant body of evidence supported its use in reducing the high level of postoperative septic complications associated with colorectal surgery [3–6]. Common practice in North America at that time was aligned with available best evidence.

It seems that 3 factors challenged this prevailing practice in the 1990s and early 2000s: (1) the drive towards preoperative intravenous (IV) antibiotic use, (2) evidence demonstrating a lack of effectiveness of MBP alone, and (3) concerns regarding the emergence of resistant bacterial strains or *Clostridium difficile*. With the trend towards the omission of bowel preparation altogether and administering IV antibiotics at induction, it seems oral antibiotics were thought perhaps unnecessary, ineffective in a loaded colon, or even harmful.

Recent retrospective observational studies using national multi-institutional surgical outcomes data have clearly shown a benefit for oral antibiotics and MBP over and above IV antibiosis, and greater still than without mechanical cleansing at all [7–10]. In addition, there is decent evidence to refute any significant increase in *C difficile* rates [10]. The questions remaining to be answered are: do oral antibiotics act effectively, even in a loaded colon, and are different regimens required for colonic versus rectal resections or for minimally invasive versus open surgery? There is no recent level I evidence evaluating the role of oral antibiotics in preparation, mechanical or otherwise.

SIGNIFICANCE

Intraoperative manipulation of the colon presents a significant risk for bowel flora contamination and, for this reason, colorectal surgery is a high outlier for surgical site infection (SSI) [11]. Reducing rates is a priority for both patients and physicians because SSI is associated with significant morbidity, increased length of stay, intensive care admission, hospital-associated costs, and death [12]. Effective preoperative preparation of the colon has the potential to significantly reduce septic complications, including SSI and anastomotic leak.

MECHANICAL BOWEL PREPARATION ALONE

For more than a century, surgeons believed that efficient MBP and the reduction of fecal loading reduced the risk of septic complications, specifically the incidence and the clinical consequences of anastomotic leak after colorectal surgery. An empty colon is also appealing because there are several perceived technical benefits for the colorectal surgeon, including easier bowel handling, better ability to palpate small tumors and polyps, and facilitation of on-table endoscopy [13]. In 1972, Hughes [14] disrupted prevailing dogma and published results of 97 subjects undergoing elective colorectal resection, of whom 46 underwent vigorous mechanical preparation and the remainder did not. There was no difference in wound infection rates between the 2 groups.

A convincing body of evidence currently suggests that MBP alone does not exert any beneficial effects on postoperative outcomes and, in some cases, there are concerns that it may cause harm [15–18].

Liquid contents may increase the chance of spillage; however, when this has been found, it did not affect subsequent infection rates [19,20]. MBP has also been shown to be poorly tolerated, with adverse gastrointestinal symptoms as well as rare reports of metabolic disturbances (ie, hyperphosphatemia, hypocalcemia, hyponatremia) and, sometimes, acute renal failure, tetany, or seizure [21–23]. Thus, many investigators recommended that it be completely abandoned [24–26].

MBP has been found to increase [15] or have no effect on postoperative complications [26]. In 1994, a randomized controlled trial (RCT) of 149 subjects admitted for colorectal surgery showed that MBP and IV antibiotics compared with no MBP with IV antibiotics increased surgical wound infection (SWI) but anastomotic leak remained unaffected [27]. An RCT of 153 subjects undergoing left-sided resections in 2005 echoed these poorer outcomes whereby MBP increased overall complications, abdominal complications, extra-abdominal morbidity, and length of stay but, again, with no effect on anastomotic leak [15].

Contant and colleagues [17] conducted a multicentre randomised non-inferiority study regarding the benefit of MBP versus no MBP and reported that there were fewer abscesses if anastomotic leak developed in the MBP group but anastomotic leak rate, septic complications, length of stay, postoperative ileus, reoperation, and mortality remained the same. Other trials also showed no difference between MBP and no MBP in regard to SWI, postoperative ileus, anastomotic leak [26], general infection, cardiovascular complications, reoperation, and death [16].

A Cochrane Review last updated in 2011 concluded that MBP for colonic resection provided no benefit and was unnecessary; however, the evidence was less clear for rectal operations and, therefore, selective use was still appropriate. Most of this evidence was based on studies that administered IV antibiotic prophylaxis routinely with MBP, and the role or effect of oral antibiotics (present in only a small minority of trials) was not considered [28] (Fig. 1).

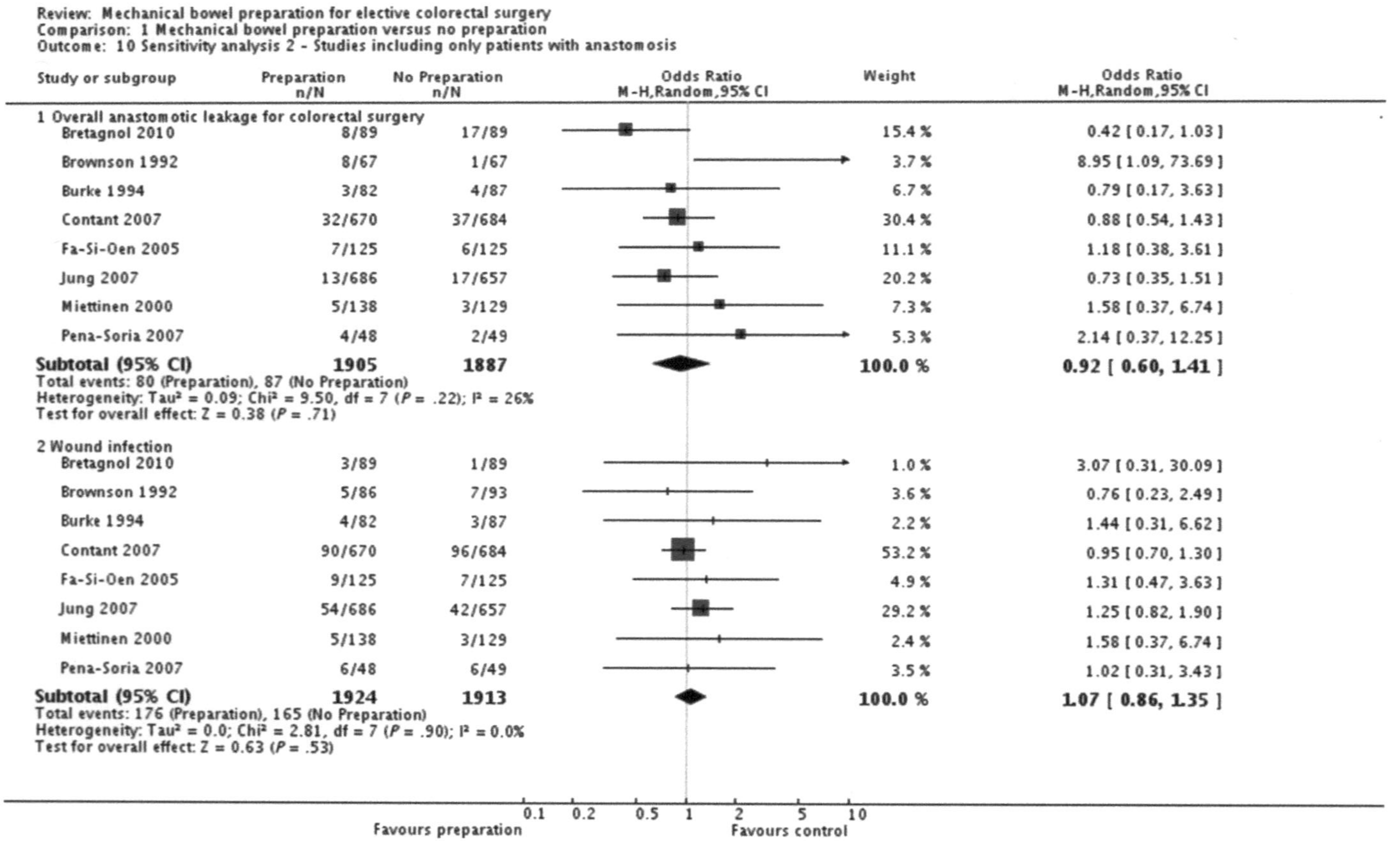

Fig. 1. Meta-analysis of trials comparing MBP versus no preparation for anastomotic leak and wound infection in colorectal surgery. (*From* Güenaga KF, Matos D, Wille-Jørgensen P. Mechanical bowel preparation for elective colorectal surgery. Cochrane Database Syst Rev 2011;(9):CD001544; with permission.)

Most national surgical guidelines have followed this advice recommending a general abandonment of MBP [29,30]. The Enhanced Recovery After Surgery (ERAS) protocol also recommends either no or selective use of MBP to minimize physiologic disturbances that may delay return of bowel function (Fig. 1) [31]. No further trials of MBP versus no MBP are required, the question is whether the role of oral antibiosis should be provided in combination, or alone.

Despite evidence against its use, a significant proportion of surgeons continue to prescribe MBP. Practice varies according to country of origin, whether used before colon or rectal resections, and according to surgical approach. Surveys certainly show that there is no consensus. In 1990, 51% of 300 American Society of Colon and Rectal Surgeons (ASCRS) surgeons surveyed used some form of cathartic [32]. In 1990, Solla and Rothenberger [33] found that all of the board-certified colorectal surgeons surveyed used MBP and the majority (88%) used oral and IV antibiotics in combination. In 1997, Nichols and colleagues [34] surveyed current practices in North American colorectal surgeons and found similar results: 100% of surgeons who responded used MBP and the majority (86.5%) with oral and IV antibiotics. The use of MBP declined in time; however, in 2011, a survey of the Dutch Association for Endoscopic Surgery reported 20% of respondents prescribed MBP before colonic resections, whereas 63% prescribed MBP before rectal resections [35]. In the United Kingdom, in 2011, of 199 Association of Coloproctology of Great Britain and Ireland (ACPGBI) members surveyed, the percentage using MBP for open versus laparoscopic surgery was 9.5% versus 16.8% for right hemicolectomy, 43.4% versus 40.2% for left hemicolectomy, 20.5% versus 22.5% for an abdominoperineal resection, and 72.2% versus 63.6% for low anterior resection [36]. In a recent 2011 survey of ASCRS members on SSI prevention strategies, 76% of respondents reported routine use of MBP, 19% selective use, 4% no preparation, and 36% oral antibiotics with MBP (OAMBP) [37].

Research to date has focused on septic complications following the use of MBP; however, there may still be benefits to MBP that are less well understood. A survival benefit has been shown in a recent follow-up study by Collin and colleagues [38], which looked at the long-term effects of MBP in subjects with colorectal cancer. Subjects who received MBP preoperatively had significantly better cancer-specific and overall survival outcomes at 10 years.

Why surgeons continue to use MBP alone or with oral antibiotics may well be because of its long-standing and historical association with improved outcomes, the idea that cleansing the colon to reduce infection is entirely intuitive, and because no clear and consistent guidelines exist.

COLONIC BACTERIA

The colon contains the largest number of microbes per unit volume of the entire intestine, with a complex community of bacterial organisms within the lumen, feces, and mucosa. Human fecal flora is thought to consist of 400 different species at a concentration of 10^{11} viable microorganisms per gram of contents and consisting of both aerobic and anaerobic bacteria [39,40].

Numerous studies in the 1970s provided a causal link between the endogenous anaerobic colonic microflora and postoperative infection [41] and, more recently, bacteria isolated from wound fat at operation and then subsequent wound infections have been shown to be similar to those found in the colon [42]. The question of antibiotic use was settled in 1981 when Baum and colleagues [43] conducted a systematic review of 26 trials published between 1965 and 1980. They concluded there was unequivocal evidence in favor of antibiotics alongside MBP in colorectal surgery. The antibiotic regimens were heterogeneous but it was suggested that no further controlled studies omitting antibiotics could ethically be performed in light of these findings.

MECHANICAL BOWEL PREPARATION PLUS ORAL ANTIBIOTICS

It seems logical that to have maximal effect on colonic bacterial concentration, and thus a beneficial effect on postoperative infectious complications, a complete cleanse of the colon and then the addition of nonabsorbable antibiotics would be required, with potential role for systemic antibiosis to further reduce mucosal-associated flora [44]. A complete sterilization of the bowel is an unlikely outcome; however, more realistic would be a method of transiently reducing the concentration of viable bacteria.

In 1955, Cohn and Rives [45], and again in 1957, Cohn and Longacre [46], had shown that oral neomycin and nystatin decreased aerobic bacteria in humans and, furthermore, that in dogs oral antibiotics reduced the number of anastomotic leaks. However, Nichols and colleagues [47] pioneered research into what is now thought of as preoperative preparation of the bowel in colorectal surgery, building on an already significant bulk of data espousing the beneficial effects of colonic antisepsis. In 1972, they published an article showing that although mechanical cleansing reduced gross fecal mass within the colon, there was no role in suppressing bacterial growth and that the concentrations of obligate anaerobes, aerobes, and facultative organisms remained unchanged.

Due to the polymicrobial nature of the gut, both anaerobic and aerobic cover is required to reduce luminal and mucosal bacteria. Nichols and colleagues [47] showed that the optimum regimen of neomycin and erythromycin combined and given the day before surgery (19 hours prior) significantly reduced fecal aerobic and anaerobic bacterial concentrations. Later, Nichols and colleagues [48] also found that mechanical bowel cleansing had the effect of increasing the concentration of intraluminal erythromycin (Fig. 2).

More recently, intraoperative mucosal swabs taken from subjects who had oral antibiotics and MBP have been shown to yield a lower concentration of gram-negative and anaerobic bacteria compared with those who had IV antibiotics alone, with peritoneal fluid positive culture rates also lower [49]. In animals, oral antibiotics and MBP result in a decrease in mucosa-associated microflora compared with clear liquid diet or preparation without antibiotics [50].

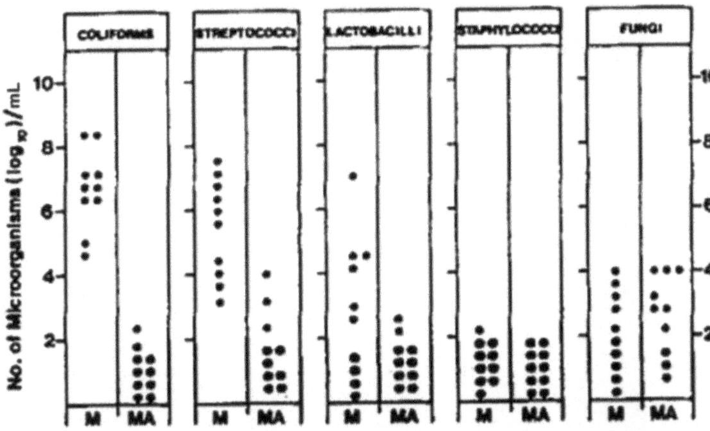

Fig. 2. The effect of neomycin-erythromycin on the aerobic colonic microflora. M, mechanical preparation; MA, mechanical preparation and neomycin-erythromycin base. (*From* Nichols RL, Broido P, Condon RE, et al. Effect of preoperative neomycin-erythromycin intestinal preparation on the incidence of infectious complications following colon surgery. Ann Surg 1973;178(4):454; with permission.)

In 1973, the theory behind the preparation proposed by Nichols and Condon [2] was put into practice with both a randomized prospective trial and an additional retrospective analysis [51]. In the first trial, 20 subjects received either MBP with oral antibiotics or MBP alone before colorectal resection and no parenteral antibiotics were administered preoperatively or intraoperatively. They found that clinical sepsis (wound abscess and anastomotic leak) was absent in the group assigned oral antibiotics but present in 3 out of 10 in those with MBP. In the retrospective study, 0% of 69 subjects treated with MBP and oral antibiotics developed postoperative infectious complications compared with 17% of 29 subjects in the MBP alone arm (Table 1).

In 1977, Clarke and colleagues [3] led a larger Veterans Administration randomized placebo-controlled double-blind study of 116 subjects, who received either oral antibiotics or placebo, and both groups were given preoperative MBP. At that time, MBP was started 3 days preoperatively and consisted of a clear liquid diet throughout. In addition, their regimen consisted of: day 1, bisacodyl 1 capsule 6 PM; day 2, magnesium sulfate, 30 mL, 50% solution (15 gm) orally at 10:00 AM, 2:00 PM, and 6:00 PM, with a first enema at 7:00 PM, second enema at 8:00 PM, and subsequent enemas continued hourly until no solid feces returned; and day 3 magnesium sulfate at 10:00 AM and 2:00 PM with neomycin sulfate (1.0 gm) and erythromycin (1 gm) at 1:00 PM, 2:00 PM, and 11:00 PM. The overall rate of directly related septic complications was 43% in the placebo group and 9% in the antibiotic group ($P<.001$), which included a statistically significant difference in rates of wound complications (35% vs 9%), intra-abdominal abscess (17% vs 4%), anastomotic leak (17% vs 4%), nonlocalized peritonitis, and death due to sepsis.

Table 1
Septic complications related to colorectal operations

Operation strata	Treatment	Number of subjects	Wound infection	Abscess or peritonitis	Anastomotic major	Leak minor	Septicemia	Death	Total septic subjects[a]	Wilcoxon 2-sample rank test[b]	Chi-square test[c]
Intraperitoneal	Placebo	35	10	6	3	2	1	0	12	0.002	0.003
	Antibiotic	33	5	2	1	0	1	0	5	—	—
Extraperitoneal	Placebo	10	4	3	4	1	4	1	5	0.012	0.179
	Antibiotic	6	0	0	0	1	0	0	0	—	—
Abdominoperineal resection	Placebo	13	7	1	0	0	1	1	9	0.003	0.004
	Antibiotic	12	0	0	0	0	0	0	0	—	—
Other	Placebo	2	0	0	0	0	0	0	0	—	—
	Antibiotic	5	0	0	0	0	0	0	0	—	—
Total	Placebo	60	21	10	7	3	6	2	26	0.0001	0.001
	Antibiotic	56	5	2	1	1	1	0	5	—	—

[a]Some subjects developed more than 1 septic complication but are counted only once.
[b]P values for difference in all septic complications between treatment groups with each subject assigned a weighted score.
[c]P values for difference between treatment groups in those septic complications directly related to the colorectal operation and all other outcomes.

From Clarke JS, Condon RE, Bartlett JG, et al. Preoperative oral antibiotics reduce septic complications of colon operations: results of prospective, randomized, double-blind clinical study. Ann Surg 1977;186(3):255; with permission.

These results were in agreement with those of Goldring and colleagues [52] who published a controlled trial in the *Lancet* 2 years earlier. They demonstrated a significant reduction of both aerobic and anaerobic colonic microflora in the group receiving prophylactic antimicrobial agents with MBP, and this was reflected in an observed significant reduction in postoperative wound infections.

The efficacy of oral prophylactic antimicrobial agents had been established only when used in combination with MBP. There are still very few data examining the use of oral antibiotics alone. This question of whether oral antibiotics should be administered with or without MBP has only recently been addressed.

What followed from this considerable research demonstrating the benefits of OAMBP were a large number of prospective trials, multicenter studies, Cochrane Reviews, as well as further systematic reviews and meta-analyses on the topic of the optimal preparation of the colon. Trials moved from comparing MBP with or without oral antibiotics, to focusing on the role of IV antibiotics and whether there was any need for MBP at all. During this period, MBP fell out of favor and parenteral antibiotics became increasingly popular and part of standard practice.

MECHANICAL BOWEL PREPARATION PLUS IV ANTIBIOTICS (WITH OR WITHOUT ORAL)

In 1973, Evans and Pollock [53] at Scarborough hospital published a series of 762 general surgical wounds, where patients were randomized to receive prophylactic parenteral cephaloridine or remain as a control. The findings that wound infections were reduced in all but vascular operations on the lower extremity was the first study that prompted a surge in interest in the use of prophylactic IV antibiotics.

Surgeons were clearly beginning to use combined antibiotic prophylaxis as shown by a survey of surgeons' practice presented at the 1978 annual meeting of the Society for Surgery of the Alimentary Tract, which found that the most commonly prescribed regimen was MBP with oral and IV antibiotics (49% of respondents); however, 31% of those delivered parenteral antibiotics postoperatively as well [4,54].

Currently, the standard accepted approach is for the administration of appropriate IV antibiotics within 1 hour of the incision to achieve systemic therapeutic levels and this is reflected in most surgical guidelines and hospital payment initiatives [55,56].

Oral and IV antibiotics combined have been shown to have the greatest quantitative and qualitative effect on suppressing mucosal-associated flora compared with oral antibiotics alone [57]. Ultimately, a combination of IV and oral antibiotics has also been shown superior in regard to postoperative septic complications, reducing SWIs, and anastomotic leak in colorectal surgery. Several RCTs have demonstrated clear benefit to combined oral and IV prophylaxis in reducing SWI [3,52,57–60]. A 3-arm clinical trial of preoperative oral antibiotics alone (neomycin plus erythromycin) compared with oral and IV cephalothin, versus IV antibiotics alone, in which all subjects received MBP, was terminated prematurely because of clear data to show that the latter group (parenteral antibiotics) was the least effective [4]. Lewis [42] conducted a RCT and meta-analysis comparing infection rate in subjects given MBP and oral antibiotics versus IV antibiotics alone. The occurrence of infections was reduced when oral antibiotics were added to MBP. Recently, Bellows and colleagues [61] conducted a meta-analysis of 16 RCTs that showed a 43% decrease in postoperative SWIs when nonabsorbable oral antibiotics were combined with IV prophylaxis compared with IV alone. This has been confirmed in a recent Cochrane Review, which not only showed IV and oral antibiotics in combination to be beneficial in regard to SWI but also showed improved outcomes for anaerobic and aerobic joint cover [62]. There was, however, no information regarding the use of MBP or its effect on infectious outcomes. However, Barber and colleagues [63] showed that IV (gentamicin and clindamycin) in combination with oral antibiotics (neomycin and erythromycin), and with the use of MBP, demonstrated no benefit on the reduction of wound complications over and above oral antibiotics alone. Data on the use of oral antibiotics alone are lacking and recent studies have had too few subjects in these groups to provide robust analyses (Table 2) [7,10,64].

IV antibiotics are now routinely used prophylactically in all colorectal operations, both in the United States and abroad. Payments in the United States are linked to adherence to antibiotic guidelines with the aim of reducing preventable SSIs. The Surgical Care Improvement Project (SCIP) guidelines as of 2004 mandate use of appropriate prophylactic IV antibiotics within 60 minutes of the start of all colorectal procedures and most operations classified as clean-contaminated or more [55]. Recent evidence and retrospective data must now be interpreted with this knowledge in mind because studies are carried out on subjects who naturally have IV antibiotics administered.

CURRENT EVIDENCE

Several recent retrospective studies based on good quality multi-institutional clinical data and according to standardized definitions have been published. The unified message is that MBP alongside oral and IV antibiotics provides optimal outcomes following colorectal resection [7–10].

The Michigan Surgical Quality Collaborative statewide colectomy project has published studies showing that there is a reduction in SSI with OAMBP and, as such, recommends full bowel preparation for all eligible elective colorectal surgery patients [10,65]. In a study using the American College of Surgeons National Surgical Quality Improvement Program (NSQIP) data, the combined use of oral antibiotics and MBP compared with MBP with IV antibiotics or no preparation at all, reduced all colectomy-specific complications, including SSI, postoperative ileus, and anastomotic leak, as well as 30-day medical morbidity [7]. In both studies, the oral antibiotic group alone (minus MBP) was too small for any valid statistical analysis (Fig. 3).

Table 2
Combined oral and intravenous compared with oral or intravenous alone for colorectal surgery

Subject or population: colorectal surgery
Settings:
Intervention: combined oral and IV
Comparison: oral or IV alone

Outcomes	Illustrative comparative risks[a] (95% CI)		Relative effect (95% CI)	Number of participants (studies)	Quality of the evidence (GRADE)
	Assumed risk Oral or IV alone	Corresponding risk Combined oral and IV			
SWI: oral and IV versus IV alone	Study population		RR 0.55 (0.43 to 0.71)	2929 high (15 RCTs)	High
	128 per 1000	70 per 1000 (55 to 91)			
	Moderate				
	230 per 1000	126 per 1000 (99 to 163)			
SWI: combined oral and iv versus oral alone	Study population		RR 0.52 (0.35 to 0.76)	1880 high (9 RCTs)	High
	79 per 1000	41 per 1000 (28 to 60)			
	Moderate				
	146 per 1000	76 per 1000 (51 to 111)			

GRADE Working group grades of evidence: high quality, further research is very unlikely to change the confidence in the estimate of effect; moderate quality, further research is likely to have an important impact on the confidence in the estimate of effect and may change the estimate; low quality, further research is very likely to have an important impact on the confidence in the estimate of effect and is likely to change the estimate; very low quality, very uncertain about the estimate.

Abbreviations: CI, confidence interval; RR, risk ratio.

[a]The basis for median control group risk across studies. The corresponding risk (and its 95% CI) is based on the assumed risk in the comparison group and the relative effect of the intervention (and its 95% CI).

From Nelson RL, Gladman E, Barbateskovic M. Antimicrobial prophylaxis for colorectal surgery. Cochrane Database Syst Rev 2014;(5):CD001181; with permission.

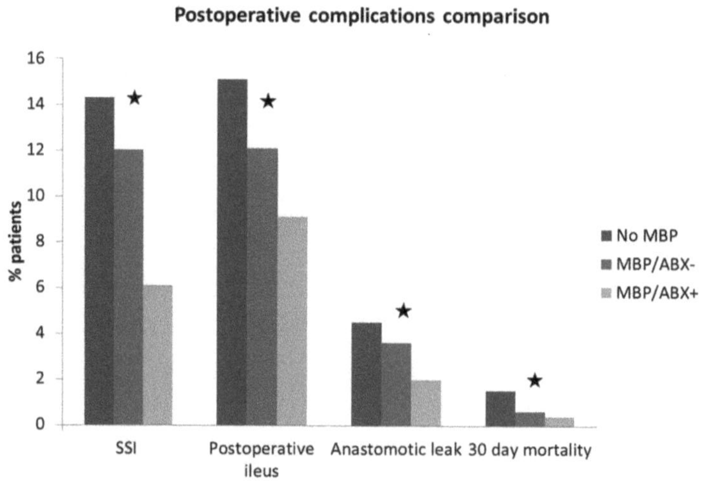

Fig. 3. Postoperative complications: SSI, postoperative ileus, anastomotic leak, and 30-day mortality according to type of bowel preparation. MBP+/ABX-, MBP with no antibiotics; MBP+/ABX+, MBP and oral antibiotics, No MBP, no MBP. * Statistical significance at $P < 0.0001$. (*From* Kiran RP, Murray AC, Chiuzan C, et al. Combined preoperative mechanical bowel preparation with oral antibiotics significantly reduces surgical site infection, anastomotic leak, and ileus after colorectal surgery. Ann Surg 2015;262(3):418; with permission.)

In a propensity score analysis matching OAMBP and non-MBP patients, Kim and colleagues [66] similarly found that oral antibiotics in combination with MBP had superior outcomes in relation to septic complications, including any SSI, organ space SSI, and superficial SSI, but with similar rates of postoperative ileus. Morris and colleagues [8] looked at colorectal operations with a large proportion of minimally invasive resections and showed that OAMBP significantly reduced length of stay and readmission. Also, on multivariable analysis the addition of antibiotics was independently associated with reduced SSI. Scarborough and colleagues [9], using NSQIP, confirm these findings with lower SSI, anastomotic leak, procedure-related readmission, and postoperative hospitalization.

The main limitation with these retrospective data is a lack of information regarding the type of MBP given, quality of resulting preparation, and the specific oral antibiotics used. In addition, whether or not subjects received IV systemic antibiotics at induction is not included. However, in accordance with evidence that 96% of United States hospitals adhere to the Joint Commission's SCIP Inf-1 guideline (prophylactic antibiotic received within 1 hour before surgical incision), the authors propose that the most patients did [67].

One concern regarding the use of oral antibiotics is the potential for bacterial overgrowth and increase in rates of *C difficile.* A review of 8000 VASQIP subjects found that readmission for *C difficile* was greater in the OAMBP group versus MBP alone (0.5% vs 0.3%) [68]. However, this has been refuted and, in fact, there is a suggestion that because MBP and oral antibiotics reduce infectious complications and hence the need for postoperative antibiotics, it may actually be beneficial (Table 3) [10].

RECTUM VERSUS COLON

Extraperitoneal rectal resections have a greater risk of anastomotic leak and SSI and, therefore, may benefit more from MBP than colon resection.

In addition, there is some thought that stool in the proximal and distal colon may prevent manipulation and safe firing of the circular stapler [15].

A propensity score analysis matching MBP and non-MBP subjects undergoing right, left, or rectal resections for cancer, in which non-MBP subjects undergoing left-sided or rectal operations were given 1 rectal enema, concluded that an enema in the latter group seemed dangerous, citing the higher rate of postoperative complications (Clavien Dindo III–IV) [66]. A further study of 96 matched subjects undergoing rectal resection and primary anastomosis with protective ileostomy with either MBP or rectal enema found there was no difference in anastomotic leak, pelvic abscess, wound infection, ileus, and bleeding. Because the enema was better tolerated and less invasive, this was then recommended [69]. A subgroup analysis of 449 subjects undergoing rectal resection, performed by van't Sant and colleagues [18], showed that MBP had no influence on anastomotic leak rate. In 2010, the French Research Group of Rectal Cancer Surgery (GRECCAR) III trial, compared MBP and IV antibiotics with no MBP and IV antibiotics for subjects undergoing rectal resection for cancer. The investigators concluded that no MBP was associated with

Table 3
The use of mechanical bowel preparation and *Clostridium difficile* infection at the subject level

	C difficile infection N (%)	No *C difficile* infection N (%)	*P*
No bowel preparation, n = 578	14 (2.4)	564 (97.6)	.95
Yes bowel preparation, n = 1685	40 (2.4)	1645 (97.6)	
Without oral antibiotics, n = 1001	29 (2.9)	972 (97.1)	.09
With oral antibiotics, n = 684	11 (1.6)	673 (98.4)	

Variable	Unadjusted OR (95% CI)	Adjusted[a] OR (95% CI)
No MBP	Reference	—
Yes MBP	0.98 (0.53–1.81)	0.96 (0.50–l.83)
Without oral antibiotics[b]	Reference	—
With oral antibiotics[b]	0.55 (0.27–1.10)	0.60 (0.29–1.23)

Abbreviations: n, size of subsample; N, total sample size; OR, odds ratio.

[a]Adjustment for patient factors found to be significant on univariate analysis. Hospital median rate of mechanical bowel infection, 2.8%; range, 0–14.7%.

[b]Cohort that used mechanical bowel preparation.

From Krapohl GL, Phillips LR, Campbell DA Jr, et al. Bowel preparation for colectomy and risk of *Clostridium difficile* infection. Dis Colon Rectum 2011;54(7):810–7; with permission.

increased infectious complications and overall morbidity, as well as higher rates of leaks and peritonitis, but with no difference in overall morbidity or length of stay. As a result, some form of MBP was recommended [21]. A recent meta-analysis demonstrated no beneficial effect for MBP on all 30-day morbidity, anastomotic leak, and SSI in proctectomy [70]. Two further meta-analyses stratified for colon and rectal surgery; one showing no trend in either direction and another favoured no MBP, but this was not statistically significant [28,71]. Again, the question about antibiotic use has not been addressed.

ROLE OF ENEMA

Two RCTs have evaluated the effect of bowel preparation versus a single enema before colorectal surgery. Neither trial found a difference between the 2 groups with regard to anastomotic leak; however, the second noted an increased risk of leak requiring reoperation following a phosphate enema and, therefore, the trial was terminated prematurely [72,73].

LAPAROSCOPIC VERSUS OPEN

The potential benefits of MBP in laparoscopic surgery include easier bowel maneuverability, ability to identify small tumors, the facilitation of on-table endoscopy, and increased workspace with pneumoperitoneum. However, some investigators say that the additional weight of the colon and resultant effects of gravity aid exposure. Experiments on pigs using measurements of the pneumoperitoneal abdominal volume on computed tomography have shown significantly increased available space associated with MBP [74]. Recent studies using multi-institutional data have a large proportion of subjects undergoing minimally invasive surgery and clearly show a benefit to OAMBP. However, no trials have specifically looked at the role of OAMBP in laparoscopic versus open operations.

PRESENT RELEVANCE AND FUTURE AVENUES

Although current evidence based on retrospective data supports the use of a combined preparation with MBP and oral antibiotics versus no preparation on MBP alone, level I evidence relating to this question, particularly in the era of routine prophylactic IV antibiotics before surgery, is lacking. Questions regarding the optimal pre-operative regimen for laparoscopic versus open surgery and colon versus rectal anatomical location with sufficient power to detect differences in outcomes are required. Research should no longer continue to focus on the use or non-use of MBP unless antibiotics are used in conjunction. A multicenter RCT on the topic would be very timely.

SUMMARY

The best postoperative surgical outcomes can be achieved when oral antibiotic and MBP are used in conjunction with appropriate IV antibiotics at induction. A well-planned randomized placebo-controlled trial will provide the level of evidence required to bring colorectal surgical guidelines into line with current best evidence.

References

[1] Garlock JH, Seley GP. The use of sulfanilamide in surgery of the colon and rectum. Preliminary report. Surgery 1939;5(5):787–90.
[2] Nichols RL, Condon RE. Preoperative preparation of the colon. Surg Gynecol Obstet 1971;132:323–37.
[3] Clarke JS, Condon RE, Bartlett JG, et al. Preoperative oral antibiotics reduce septic complications of colon operations: results of prospective, randomized, double-blind clinical study. Ann Surg 1977;186:251–9.
[4] Condon RE, Bartlett JG, Nichols RL, et al. Preoperative prophylactic cephalothin fails to control septic complications of colorectal operations: results of controlled clinical trial: a Veterans Administration cooperative study. Am J Surg 1979;137:68–74.
[5] Condon RE, Bartlett JG, Greenlee H, et al. Efficacy of oral and systemic antibiotic prophylaxis in colorectal operations. Arch Surg 1983;118:496–502.
[6] Matheson DM, Arabi Y, Baxter-Smith D, et al. Randomized multicentre trial of oral bowel preparation and antimicrobials for elective colorectal operations. Br J Surg 1978;65: 597–600.
[7] Kiran RP, Murray AC, Chiuzan C, et al. Combined preoperative mechanical bowel preparation with oral antibiotics significantly reduces surgical site infection, anastomotic leak, and ileus after colorectal surgery. Ann Surg 2015;262(3):416–25 [discussion: 423–5].
[8] Morris MS, Graham LA, Chu DI, et al. Oral antibiotic bowel preparation significantly reduces surgical site infection rates and readmission rates in elective colorectal surgery. Ann Surg 2015;261(6):1034–40.
[9] Scarborough JE, Mantyh CR, Sun ZS, et al. Combined mechanical and oral antibiotic bowel preparation reduces incisional surgical site infection and anastomotic leak rates after elective colorectal resection. Ann Surg 2015;262:1–7.
[10] Kim EK, Sheetz KH, Bonn J, et al. A statewide colectomy experience: the role of full bowel preparation in preventing surgical site infection. Ann Surg 2014;259:310–4.
[11] Wick EC, Vogel JD, Church JM, et al. Surgical site infections in a "high outlier" institution: are colorectal surgeons to blame? Dis Colon Rectum 2009;52(3):374–9.
[12] Kirkland KB, Briggs JP, Trivette SL, et al. The impact of surgical-site infections in the 1990s: attributable mortality, excess length of hospitalization, and extra costs. Infect Control Hosp Epidemiol 1999;20(11):725–30.
[13] Rovera F, Dionigi G, Boni L, et al. Mechanical bowel preparation for colorectal surgery. Surg Infect (Larchmt) 2006;7:S61–3.
[14] Hughes ESR. Asepsis in large-bowel surgery. Ann R Coll Surg Engl 1972;51:347–56.
[15] Bucher P, Gervaz P, Soravia C, et al. Randomized clinical trial of mechanical bowel preparation versus no preparation before elective left-sided colorectal surgery. Br J Surg 2005;92:409–14 [Erratum appears in Br J Surg 2005;92:1051].
[16] Jung B, Påhlman L, Nyström PO, et al, Mechanical Bowel Preparation Study Group. Multicentre randomized clinical trial of mechanical bowel preparation in elective colonic resection. Br J Surg 2007;94:689–95.
[17] Contant CM, Hop WC, van't Sant HP, et al. Mechanical bowel preparation for elective colorectal surgery: a multicentre randomised trial. Lancet 2007;370:2112–7 [Erratum appears in Lancet 2008;371:1664].
[18] Van't Sant HP, Slieker JC, Hop WC, et al. The influence of mechanical bowel preparation in elective colorectal surgery for diverticulitis. Tech Coloproctol 2012;16:309–14.
[19] Zmora O, Pikarsky AJ, Wexner SD. Bowel preparation for colorectal surgery [Review]. Dis Colon Rectum 2001;44(10):1537–49.
[20] Mahajna A, Krausz M, Rosin D, et al. Bowel preparation is associated with spillage of bowel contents in colorectal surgery. Dis Colon Rectum 2005;48(8):1626–31.
[21] Bretagnol F, Panis Y, Rullier E, et al, French Research Group of Rectal Cancer Surgery (GRECCAR). Rectal cancer surgery with or without bowel preparation: The French GRECCAR III multicenter single-blinded randomized trial. Ann Surg 2010;252(5):863–8.

[22] Orias M, Mahnensmith RL, Perazella MA. Extreme hyperphosphatemia and acute renal failure after a phosphorus-containing bowel regimen. Am J Nephrol 1999;19(1):60–3.
[23] Hookey LC, Vanner S. A review of current issues underlying colon cleansing before colonoscopy [Review]. Can J Gastroenterol 2007;21(2):105–11.
[24] Slim K, Vicaut E, Launay-Savary MV, et al. Updated systematic review and meta-analysis of randomized clinical trials on the role of mechanical bowel preparation before colorectal surgery. Ann Surg 2009;249:203–9.
[25] Bucher P, Mermillod B, Gervaz P, et al. Mechanical bowel preparation for elective colorectal surgery: a meta-analysis. Arch Surg 2004;139:1359–64.
[26] Fa-Si-Oen P, Roumen R, Buitenweg J, et al. Mechanical bowel preparation or not? Outcome of a multicenter, randomized trial in elective open colon surgery. Dis Colon Rectum 2005;48:1509–16.
[27] Santos JC Jr, Batista J, Sirimarco MT, et al. Prospective randomized trial of mechanical bowel preparation in patients undergoing elective colorectal surgery. Br J Surg 1994;81:1673–6.
[28] Guenaga KK, Matos D, Wille-Jørgensen P. Mechanical bowel preparation for elective colorectal surgery. Cochrane Database Syst Rev 2009;(1):CD001544.
[29] Eskicioglu C, Forbes SS, Fenech DS, et al, Best Practice in General Surgery Committee. Preoperative bowel preparation for patients undergoing elective colorectal surgery: a clinical practice guideline endorsed by the Canadian Society of Colon and Rectal Surgeons. Can J Surg 2010;53(6):385–95.
[30] National Institute of Clinical Excellence (NICE). Available at: https://www.nice.org.uk/guidance/cg74/chapter/guidance#preoperative-phase. Accessed October 25, 2015.
[31] ERAS protocol. Available at: http://www.erassociety.org/index.php/eras-care-system/eras-protocol. Accessed October 25, 2015.
[32] Beck DE, Fazio VW. Current preoperative bowel cleansing methods. Results of a survey. Dis Colon Rectum 1990;33(1):12–5.
[33] Solla JA, Rothenberger DA. Preoperative bowel preparation. A survey of colon and rectal surgeons [Review]. Dis Colon Rectum 1990;33(2):154–9.
[34] Nichols RL, Smith JW, Garcia RY, et al. Current practices of preoperative bowel preparation among North American colorectal surgeons. Clin Infect Dis 1997;24(4):609–19.
[35] Slieker JC, van't Sant HP, Vlot J, et al. Bowel preparation prior to laparoscopic colorectal resection: what is the current practice? J Laparoendosc Adv Surg Tech A 2011;21(10):899–903.
[36] Drummond RJ, McKenna RM, Wright DM. Current practice in bowel preparation for colorectal surgery: a survey of the members of the Association of Coloproctology of GB & Ireland. Colorectal Dis 2011;13(6):708–10.
[37] Markell KW, Hunt BM, Charron PD, et al. Prophylaxis and management of wound infections after elective colorectal surgery: a survey of the American Society of Colon and Rectal Surgeons membership. J Gastrointest Surg 2010;14(7):1090–8.
[38] Collin Å, Jung B, Nilsson E, et al. Impact of mechanical bowel preparation on survival after colonic cancer resection. Br J Surg 2014;101(12):1594–600.
[39] Matsuda K, Tsuji H, Asahara T, et al. Sensitive quantitative detection of commensal bacteria by rRNA-targeted reverse transcription-PCR. Appl Environ Microbiol 2007;73(1):32–9.
[40] Smith HW, Crabb WE. The fæcal bacterial flora of animals and man: its development in the young. J Pathol 1961;82:53–66.
[41] Nichols RL, Condon RE. Role of the endogenous gastrointestinal microflora in postoperative wound sepsis [Review]. Surg Annu 1975;7:279–93.
[42] Lewis RT. Oral versus systemic antibiotic prophylaxis in elective colon surgery: a randomized study and meta-analysis send a message from the 1990s. Can J Surg 2002;45:173–80.
[43] Baum ML, Anish DS, Chalmers TC, et al. A survey of clinical trials of antibiotic prophylaxis in colon surgery: evidence against further use of no-treatment controls. N Engl J Med 1981;305(14):795–9.

[44] Poth EJ. Historical development of intestinal antisepsis. World J Surg 1982;6:153–9.
[45] Cohn I Jr, Rives JD. Antibiotic protection of colon anastomoses. Ann Surg 1955;141(5): 707–17.
[46] Cohn I Jr, Longacre AB. Erythromycin and erythromycin-neomycin for intestinal antisepsis. Am J Surg 1957;94(3):402–8.
[47] Nichols RL, Condon RE, Gorbach SL, et al. Efficacy of preoperative antimicrobial preparation of the bowel. Ann Surg 1972;176(2):227–32.
[48] Nichols RL, Condon RE, DiSanto AR. Preoperative bowel preparation: erythromycin base serum and fecal levels following oral administration. Arch Surg 1977;112:1493–6.
[49] Takesue Y, Yokoyama T, Akagi S, et al. A brief course of colon preparation with oral antibiotics. Surg Today 2000;30(2):112–6.
[50] Groner JI, Edmiston CE Jr, Krepel CJ, et al. The efficacy of oral antimicrobials in reducing aerobic and anaerobic colonic mucosal flora. Arch Surg 1989;124(3):281–4.
[51] Nichols RL, Broido P, Condon RE, et al. Effect of preoperative neomycin-erythromycin intestinal preparation on the incidence of infectious complications following colon surgery. Ann Surg 1973;178(4):453–62.
[52] Goldring J, McNaught W, Scott A, et al. Prophylactic oral antimicrobial agents in elective colonic surgery. A controlled trial. Lancet 1975;2(7943):997–1000.
[53] Evans C, Pollock AV. The reduction of surgical wound infections by prophylactic parenteral cephaloridine: a controlled clinical trial. Br J Surg 1973;60:434.
[54] CDC guidelines. Available at: http://www.cdc.gov/hicpac/pdf/guidelines/SSI_1999.pdf. Accessed October 25, 2015.
[55] SCIP guidelines. Available at: http://www.jointcommission.org/assets/1/6/SCIP-Measures-012014.pdf. Accessed October 25, 2015.
[56] Arabi Y, Dimock F, Burdon DW, et al. Influence of bowel preparation and antimicrobials on colonic microflora. Br J Surg 1978;65:555–8.
[57] Coppa GF, Eng K, Gouge TH, et al. Parenteral and oral antibiotics in elective colon and rectal surgery. A prospective, randomized trial. Am J Surg 1983;145:62–5.
[58] Khubchandani IT, Karamchandani MC, Sheets JA, et al. Metronidazole vs. erythromycin, neomycin, and cefazolin in prophylaxis for colonic surgery. Dis Colon Rectum 1989;32: 17–20.
[59] Ishida H, Yokoyama M, Nakada H, et al. Impact of oral antimicrobial prophylaxis on surgical site infection and methicillin-resistant Staphylococcus aureus infection after elective colorectal surgery. Results of a prospective randomized trial. Surg Today 2001;31:979–83.
[60] Washington JA 2nd, Dearing WH, Judd ES, et al. Effect of preoperative antibiotic regimen on development of infection after intestinal surgery: prospective, randomized, double-blind study. Ann Surg 1974;180:567–72.
[61] Bellows CF, Mills KT, Kelly TN, et al. Combination of oral non-absorbable and intravenous antibiotics versus intravenous antibiotics alone in the prevention of surgical site infections after colorectal surgery: a meta-analysis of randomized controlled trials. Tech Coloproctol 2011;15:385–95.
[62] Nelson RL, Gladman E, Barbateskovic M. Antimicrobial prophylaxis for colorectal surgery. Cochrane Database Syst Rev 2014;(5):CD001181.
[63] Barber MS, Hirschberg BC, Rice CL, et al. Parenteral antibiotics in elective colon surgery? A prospective, controlled clinical study. Surgery 1979;86(1):23–9.
[64] Cannon JA, Altom LK, Deierhoi RJ, et al. Preoperative oral antibiotics reduce surgical site infection following elective colorectal resections. Dis Colon Rectum 2012;55:1160–6.
[65] Englesbe MJ, Brooks L, Kubus J, et al. Campbell DA Jr.A statewide assessment of surgical site infection following colectomy: the role of oral antibiotics. Ann Surg 2010;252(3):514–9 [discussion: 519–20].
[66] Kim YW, Choi EH, Kim IY, et al. The impact of mechanical bowel preparation in elective colorectal surgery: a propensity score matching analysis. Yonsei Med J 2014;55(5): 1273–80.

[67] Munday GS, Deveaux P, Roberts H, et al. Impact of implementation of the Surgical Care Improvement Project and future strategies for improving quality in surgery. Am J Surg 2014;208:835–40.
[68] Toneva GD, Deierhoi RJ, Morris M, et al. Oral antibiotic bowel preparation reduces length of stay and readmissions after colorectal surgery. J Am Coll Surg 2013;216(4):756–62 [discussion: 762–3].
[69] Pittet O, Nocito A, Balke H, et al. Rectal enema is an alternative to full mechanical bowel preparation for primary rectal cancer surgery. Colorectal Dis 2015;17(11):1007–10.
[70] Courtney DE, Kelly ME, Burke JP, et al. Postoperative outcomes following mechanical bowel preparation before proctectomy: a meta-analysis. Colorectal Dis 2015;17(10):862–9.
[71] Wille-Jørgensen P, Guenaga KF, Matos D, et al. Pre-operative mechanical bowel cleansing or not? an updated meta-analysis. Colorectal Dis 2005;17(4):304–10.
[72] Bertani E, Chiappa A, Biffi R, et al. Comparison of oral polyethylene glycol plus a large volume glycerine enema with a large volume glycerine enema alone in patients undergoing colorectal surgery for malignancy: a randomized clinical trial. Colorectal Dis 2011;13(10):e327–34.
[73] Platell C, Barwood N, Makin G. Randomized clinical trial of bowel preparation with a single phosphate enema or polyethylene glycol before elective colorectal surgery. Br J Surg 2006;93(4):427–33.
[74] Vlot J, Slieker JC, Wijnen R, et al. Optimizing working-space in laparoscopy: measuring the effect of mechanical bowel preparation in a porcine model. Surg Endosc 2013;27(6): 1980–5.

Advances in Surgery 50 (2016) 67–78
ADVANCES IN SURGERY

Incarcerated/Strangulated Hernia: Open or Laparoscopic?

James G. Bittner IV, MD
Virginia Commonwealth University, Medical College of Virginia, Department of Surgery, VCU Comprehensive Hernia Center, PO Box 980519, Richmond, VA 23298, USA

Keywords
• Incarceration • Strangulation • Inguinal hernia • Laparoscopic

Key points

- Incarceration and strangulation represent significant challenges in the management of adult and pediatric patients with inguinal hernia.
- Surgeons who care for adult and pediatric patients must be well versed in the literature to ensure evidence-based decision-making and management strategies that will yield the best possible outcomes.
- Ultimately, despite advances in minimally invasive approaches and published practice guidelines, surgeons most often seem to assess patient risk factors, choose the appropriate timing for intervention, and perform the operation that they are most comfortable with and that matches the acute need of the patient with incarcerated or strangulated inguinal hernia.

INTRODUCTION

In general, hernia repair remains one of the most common operations performed in the United States, in particular inguinal hernia repair, with more than 800,000 procedures performed annually [1]. When hernias present as incarcerated or strangulated, decision-making and management strategies may vary. Unlike elective repair of a reducible hernia wherein the primary goal is long-lasting closure and prevention of hernia recurrence, the goals of emergent repair of a strangulated hernia may be to alleviate bowel obstruction, debride devitalized tissue, and/or mitigate the risk of abdominal catastrophe. As such, thoughtful, evidence-based decision-making and sound surgical technique

The author has nothing to disclose.

E-mail address: jgbittner@vcu.edu

0065-3411/16/$ – see front matter
http://dx.doi.org/10.1016/j.yasu.2016.03.006

play crucial roles in the successful management of incarcerated and strangulated inguinal hernia. The purpose of this article is to review the diagnosis of incarcerated and strangulated hernias, discuss the available evidence that supports clinical decision-making, and examine the various surgical approaches–open and laparoscopic–for repair of these complex hernias.

DIAGNOSIS

The diagnosis of incarcerated or strangulated inguinal hernia begins with a thorough history and physical examination, with particular attention paid to the duration and severity of symptoms, the presence of comorbid conditions, and the surgical history. One important goal of history-taking is to identify modifiable risk factors (Table 1), and through patient engagement, counseling, and medical treatment, lower the risk of recurrence and morbidity following hernia repair. Lowering the risk of recurrence and morbidity is particularly significant for patients who present with incarcerated hernia but initially may be amenable to nonoperative management. Other components of the history that warrant attention with regard to incarcerated and strangulated hernia are the location, duration, severity of pain, the presence of gastrointestinal signs and symptoms, and the noted period since the herniated contents were no longer reducible.

The diagnosis of incarcerated and strangulated hernia is based on physical examination. It is important to detail clinical examination findings specific to incarcerated and strangulated hernia. Pertinent findings on examination in both standing and supine positions include a palpable bulge and/or nonreducible mass of the abdominal wall, inguinal region, scrotum, or medial thigh caudad to the inguinal ligament, depending on the location of the hernia defect and amount of contents within the hernia sac. Patients with acutely incarcerated and strangulated hernia frequently report localized tenderness or pain on examination as well. Patients with strangulated hernia in particular may present with pain out of proportion to examination, erythema of skin overlying herniated contents, hyperesthesia, and/or wound drainage prompting immediate investigation. Additional clinical and laboratory findings can include signs of dehydration, alkalosis, leukocytosis, lactic acidosis, and/or other evidence of systemic inflammatory response syndrome.

Radiologic imaging may be used in some cases to identify precisely the location, size, and shape of the defect as well as the type and viability of contents within the hernia sac. Various options are available, including ultrasonography, MRI, and herniogram, but the most commonly used imaging study for evaluating incarcerated and strangulated hernia is computed tomography (CT). Given the rapidity with which CT can be obtained in the United States, and the valuable information it may provide before surgical intervention, this author is of the opinion that CT of the abdomen and pelvis should usually precede elective and urgent repair of incarcerated and strangulated hernia.

Table 1
Published outcomes of open mesh repair for incarcerated and strangulated inguinal hernia

Authors	Patients (n)	Resection of nonviable intestine (%)	Surgical site infection (%)	Mesh infection (%)	Recurrence (%)	Mean/median follow-up (mo)
Pans et al [28], 1997	35	2.6	5.7	0	2.9	50.4
Wysocki et al [29], 2001	20	5	0	0	N/A	15.3
Wysocki et al [30], 2002	27	3.7	0	0	0	18
Papaziogas et al [31], 2005	33	12.1	6.1	0	3	84
Wysocki et al [32], 2006	56	3.6	3.6	0	N/A	35.8
Bessa et al [33], 2007	25	16	0	0	0	11.4
Atila et al [16], 2010	95	14.7	1.1	0	2.1	47
Derici et al [34], 2010	29	20.7	10.3	0	3.4	48.7
Elsebae et al [35], 2008	27	0	3.7	0	0	22
Ueda et al [36], 2012	10	100	20	0	0	20
Lohsiriwat et al [37], 2013	20	0	0	0	5	72
Sawayam et al [38], 2014	74	13.5	2.7	0	N/A	N/A
Totals	451	13.5	3.3	0	2	

Abbreviation: N/A, not applicable as these data were not reported.

Data from Bessa SS, Abdel-fattah MR, Al-Sayes A, et al. Results of prosthetic mesh repair in the emergency management of the acutely incarcerated and/or strangulated groin hernias: a 10-year study. Hernia 2015;19(6):909–14.

DECISION-MAKING

The approach to incarcerated and strangulated hernias differs depending on the patient's symptoms, comorbidities, diagnosis, resource availability, and surgeon training and experience. Regardless of surgeon experience with complex abdominal wall reconstruction and hernia repair, a primary goal is to provide safe, timely management of the acute process. Subsequently, surgeon knowledge of techniques, prostheses, and expected outcomes permits delayed or definitive repair of the hernia defect at the index operation.

Incarcerated/strangulated inguinal hernia

The reported incidence of emergent operation for incarcerated and strangulated inguinal hernia in the United States seems to be decreasing according to a population-based study from the Mayo Clinic [2]. Within this population followed for almost 20 years, the incidence of emergent operation for incarcerated and strangulated inguinal hernia decreased from 18.2 to 12.4 per 100,000 person-years in men and from 6.4 to 2.4 per 100,000 person-years in women [2]. Two prospective randomized trials lend further support to the low incidence of incarcerated and strangulated inguinal hernia among patients diagnosed with an inguinal hernia. In the North American trial, the overall incidence of hernia accident (incarceration and strangulation) was 2.4% (0.2 per 100 person-years) among men with asymptomatic or mildly symptomatic inguinal hernia over a period of 10 years [3]. The trial conducted in the United Kingdom confirmed a similar finding, that is, a low (2.5%) overall incidence of incarceration and strangulation among men at least 55 years old with a reducible inguinal hernia over a 7.5-year period [4].

Despite the safety of watchful waiting as a management strategy for patients with asymptomatic or minimally symptomatic inguinal hernia based on 2 randomized trials, the low incidence of incarcerated and strangulated inguinal hernia overall [3,4], and the improved outcomes of emergency intervention over the years [5], elective repair remains a recommended management strategy for medically fit patients with asymptomatic inguinal hernia [6]. Older men with asymptomatic or minimally symptomatic reducible inguinal hernia or those with severe comorbidity may be selected for watchful waiting [6]. The presence of an incarcerated or strangulated inguinal hernia is an indication for repair.

Patients with asymptomatic or minimally symptomatic yet chronically incarcerated inguinal hernia may be managed by watchful waiting or elective repair. In medically fit patients with incarcerated inguinal hernia, both open and minimally invasive approaches are safe and effective options for repair. Two recent studies with long-term follow-up and a meta-analysis reported similar rates of hernia recurrence between open Lichtenstein tension-free repair and laparoscopic totally extraperitoneal repair for patients mostly with primary unilateral inguinal hernia [6–8]. Randomized controlled trials and meta-analysis of patients with recurrent inguinal hernia after open repair showed that a laparoscopic approach yielded significantly less postoperative pain and no difference in recurrence rates compared with an open approach [6,9,10]. These findings led to the recommendation that recurrent inguinal hernia after open repair is best managed using a minimally invasive technique [6]. The data are less clear when considering incarcerated and strangulated inguinal hernia repair.

SURGICAL APPROACHES—LAPAROSCOPY

Laparoscopic repair for adults

One systematic review including 7 articles published between 1996 and 2007 reported on the use of laparoscopy for the management of incarcerated and strangulated inguinal hernia. Of 328 patients, there were 6 conversions to an open procedure, 34 complications (mostly minor), and 17 bowel resections [11]. Most incarcerated and strangulated hernias were reduced using a combination of manual and laparoscopic manipulation under general anesthesia. Conversions occurred due to findings or situations at the time of operation. The reasons for conversion included an obturator hernia, iatrogenic bowel injury, need for omentectomy, bowel distention making visualization difficult, and dense intraperitoneal adhesions [11–13]. Complications related to a laparoscopic approach included a left colon injury during Veress needle insufflation and 3 intraperitoneal mesh infections, 2 of which required reoperation [11]. The largest series included in this systematic review comprised 194 patients who underwent laparoscopic transabdominal preperitoneal repair. The investigators reported no conversions and an overall morbidity of 3.8% [14]. One patient sustained an injury to the cecum from Veress needle insertion without sequelae, and one patient required reoperation for removal of infected synthetic mesh placed during the index operation [14].

A randomized controlled trial of 41 patients with strangulated inguinal hernia was conducted to compare hernia sac laparoscopy to open inspection of the hernia sac with or without laparotomy. Patients were randomized to either hernia sac laparoscopy plus open inguinal hernia repair or to open inspection of the hernia sac with or without laparotomy followed by open inguinal hernia repair if their strangulated inguinal hernia reduced spontaneously on induction of general anesthesia. Regardless of whether the patient initially underwent laparoscopy or open exploration of the hernia sac with or without laparotomy, all hernias were repaired using an open technique with implantation of permanent synthetic mesh. Both patient cohorts were similar with respect to age, duration of incarceration or strangulation, and comorbidities. Of the 21 patients in the hernia sac laparoscopy group, 2 required laparoscopic bowel resection before open inguinal hernia repair with mesh. In the open group, 4 of 20 patients underwent laparotomy at the surgeons' discretion and 2 of those required bowel resection. One patient in the open group had a delayed laparotomy for missed bowel ischemia. Minor complication rates were similarly low (14% and 15%) in both cohorts; however, major complications were 20% higher in the open exploration group. Zero patients in the hernia sac laparoscopy group and 2 patients in the open exploration group died, although the study was underpowered to detect a difference in mortalities between cohorts. The sensitivity, specificity, positive predictive value, and negative predictive value (all 100%) for hernia sac laparoscopy were greater than for open exploration of the hernia sac with or without laparotomy [15]. The investigators concluded that laparoscopy is a safe and accurate method to prevent unnecessary laparotomy after spontaneous reduction of strangulated inguinal hernia, particularly in high-risk patients who suffer greater morbidity [15].

A recent study of patients undergoing laparoscopic bowel resection and concomitant repair of acutely incarcerated inguinal hernia showed a low rate of mesh infection when the mesh was placed in the preperitoneal space [16]. A subsequent systematic review analyzed the risk of surgical site infection (SSI) and hernia recurrence among patients with acutely incarcerated inguinal hernia treated by open Lichtenstein repair with polypropylene mesh and those who received a pure tissue repair. In total, 9 of 232 publications were analyzed, of which 2 were randomized controlled trials and 3 were prospective nonrandomized studies. Only 5 studies (413 patients) reported rates of SSI. Interestingly, the SSI rate was almost 50% lower in the mesh repair group, although the difference failed to reach statistical significance. When the study with highest heterogeneity was excluded from analysis, the heterogeneity was good (I^2 0%) and the lower risk of SSI after mesh repair achieved statistical significance (odds ratio 0.25, 95% confidence interval 0.08–0.72). When 221 patients in the Lichtenstein repair group were categorized according to whether or not they underwent concomitant bowel resection, there was no significant difference in SSI rates. Three studies (260 patients) with low heterogeneity were analyzed for hernia recurrence rates. Mesh repair was found to have a significantly lower rate of hernia recurrence across all studies [17].

Elderly patients are not immune from incarcerated and strangulated inguinal hernia. A retrospective review compared open and laparoscopic approaches to the management of inguinal hernia in octogenarians [18]. Patients at least 80 years old who underwent inguinal hernia repair between 2006 and 2009 at a single center were included. In all, 81 patients underwent open (72%) and laparoscopic (28%) repair. Both groups had a similar number of operations performed for incarcerated inguinal hernia (open 17% and laparoscopic 13%). In the subset of patients with incarcerated inguinal hernia who underwent laparoscopic repair, concomitant procedures included diagnostic laparoscopy and umbilical hernia repair. The open repair group required appendectomy for necrotic appendix in a strangulated femoral hernia and a pelvic floor reconstruction. There were no statistical differences between open and laparoscopic groups with regard to postoperative urinary retention, overall morbidity, and mortality. Of note, the laparoscopic group had a statistically significantly shorter average hospital length of stay compared with the open group (0 vs 1 day). During the mean follow-up of 31 months for the laparoscopic group and 19 months for the open group, only one hernia recurrence was noted in the open group. The investigators concluded that factors including the patient condition, the presence of bilateral or recurrent inguinal hernia, and patient preference may favor a laparoscopic approach, although an individualized approach is advisable when considering inguinal hernia repair in octogenarians [18].

Published results led to the recommendation that a laparoscopic approach to incarcerated and strangulated inguinal hernia is feasible, facilitates bowel resection as needed, and exhibits an overall morbidity similar to an open approach [11,19]. In the case of strangulated inguinal hernia, diagnostic laparoscopy is preferred to open exploration [15,19]. The use of synthetic mesh in the preperitoneal space is possible with a relatively low risk of morbidity in clean-contaminated situations such as bowel resection [16–19]. It should be noted that only 69% of 150 expert panelists from the European Association for Endoscopic Surgery agreed with the recommendation for mesh placement in clean-contaminated cases [19].

Despite these data and guidelines, a recent population-based cohort study from Quebec, Canada revealed infrequent use of laparoscopy for repair of incarcerated inguinal hernia between 2007 and 2011. Of 49,657 inguinal hernias repaired by 478 surgeons, laparoscopy was used for 8% of repairs. For incarcerated inguinal hernia, only 4% were managed with laparoscopic repair [20]. It is possible that such low penetrance of laparoscopy is due in part to the fact that only 44% of surgeons performed any laparoscopic inguinal hernia repair [20]. It seems as though in Quebec at least there is a difference between clinical practice and published guidelines with regard to management of incarcerated and strangulated inguinal hernia. To expand on that, Canadian researchers fielded a survey of 697 practicing general surgeon members of North American surgical societies and found that a minority of respondents preferred laparoscopic repair for nonobstructing (10%) and obstructing (7%) incarcerated inguinal hernia [21]. The respondents (46%) who did not perform any laparoscopic inguinal hernia repair cited lack of benefit from laparoscopy, lack of training or prolonged learning curve, and increased operative time as perceived barriers to adoption of a minimally invasive approach [21]. These 2 studies speak to the need for greater education about current management strategies and guidelines as well as methods of technical skills training for laparoscopic inguinal hernia repair.

Laparoscopic repair for children

Management of incarcerated and strangulated inguinal hernia in children is both challenging and associated with potential complications. A retrospective study of 63 incarcerated inguinal hernia repairs compared open and laparoscopic techniques. The 2 cohorts were similar demographically, but the length of operation was significantly longer in the laparoscopy group. At 3.5-months follow-up, more children in the open group suffered serious complications [22]. A much larger retrospective study of children with failed manual reduction of an incarcerated inguinal hernia under sedation was performed to assess the seriousness of irreducible inguinal hernia [23]. Of 2184 children, only 1.6% presented with a nonreducible inguinal hernia over a 10-year period. In those 34 children with incarcerated or strangulated inguinal hernia, laparoscopic repair was performed in 62% and 2 required conversion. In this patient subgroup, laparoscopy allowed for identification of hernia sac contents (small intestine, omentum, and ovary) and resection of small intestine (4%) and omentum (6%). There were no hernia recurrences. These data suggest the safety and durability of laparoscopy for management of incarcerated inguinal hernia in children [23].

Published literature relays other potential benefits of laparoscopy for pediatric patients with incarcerated inguinal hernia. From a retrospective cohort of 601 children who underwent laparoscopic inguinal hernia repair over a 2-year period, 46 children presented with incarcerated inguinal hernia [24]. Of these patients, 45.6% had an incarcerated hernia that reduced preoperatively and subsequently underwent laparoscopic repair. The remaining group of children (54.4%) had nonreducible inguinal hernia that failed manual reduction and required urgent laparoscopic repair. Short-term outcomes demonstrated no conversion to an open procedure, short average operative time, variable hospital length of stay (median 36 hours), and few (4.3%) recurrences with a minimum follow-up of 14 months. The investigators thought laparoscopy offered the advantages of direct visualization during reduction of hernia contents and inspection of incarcerated tissue at the index operation [24].

A smaller series of 275 laparoscopic inguinal hernia repairs in 187 children was assessed retrospectively for clinical outcomes [25]. Fifteen hernia repairs were performed in children with nonreducible inguinal hernia after failed manual reduction. With a minimum follow-up of 2 years, the overall recurrence rate was 1.5% with no spermatic cord injuries, testicular atrophy, or symptoms of ilioinguinal nerve injuries. The laparoscopic approach minimizes the manipulation of the spermatic cord structures and provides excellent cosmesis according to the investigators [25].

Despite the shortage of high-level studies comparing laparoscopic and open approaches to inguinal hernia repair in children, publications to date highlight several advantages of laparoscopy. In general, studies suggest potential benefits of laparoscopy for inguinal hernia repair, which include the ability to detect and simultaneously repair a contralateral patent processus vaginalis or hernia and may even yield a lower recurrence rate compared with a traditional open approach. In addition, the ability to identify and manage intraperitoneal contents reduced from the hernia sac may be improved with laparoscopy. Although rates of injury to spermatic cord structures and testicular atrophy are low and cosmesis is good after laparoscopic repair, little evidence supports that any of these outcomes are improved over open repair.

SURGICAL APPROACHES—OPEN

Open repair for adults

Open repair often is considered the gold standard for operative management of incarcerated and strangulated inguinal hernia. Some debate exists about the utilization of synthetic mesh during emergent repair of such hernias, especially when a concomitant procedure is required. A recent prospective study conducted in Egypt investigated outcomes of 234 adult patients (90.6% male) who presented with acutely incarcerated or strangulated inguinal hernia between 2003 and 2013 at a single center [26]. Patients were excluded from analysis if they presented with generalized peritonitis or gross contamination (feculent material) within the hernia sac. All patients underwent open Lichtenstein tension-free repair using heavyweight polypropylene mesh. In most patients, the hernia sac contained viable contents (82.5%), most often small intestine (75.2%). In total, 13.7% of patients required enterectomy with anastomosis and 3.8% underwent partial omentectomy. At a mean follow-up of 62.5 months, with 86.3% of patients available for assessment at 10 years, only 2 patients developed hernia recurrence and one individual suffered mesh infection. In this patient, the mesh was removed during the sixth postoperative month. There was no significant difference in rates of wound infection, hematoma, deep venous thrombosis, transient liver dysfunction, or mesh infection between patients with viable and nonviable contents within the hernia sac [26].

Preceding studies also reported on the safety and efficacy of open repair for incarcerated and strangulated inguinal hernia. Sixteen studies representing 535 patients detailed the use of mesh repair for management of acutely incarcerated and strangulated inguinal hernia (mean/median follow-up ranging from 11.3 to 84 months). Within these studies, 451 patients underwent open repair with mesh (see Table 1). Of those who had an open mesh repair, 61 (13.5%) required enterectomy with anastomosis for nonviable intestine, 15 (3.3%) developed an SSI, none suffered mesh infection, and 6 patients developed recurrent inguinal hernia [26]. Although chronic mesh infection may present months to years postoperatively [27], the homogeneous outcomes reported in the available literature suggest a low rate of permanent synthetic mesh infection following open mesh repair for incarcerated and strangulated inguinal hernia, even in clean-contaminated situations at short- and long-term follow-up [16,26,28–38].

Open repair for children

A large study of 3776 pediatric patients who underwent open inguinal hernia repair between 2005 and 2009 at a single center reported on outcomes [39]. Within this group, a subset of 83 (2.2%) patients presented with nonreducible inguinal hernia that failed manual reduction and required urgent operation. The postoperative complication rate for patients with incarcerated inguinal hernia that failed manual reduction was 3.6%. Twelve of these patients required concomitant operation, including bowel resection for intestinal perforation, oophorectomy, omentectomy, and Meckel diverticulectomy. The rates of hernia recurrence requiring reoperation were low in this subset (1.2%) and overall (0.4%). These results support the safety and efficacy of open inguinal hernia repair for pediatric patients and the low rates of complications and recurrence in the setting of nonreducible inguinal hernia that failed manual reduction and required urgent operation [39].

Open repair of incarcerated and strangulated inguinal hernia is a standard approach used throughout the world. Comparative studies of open and laparoscopic repair are too few and the data equivocal to conclude definitively that one approach is superior to the other. Guidelines on the management of inguinal hernia in children continue to support open repair as the gold standard. The guidelines also discuss various laparoscopic techniques for pediatric hernia repair, including transperitoneal and preperitoneal approaches as well as hernioscopy, which can augment open repair [40].

SUMMARY

Incarceration and strangulation represent significant challenges in the management of adult and pediatric patients with inguinal hernia. Surgeons who care for adult and pediatric patients must be well versed in the literature to ensure evidence-based decision-making and management strategies that will yield the best possible outcomes. This article reviewed the diagnosis of incarcerated and strangulated hernias, discussed the available evidence that supports clinical decision-making, and examined the various surgical approaches for repair. Ultimately, despite advances in minimally invasive approaches and published practice guidelines, surgeons most often seem to assess patient risk factors, choose the appropriate timing for intervention, and perform the operation that they are most comfortable with and that matches the acute need of the patient with incarcerated or strangulated inguinal hernia.

References

[1] Towfigh S, Neumayer L. Inguinal hernia. In: Cameron JL, Cameron AM, editors. Current surgical therapy. 11th edition. New York: Saunders Publishing; 2014. p. 531–6.

[2] Hernandez-Irizarry R, Zendejas B, Ramirez T, et al. Trends in emergent inguinal hernia surgery in Olmstead County, MN: a population-based study. Hernia 2012;16:397–403.

[3] Fitzgibbons RJ, Ramanan B, Arya S, et al. Long-term results of a randomized controlled trial of a nonoperative strategy (watchful waiting) for men with minimally symptomatic inguinal hernias. Ann Surg 2013;258:508–15.

[4] Chung L, Norrie J, O'Dwyer P. Long-term follow-up of patients with a painless inguinal hernia from a randomized clinical trial. Br J Surg 2011;98:596–9.

[5] Turaga K, Fitzgibbons RJ, Puri V. Inguinal hernias: should we repair? Surg Clin North Am 2008;88:127–38.

[6] Miserez M, Peeters E, Aufenacker T, et al. Update with level 1 studies of the European Hernia Society guidelines on the treatment of inguinal hernia in adult patients. Hernia 2014;18:151–63.

[7] Eklund AS, Montgomery AK, Rasmussen IC, et al. Low recurrence rate after laparoscopic (TEP) and open (Lichtenstein) inguinal hernia repair: a randomized, multicenter trial with 5-year follow-up. Ann Surg 2009;249:33–8.

[8] Langeveld HR, van't Riet M, Weidema WF, et al. Total extraperitoneal inguinal hernia repair compared with Lichtenstein (the LEVEL-Trial): a randomized controlled trial. Ann Surg 2010;251:819–24.

[9] Demetrashvili Z, Qerqadze V, Kamkamidze G, et al. Comparison of Lichtenstein and laparoscopic transabdominal preperitoneal repair of recurrent inguinal hernias. Int Surg 2011;96:233–8.

[10] Eklund A, Montgomery A, Bergkvist L, et al. Chronic pain 5 years after randomized comparison of laparoscopic and Lichtenstein inguinal hernia repair. Br J Surg 2010;97:600–8.

[11] Deeba S, Purkayastha S, Paraskevas P, et al. Laparoscopic approach to incarcerated and strangulated inguinal hernia. JSLS 2009;13:327–31.
[12] Ferzli G, Shapiro K, Chaudry G, et al. Laparoscopic extra-peritoneal approach to acutely incarcerated inguinal hernia. Surg Endosc 2004;18:228–31.
[13] Rebuffat C, Galli A, Scalambra MS, et al. Laparoscopic repair of strangulated hernias. Surg Endosc 2006;20:13113–4.
[14] Leibl BJ, Schmedt CG, Kraft K, et al. Laparoscopic transperitoneal hernia repair of incarcerated hernias: is it feasible? Results of a prospective study. Surg Endosc 2001;15:1179–83.
[15] Sgourakis G, Radtke A, Sotiropoulos G, et al. Assessment of strangulated content of the spontaneously reduced inguinal hernia via hernia sac laparoscopy: preliminary results of a prospective randomized study. Surg Laparosc Endosc Percutan Tech 2009;19:133–7.
[16] Atila K, Guler S, Inal A, et al. Prosthetic repair of acutely incarcerated groin hernias: a prospective clinical observational cohort study. Langenbecks Arch Surg 2010;395:563–8.
[17] Hentati H, Dougaz W, Dziri C. Mesh repair versus non-mesh repair for strangulated inguinal hernia: systematic review with meta-analysis. World J Surg 2014;38:2784–90.
[18] Hope WW, Bools L, Menon A, et al. Comparing laparoscopic and open inguinal hernia repair in octogenarians. Hernia 2013;17:719–22.
[19] Poelman MM, van den Heuvel B, Deelder JD, et al. EAES Consensus Development Conference on endoscopic repair of groin hernias. Surg Endosc 2013;27:3505–19.
[20] Trevisonno M, Kaneva P, Watanabe Y, et al. Current practices of laparoscopic inguinal hernia repair: a population-based analysis. Hernia 2015;19:725–33.
[21] Trevisonno M, Kaneva P, Watanabe Y, et al. A survey of general surgeons regarding laparoscopic inguinal hernia repair: practice patterns, barriers, and educational needs. Hernia 2015;19:719–24.
[22] Nah SA, Giacomello L, Eaton S, et al. Surgical repair of incarcerated inguinal hernia in children: laparoscopic or open? Eur J Pediatr Surg 2011;21:8–11.
[23] Houben CH, Chan KW, Mou JW, et al. Irreducible inguinal hernia in children: how serious is it? J Pediatr Surg 2015;50:1174–6.
[24] Esposito C, Turial S, Alicchio F, et al. Laparoscopic repair of incarcerated inguinal hernia: a safe and effective procedure to adopt in children. Hernia 2013;17:235–9.
[25] Dutta S, Albanese C. Transcutaneous laparoscopic hernia repair in children: a prospective review of 275 hernia repairs with minimum 2-year follow-up. Surg Endosc 2009;23:103–7.
[26] Bessa SS, Abdel-fattah MR, Al-Sayes A, et al. Results of prosthetic mesh repair in the emergency management of the acutely incarcerated and/or strangulated groin hernias: a 10-year study. Hernia 2015;19(6):909–14.
[27] Delikoukos S, Tzovaras G, Liakou P, et al. Late-onset deep mesh infection after inguinal hernia repair. Hernia 2007;11:15–7.
[28] Pans A, Desaive C, Jacquet N. Use of preperitoneal prosthesis for strangulated groin hernia. Br J Surg 1997;84:310–2.
[29] Wysocki A, Pozniczek M, Krzywon J, et al. Use of polypropylene prosthesis for strangulated inguinal and incisional hernias. Hernia 2001;5:105–6.
[30] Wysocki A, Pozniczek M, Krzywon J, et al. Lichtenstein repair for incarcerated groin hernias. Eur J Surg 2002;168:452–4.
[31] Papaziogas B, Lazaridis CH, Makria J, et al. Tension-free repair versus modified Bassini technique (Andrews technique) for strangulated inguinal hernia: a comparative study. Hernia 2005;9:156–9.
[32] Wysocki A, Kulawik J, Poźniczek M, et al. Is the Lichtenstein operation of strangulated groin hernia a safe procedure? World J Surg 2006;30:2065–70.
[33] Bessa SS, Katri KM, Abdel-Salam WN, et al. Early results from the use of the Lichtenstein repair in the management of strangulated groin hernia. Hernia 2007;11:239–42.
[34] Derici H, Unalp HR, Nazli O, et al. Prosthetic repair of incarcerated inguinal hernias: is it a reliable method? Langenbecks Arch Surg 2010;395:575–9.

[35] Elsebae MM, Nasr M, Said M. Tension-free repair versus Bassini technique for strangulated inguinal hernia: a controlled randomized study. Int J Surg 2008;6:302–5.
[36] Ueda J, Nomura T, Sasaki J, et al. Prosthetic repair of an incarcerated groin hernia with small intestinal resection. Surg Today 2012;42:359–62.
[37] Lohsiriwat D, Lohsiriwat V. Long-term outcomes of emergency Lichtenstein hernioplasty for incarcerated inguinal hernia. Surg Today 2013;43:990–4.
[38] Sawayama H, Kanemitsu K, Okuma T, et al. Safety of polypropylene mesh for incarcerated groin and obturator hernias: a retrospective study of 110 patients. Hernia 2014;18: 399–406.
[39] Erdogan D, Karaman I, Aslan MK, et al. Analysis of 3776 pediatric inguinal hernia and hydrocele cases in a tertiary center. J Pediatr Surg 2013;48:1767–72.
[40] International Pediatric Endosurgery Group Standards and Safety Committee. IPEG guidelines for inguinal hernia and hydrocele. J Laparoendosc Adv Surg Tech A 2010;20:x–xiv.

Advances in Surgery 50 (2016) 79–91

ADVANCES IN SURGERY

Strategies to Reduce Postoperative Urinary Tract Infections

Christina M. Papageorge, MD,
Gregory D. Kennedy, MD, PhD*

Department of Surgery, University of Wisconsin School of Medicine and Public Health, 600 Highland Avenue, BX7375 Clinical Science Center – H4, Madison, WI 53792, USA

Keywords

• Urinary tract infection • Postoperative complications • Urinary retention • Catheter-associated urinary tract infection • Hospital-acquired infection • Quality improvement

Key points

- Postoperative urinary tract infection (UTI) is common and is associated with significant morbidity and cost.
- Urinary catheters are the most common cause of postoperative UTI, and interventions to reduce catheter use and duration are effective in preventing this complication.
- Multiple strategies have been demonstrated to reduce the incidence of UTI, including sterile catheter insertion technique, provider reminder systems, and early postoperative removal of catheters.
- Multifaceted and multidisciplinary approaches are necessary to change the culture of safety surrounding urinary catheter use.

INTRODUCTION

Urinary tract infection (UTI) is an important cause of postoperative morbidity in surgical patients. As the second leading cause of postoperative infections following surgical site infection, postoperative UTI contributes to increased costs, longer hospital stays, and increased mortality. Postoperative UTI has been shown to occur in association with other postoperative

Disclosure Statement: The authors have nothing to disclose.

*Corresponding author. *E-mail address:* kennedyg@surgery.wisc.edu

0065-3411/16/$ – see front matter
http://dx.doi.org/10.1016/j.yasu.2016.03.007

complications, thereby acting as a marker, if not a cause, of increased postoperative morbidity. Furthermore, treatment of UTI necessitates antibiotic use, which exposes patients to an array of risks and potential complications, such as antibiotic resistance and *Clostridium difficile* infection. In addition to these adverse consequences for the patient, there are now reimbursement penalties for hospital-acquired UTI, lending further incentive to the development and implementation of evidence-based strategies to reduce postoperative UTI.

Because emphasis on improving outcomes while controlling costs during the perioperative period remains a national priority, it is important to evaluate evidence surrounding the prevention of hospital-acquired infections (HAIs), such as postoperative UTI. This process requires a clear understanding of underlying causes, modifiable risk factors, strategies for identifying and targeting high-risk populations, development of evidence-based interventions, and effective implementation of such interventions. This article summarizes important measures and interventions in the prevention of postoperative UTI.

SIGNIFICANCE

Hospital-acquired UTI has historically been the leading cause of HAIs, previously accounting for approximately one-third of all such infections in the United States [1]. The most current prevalence survey performed by the Centers for Disease Control and Prevention (CDC) indicates that UTI now accounts for 13% of all HAIs, with an estimated 93,300 infections in the United States in 2011 [2]. Despite this relative improvement compared with other HAIs, the most recent National and State Healthcare-Associated Infections Progress Report based on data through 2013 identified a 6% increase nationally in catheter-associated UTI (CAUTI) rates between 2009 and 2013 [3]. Furthermore, this problem is particularly relevant in surgical populations because analysis of administrative data suggests that 70% of nosocomial UTIs occur in patients undergoing surgery at some point during their hospital stay [4]. In fact, UTI is the second most common type of postoperative infection following surgical site infection in patients undergoing small or large bowel resection [5]. Analysis of the American College of Surgeons National Surgical Quality Improvement Program database reveals that the crude rate of postoperative UTI within 30 days of surgery in all-comers is 1.7%, but with significantly higher incidence among certain subpopulations of surgical patients [6].

Accompanying the high prevalence of hospital-acquired UTI is significant morbidity for patients suffering this complication. In general, hospital-acquired UTI results in prolonged hospital stay, increased costs, and higher mortality [5,7–10]. In surgery patients specifically, UTI is similarly associated with worse outcomes. For example, analysis of patients undergoing colorectal resection for malignancy in the National Surgical Quality Improvement Program database demonstrated association of postoperative

UTI with an average of 5 days longer hospital stay and nearly double 30-day mortality (3.3% vs 1.7%) [9]. More than half of patients with postoperative UTI in this analysis also suffered at least one or more other postoperative complications. In a study of Medicare patients who underwent bowel resection at a single institution, CAUTI occurred in 12% of individuals aged 65 to 79 years and 36% of those aged 80 years or older [5]. Occurrence of CAUTI in this group of patients was associated with hospital costs twice those of patients who did not develop a CAUTI. In yet another analysis of colorectal surgery patients using National Inpatient Sample data, Kang and colleagues [11] identified postoperative UTI to be an independent predictor for several other complications including acute renal failure, deep vein thrombosis, ileus, anastomotic leak, pulmonary embolism, and respiratory failure.

The importance of preventing hospital-acquired UTI has been appropriately reflected in national legislation in recent years. In 2008, hospital-acquired UTI became one of several "reasonably preventable events" for which hospitals are no longer reimbursed by the Centers for Medicare and Medicaid (CMS) [12]. In 2003, the Joint Commission began publishing an annual list of National Patient Safety Goals to highlight important patient safety issues and provide guidance to accredited organizations. In 2012, the Joint Commission designated prevention of CAUTI as a National Patient Safety Goals, and it remains as such through 2015 [13].

To design interventions to prevent these infections, it is necessary to define the causes and risk factors for postoperative UTI. Common risk factors for postoperative UTI include female gender, older age, surgery of the alimentary tract (particularly colorectal resections), increased operative length of time, medical comorbidities, dependent functional status, preoperative anemia and hypoalbuminemia, open surgery, and higher American Society of Anesthesiologists class [5,6,11,14]. The single biggest modifiable risk factor, however, is indwelling catheter use and duration. It is estimated that 80% of postoperative UTIs are associated with catheter use. Therefore eliminating or reducing indwelling urinary catheters in the postoperative period would significantly reduce UTI risk. As a common indication for catheterization in the postoperative period, urinary retention may also prove to be a modifiable risk factor for UTI in surgical patients. Table 1 summarizes the modifiable and nonmodifiable risk factors for postoperative UTI that have previously been identified.

Working from an understanding of risk factors and the common underlying etiologies of postoperative UTI, it is possible to develop evidence-based prevention strategies. Many strategies have been described with varying degrees of success. Reducing postoperative UTI requires a multifaceted approach with buy-in from all members of the health care team. In the subsequent sections, we discuss the various strategies and evidence surrounding the prevention of postoperative UTI.

Table 1
Modifiable and nonmodifiable risk factors for postoperative urinary tract infection

Modifiable	Nonmodifiable
Urinary catheter use	Female gender
Urinary catheter duration	Older age
Postoperative urinary retention[a]	Multiple medical comorbidities
Open operative approach[a]	Preoperative anemia[a]
	Preoperative hypoalbuminemia[a]
	Dependent functional status
	Higher ASA class
	Operation (higher risk in gastrointestinal surgery, especially colorectal surgery)
	Longer operative length of time[a]

Abbreviation: ASA, American Society of Anesthesiologists.
[a]Indicates potentially modifiable risk factors.

PREVENTION OF CATHETER-ASSOCIATED URINARY TRACT INFECTION

The single most important cause of postoperative UTI is transurethral catheter usage. Approximately 67% to 80% of all hospital-acquired UTIs are associated with an indwelling urinary catheter [2,15,16]. Estimates suggest that for each day an indwelling bladder catheter remains in place, there is a 3% to 10% chance of developing bacteriuria [17,18]. Therefore, many interventions targeted at preventing UTI necessarily need to address reduced catheter usage and sterile catheter technique. Contamination can occur because of unsterile technique at the time of catheter insertion, reflux of contaminated urine from the catheter tubing back up into the bladder, and extraluminal entry of pathogens on the outer surface of the catheter tubing with retrograde migration up the urethra (Fig. 1) [19]. Catheter usage is a necessary exposure for CAUTI, and although many strategies have been demonstrated to reduce reliance on catheters in surgical patients, it is impossible to eliminate their use entirely. At a minimum, a catheter is often required for intraoperative bladder drainage during long procedures and intraoperative urine output monitoring. Catheters are then often used in the immediate postoperative period for urine output monitoring and collection of urine in immobile patients. Importantly, postoperative urinary retention is a common reason for intermittent catheterization or indwelling catheter insertion. Additionally, the anticipation of urinary retention in patients deemed high risk might further discourage surgeons from removing catheters early.

CAUTI has been defined by the National Healthcare Safety Network as a symptomatic UTI occurring during or within 48 hours of indwelling urinary catheter use. In general, prevention of CAUTI hinges on several important principles: (1) sterile catheter insertion technique, (2) proper catheter maintenance, (3) minimizing number of catheter days, and (4) only using catheters when absolutely necessary. The CDC has published a comprehensive

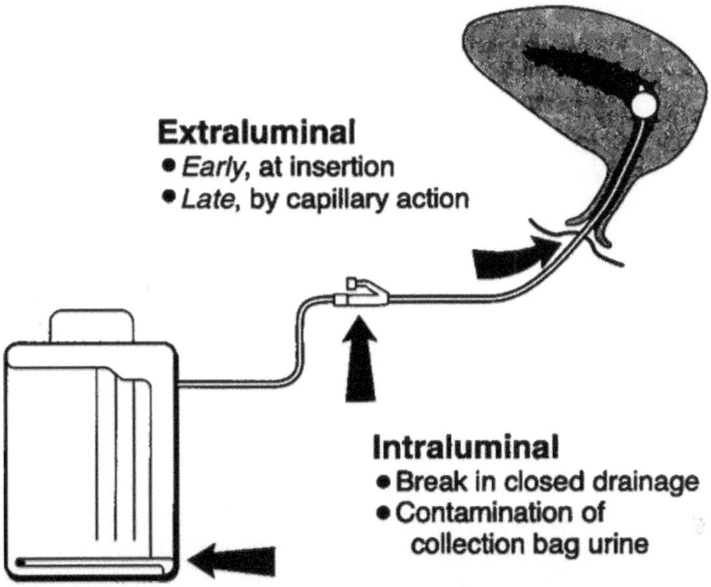

Fig. 1. Routes of entry of uropathogens to catheterized urinary tract. (*From* Maki DG, Tambyah PA. Engineering out the risk for infection with urinary catheters. Emerg Infect Dis 2001;7(2):342.)

evidence-based guideline for preventing CAUTI [20]. As long as catheters remain necessary to some extent in surgical patients, postoperative UTI is unlikely to be fully eradicated. However, there are clearly evidence-based ways to reduce this risk to patients.

Sterile catheter techniques

Proper catheter insertion technique represents the first opportunity to reduce the risk of postoperative UTI. Individuals placing urinary catheters should be trained in sterile technique for this procedure. Insertion should be performed using aseptic technique, and a sterile or aseptic solution should be used to clean the urethral meatus before catheter insertion. Sterile, single-packet lubricant jelly is then applied to the catheter tip to facilitate insertion. After insertion, the catheter tubing is secured to the patient's leg to minimize movement and urethral traction.

In the setting of elective surgery, surgeons have the opportunity to place the catheter in the controlled setting of the operating room. Nagle and colleagues [21] implemented a two-part intervention and demonstrated a significant reduction postoperative UTI rates among patients undergoing colorectal surgery. The second intervention involved a change in the conditions in which the catheter was placed in the operating room. Whereas before the intervention, a member of the operating team would perform perineal antiseptic preparation followed by catheter placement, the group then implemented a process whereby the patient was basically fully prepared and draped before placement of the catheter by a fully gowned and gloved surgeon. This intervention achieved a reduction in postoperative UTI from 2.7% to 0.8% among colorectal surgery patients at their institution. Notably, the only patient developing a UTI in the group receiving sterile intraoperative catheter placement had undergone ureteral reconstruction and double J stent placement concurrent to the colorectal operation.

Types of catheters

Several recent studies have focused on whether specific types of catheters may have an effect on rates of CAUTI. A variety of specialized catheters, such as antiseptic-coated or antimicrobial-impregnated catheters, are now commercially available and are designed to theoretically reduce infection risk. A Cochrane review published in 2014 summarized the current evidence surrounding use of such catheters [22]. The authors analyzed results from 26 randomized and quasi-randomized controlled trials comparing various types of indwelling urethral catheters for short-term catheterization in hospitalized adult patients. Silver alloy hydrogel-coated catheters do not seem to have significant benefit in reducing the incidence of symptomatic CAUTI compared with standard catheters, but may be associated with slightly lower rates of bacteriuria. In contrast, nitrofurazone-impregnated catheters were associated with a statistically significant reduction in symptomatic CAUTI (relative risk, 0.84; 95% confidence interval, 0.71–0.99) and bacteriuria when compared with standard catheters. However, antimicrobial-impregnated catheters were also associated with more patient discomfort during and following catheter usage. It is worth noting that silver alloy-coated and antimicrobial-impregnated catheters are substantially more expensive than standard catheters, and the marginal benefits may not justify the cost.

Indications for catheterization

Catheters are commonly used in surgical populations. An analysis of Medicare patients undergoing major inpatient operations including cardiac, vascular, general abdominal, colorectal surgery, and orthopedic procedures demonstrated indwelling urinary catheter use in 86% of cases [23]. In general, patients should not be catheterized for incontinence or immobility. Alternative techniques should be used whenever possible to avoid unnecessary catheter use. Such strategies include external catheters, such as condom catheters, intermittent catheterization, regular toileting, bedpans, and urinals (Table 2).

It may be tempting to rely on catheters in the perioperative period for urine output monitoring, collection of urine in patients with reduced mobility, collection of urine to avoid contamination of perineal wounds, and avoidance of issues with urinary retention. However, many of these "reasons" are inadequate given the known substantial risks of prolonged catheter use.

Timing of catheter removal

Because catheter duration is the primary determinant of risk for CAUTI, minimizing catheter duration is of the utmost importance in reducing postoperative

Table 2
Indications for perioperative indwelling catheterization with suggested alternatives

Indication	Potential alternatives
Postoperative urinary retention	Bladder management protocols using regular use of bladder scanners and intermittent catheterization
Urine output monitoring in critically ill patients	Condom catheter in male patients Daily weights
Long duration of surgery	Remove catheter at the conclusion of the case or in the recovery room
Intraoperative urine output monitoring	Remove catheter at the conclusion of the case or in the recovery room
Incontinent patient with an open sacral or perineal wound	External catheter (condom catheter)
Urologic surgery or other surgery necessitating bladder decompression	—

UTI [18]. It is well established that urinary catheter usage for greater than 48 hours is predictive of UTI. In a study of Medicare patients undergoing major surgery, half of all patients with a perioperative catheter had their catheter in situ for greater than 2 days postoperatively [23]. Notably, UTI rates were nearly double in those patients with a catheter for greater than 2 days, compared with those with shorter duration catheterization (9.4% vs 4.5%).

Implementation of reminder systems and stop orders to facilitate early catheter removal has been shown to reduce number of catheter days and CAUTI rates [18,21,24]. Nagle and colleagues [21] were able to demonstrate a reduction in postoperative UTI rates among colorectal surgery patients from nearly 7% down to 2.7% with implementation of a daily electronic order that was required to keep a catheter in place for greater than 24 hours. In this intervention, providers were required to enter an indication for continuation of the catheter before any further orders could be placed.

Reducing postoperative urinary retention

Any discussion of preventing postoperative UTI would be remiss to not discuss the prevention and management of postoperative urinary retention. Although an often-underemphasized problem in the postoperative period, urinary retention is widely prevalent and ultimately necessitates the use of catheters for temporary management until resolution. Additionally, urinary retention has been identified as an independent risk factor for postoperative UTI [11]. Risk factors for postoperative urinary retention include male gender, older age, obesity, pelvic surgery, longer operative time, and epidural use [25,26].

Several studies have aimed to evaluate the optimal amount of time to keep a urinary catheter in place following surgery. The significant risk of UTI with prolonged catheterization must be weighed against the risk of urinary retention. In a retrospective review of patients undergoing total or tumor-specific mesorectal excision for rectal cancer, the overall incidence of urinary retention was 4.8% [27]. There was no difference in urinary retention rates noted between patients catheterized for 1 day versus 2 or more days. It is worth noting that patients undergoing combined pelvic surgery and those with significant postoperative complications or known urinary disease including benign prostatic hyperplasia were excluded from this analysis, which likely eliminated some of the highest risk patients.

In a randomized controlled trial involving 126 patients comparing 1 day with 5 days of urinary catheterization following surgery for rectal cancer, there was a significantly higher incidence of urinary retention in the 1-day group compared with 5 days (25% vs 10%; $P < .05$) [28]. However, the prolonged catheter group suffered a 42% postoperative UTI rate compared with 20% in the 1-day group ($P < .01$). This study highlights the competing factors associated with early catheter removal.

Another major consideration in postoperative patients at risk for urinary retention is concomitant epidural use. It is generally accepted that epidural use in the postoperative period significantly increases the risk of urinary retention. Consequently, the decision is often made to maintain a urinary catheter until discontinuation of the epidural anesthesia. This approach results in significantly increased duration of urinary catheterization with its attendant high rates of UTI. Hu and colleagues [29] undertook a prospective trial evaluating early catheter removal in the setting of thoracic epidural anesthesia for pain control following thoracotomy. They reported a higher incidence of urinary retention in the group undergoing catheter removal on postoperative days 1 or 2, compared to a historic control group in which median catheter duration was 3 days (27% vs 12%). However, early catheter removal was associated with a reduction in UTI rate from 4% to 1%. Zaouter and colleagues [30] undertook a similar study in which they randomized patients deemed low-risk for urinary retention who underwent thoracic or abdominal surgery with thoracic epidural analgesia to either catheter removal on postoperative day 1 or catheter removal at the time of epidural discontinuation. They reported no difference in incidence of recatheterization for urinary retention, but a significant reduction in postoperative UTI rate in the early removal group (14% vs 2%; $P = .004$). Thus, although there is conflicting evidence regarding the risk of urinary retention with early catheter removal in the setting of epidural anesthesia, it is clear that prolonged catheter use results in significantly higher incidence of postoperative UTI. Given the morbidity and cost of UTI in comparison with urinary retention, surgeons should generally adhere to a policy of early catheter removal. Patients can be safely managed in this way using bladder scanners, protocols for diagnosing urinary retention, and intermittent catheterization.

Despite knowledge of specific risk factors, it remains somewhat difficult to predict which patients will develop urinary retention following surgery or catheter removal. Further research will be helpful in identifying highest risk patients before surgery and perhaps implementing interventions to prevent urinary retention. Some evidence has accumulated to suggest preoperative tamsulosin may be useful for this indication [31]. However, the data remain inconclusive. To definitively answer the question, we have initiated a randomized controlled trial of preoperative tamsulosin versus placebo to determine if postoperative urinary retention can be prevented with a simple medical intervention [32].

Prophylactic antibiotics

The evidence surrounding prophylactic antibiotics in the setting of catheter usage to reduce the risk of UTI remains equivocal. It is certainly tempting to think that use of prophylactic antibiotics may aid in reducing the risk of postoperative UTI. However, recent evidence does not support a role for prophylactic antibiotics. In a randomized, double-blind, placebo-controlled trial involving patients with catheters following pelvic reconstructive surgery, nitrofurantoin administered prophylactically during the time of catheterization was not effective in reducing the incidence of UTI within 3 weeks of surgery compared with placebo [33].

Other studies and meta-analyses have evaluated the role for prophylactic antibiotics at the time of catheter removal. This timing of antibiotic administration is based on the premise that residual bacteriuria following catheter removal may develop into a symptomatic UTI. Results of randomized controlled trials have provided conflicting evidence; however, a meta-analysis published in 2013 addressing this issue suggested at least some modest benefit to using prophylactic antibiotics [34]. In reviewing seven controlled trials with symptomatic UTI as an end point, the authors found an absolute risk reduction of 5.8% in those treated prophylactically with antibiotics compared with control subjects (4.7% vs 10.5%), yielding a number needed to treat of approximately 17. This marginal benefit must be weighed against the potential harms of liberal use of antibiotics, such as drug reactions, development of antibiotic resistance, *C difficile* infection, and cost. Furthermore, any consensus or formal recommendations are difficult to make based on variations in these trials in antibiotic choice and duration of treatment. If this strategy is to be reasonably used to reduce postoperative UTI, it will be important to target patients at particularly high risk for UTI following catheter removal.

Screening for asymptomatic bacteriuria

Ambiguous results and overtesting in the absence of clinical signs and symptoms of UTI may lead to overtreatment and inappropriate use of antibiotics. A retrospective study of inpatients at the University of Michigan revealed that 58% of patients in whom a urine culture was obtained failed to meet guideline-based criteria for the test [35]. Furthermore, a retrospective analysis of patients undergoing cardiothoracic, vascular, and orthopedic procedures at a Veterans Affairs Medical Center paradoxically found that patients treated with antibiotics preoperatively for asymptomatic bacteriuria actually had a higher postoperative UTI and wound infection rate compared with those with asymptomatic bacteriuria not receiving antibiotics [36].

Guidelines recommend against routine surveillance for asymptomatic bacteriuria in most patient populations (the most notable relevant exceptions being patients scheduled for transurethral resection of the prostate and other urologic procedures in which mucosal bleeding is anticipated) [37]. Failure to adhere to these guidelines results in increased costs and unnecessary antibiotic use with likely no added clinical benefit [38]. As long as the clinical significance of asymptomatic bacteriuria remains somewhat unclear, routine preoperative screening should be avoided.

SUMMARY

Although certainly commendable progress in specific institutions has been made as a result of targeted efforts to reduce postoperative UTI, this problem continues to be a significant source of morbidity in surgical patients. As the delivery of health care becomes more complex, it is apparent that multidisciplinary and multifaceted approaches are necessary to achieve meaningful reductions in postoperative UTI rates. As the population ages and surgical patients carry greater preoperative comorbidity, hospital-acquired UTI rates are unlikely to ever achieve the ideal "never event" status proposed by CMS. Nonetheless, it is a problem that results in significant cost, morbidity, and even mortality, and therefore must continue to be the target of quality improvement endeavors. It is inevitable that urinary catheters will continue to be a necessary part of caring for many surgical patients; however, proper catheter management is the single biggest modifiable factor related to postoperative UTI. As leaders of their care teams, surgeons should advocate for appropriate catheter use and remain constantly vigilant of removing catheters in a timely fashion.

Although it is clear that simple interventions, such as early catheter removal, are effective, it is also evident that this seemingly simple modification of practice requires a significant change in culture among hospital staff and physicians. For example, several studies have suggested that in the years following implementation of the CMS nonpayment policy for hospital-acquired CAUTI, there was no decline in rates of this type of infection [39,40]. Similarly, at one institution, increased compliance with the Surgical Care Improvement Project-9 guideline, which requires urinary catheter removal within 48 hours of surgery, an intervention that should clearly reduce UTI risk, was not associated with an associated reduction in UTI rate [41]. Both of these examples highlight the important idea that policy change itself is not adequate to improve postoperative outcomes.

The question of how to obtain lasting change in a large organization is relevant but difficult to answer. In our own institution, we found that through the implementation of a multifaceted protocol, we were able to reduce the number of catheter days but not significantly impact our CAUTI rate [42]. It was not until institutional leadership members implemented a daily walk rounds during which time they met with leaders on individual patient units that we began to see a decrease in CAUTI rates. As this example demonstrates, creation of a culture of safety, and not just the handing down of policy changes or protocols, is a critical element of quality improvement efforts [43]. Patient safety culture broadly refers to the collective values, behaviors, habits, attitudes, policies, and practices surrounding patient safety that characterize a care team, unit, or organization. A shift in this culture is possible with active engagement and a highly visible commitment to patient safety by hospital leadership, team training, and unit-based programs, and such a shift leads to improved outcomes [44–46].

Surgeons must continue to actively engage in the development of institutional protocols and standardization of practices. Surgeon participation in this process will allow for important input that ultimately yields feasible strategies and greater buy-in from key personnel. Hospitals and surgical units can benefit from the development of local protocols and systems to minimize inappropriate catheter usage and ensure proper catheter care and sterile insertion techniques. Finally, ongoing surveillance and measurement of process and outcome measures is an important step in achieving high-quality care for patients. Standardization of practices and ongoing surveillance using evidence-based guidelines, such as those reviewed in this article, should reduce the incidence of postoperative UTI.

In closing, it is worth noting the ample resources publicly available to care providers and hospitals as they tackle this problem. The CDC publishes evidence-based guidelines and guidance for implementing protocols on a hospital-level [20]. The Society for Healthcare Epidemiology of America, in conjunction with the Infectious Disease Society of America, the American Hospital Association, the Association for Professionals in Infection Control and Epidemiology, The Joint Commission, and others, have also developed comprehensive practice recommendations for the prevention of CAUTI, which were most recently updated in 2014 [18].

References

[1] Klevens RM, Edwards JR, Richards CL Jr, et al. Estimating health care-associated infections and deaths in U.S. hospitals, 2002. Public Health Rep 2007;122(2):160–6.

[2] Magill SS, Edwards JR, Bamberg W, et al. Multistate point-prevalence survey of health care-associated infections. N Engl J Med 2014;370(13):1198–208.

[3] Centers for Disease Control and Prevention. 2013 national and state healthcare-associated infections progress report. Available at: www.cdc.gov/hai/progress-report/index.html. Accessed January 14, 2015.

[4] Ricciardi R, Baxter NN, Read TE, et al. Surgeon involvement in the care of patients deemed to have "preventable" conditions. J Am Coll Surg 2009;209(6):707–11.

[5] Morse BC, Boland BN, Blackhurst DW, et al. Analysis of Centers for Medicaid and Medicare Services 'never events' in elderly patients undergoing bowel operations. Am Surg 2010;76(8):841–5.

[6] Regenbogen SE, Read TE, Roberts PL, et al. Urinary tract infection after colon and rectal resections: more common than predicted by risk-adjustment models. J Am Coll Surg 2011;213(6):784–92.

[7] Saint S. Clinical and economic consequences of nosocomial catheter-related bacteriuria. Am J Infect Control 2000;28(1):68–75.

[8] Platt R, Polk BF, Murdock B, et al. Mortality associated with nosocomial urinary-tract infection. N Engl J Med 1982;307(11):637–42.

[9] Sheka AC, Tevis S, Kennedy GD. Urinary tract infection after surgery for colorectal malignancy: risk factors and complications. Am J Surg 2016;211(1):31–9.

[10] Tambyah PA, Knasinski V, Maki DG. The direct costs of nosocomial catheter-associated urinary tract infection in the era of managed care. Infect Control Hosp Epidemiol 2002;23(1): 27–31.

[11] Kang CY, Chaudhry OO, Halabi WJ, et al. Risk factors for postoperative urinary tract infection and urinary retention in patients undergoing surgery for colorectal cancer. Am Surg 2012;78(10):1100–4.

[12] Wald HL, Kramer AM. Nonpayment for harms resulting from medical care: catheter-associated urinary tract infections. JAMA 2007;298(23):2782–4.

[13] The Joint Commission National Patient Safety Goals Effective January 1. 2015. Available at: http://www.jointcommission.org/assets/1/6/2015_NPSG_HAP.pdf. Accessed October 21, 2015.

[14] Rogers MA, Langa KM, Kim C, et al. Contribution of infection to increased mortality in women after cardiac surgery. Arch Intern Med 2006;166(4):437–43.

[15] Weber DJ, Sickbert-Bennett EE, Gould CV, et al. Incidence of catheter-associated and non-catheter-associated urinary tract infections in a healthcare system. Infect Control Hosp Epidemiol 2011;32(8):822–3.

[16] Saint S, Chenoweth CE. Biofilms and catheter-associated urinary tract infections. Infect Dis Clin North Am 2003;17(2):411–32.

[17] Chenoweth CE, Saint S. Urinary tract infections. Infect Dis Clin North Am 2011;25(1): 103–15.

[18] Lo E, Nicolle LE, Coffin SE, et al. Strategies to prevent catheter-associated urinary tract infections in acute care hospitals: 2014 update. Infect Control Hosp Epidemiol 2014;35(5): 464–79.

[19] Maki DG, Tambyah PA. Engineering out the risk for infection with urinary catheters. Emerg Infect Dis 2001;7(2):342–7.

[20] Gould CV, Umscheid CA, Agarwal RK, et al. Guideline for prevention of catheter-associated urinary tract infections 2009. Infect Control Hosp Epidemiol 2010;31(4):319–26.

[21] Nagle D, Curran T, Anez-Bustillo L, et al. Reducing urinary tract infections in colon and rectal surgery. Dis Colon Rectum 2014;57(1):91–7.

[22] Lam TB, Omar MI, Fisher E, et al. Types of indwelling urethral catheters for short-term catheterisation in hospitalised adults. Cochrane Database Syst Rev 2014;(9):CD004013.

[23] Wald HL, Ma A, Bratzler DW, et al. Indwelling urinary catheter use in the postoperative period: analysis of the national surgical infection prevention project data. Arch Surg 2008;143(6):551–7.

[24] Meddings J, Rogers MA, Krein SL, et al. Reducing unnecessary urinary catheter use and other strategies to prevent catheter-associated urinary tract infection: an integrative review. BMJ Qual Saf 2014;23(4):277–89.

[25] Changchien CR, Yeh CY, Huang ST, et al. Postoperative urinary retention after primary colorectal cancer resection via laparotomy: a prospective study of 2,355 consecutive patients. Dis Colon Rectum 2007;50(10):1688–96.

[26] Lee SY, Kang SB, Kim DW, et al. Risk factors and preventive measures for acute urinary retention after rectal cancer surgery. World J Surg 2015;39(1):275–82.

[27] Yoo BE, Kye BH, Kim HJ, et al. Early removal of the urinary catheter after total or tumor-specific mesorectal excision for rectal cancer is safe. Dis Colon Rectum 2015;58(7): 686–91.

[28] Benoist S, Panis Y, Denet C, et al. Optimal duration of urinary drainage after rectal resection: a randomized controlled trial. Surgery 1999;125(2):135–41.

[29] Hu Y, Craig SJ, Rowlingson JC, et al. Early removal of urinary catheter after surgery requiring thoracic epidural: a prospective trial. J Cardiothorac Vasc Anesth 2014;28(5): 1302–6.

[30] Zaouter C, Kaneva P, Carli F. Less urinary tract infection by earlier removal of bladder catheter in surgical patients receiving thoracic epidural analgesia. Reg Anesth Pain Med 2009;34(6):542–8.
[31] Madani AH, Aval HB, Mokhtari G, et al. Effectiveness of tamsulosin in prevention of postoperative urinary retention: a randomized double-blind placebo-controlled study. Int Braz J Urol 2014;40(1):30–6.
[32] University of Wisconsin, Madison. Prevention of post operative urinary retention (POUR). In: ClinicalTrials.gov. Bethesda (MD): National Library of Medicine (US); 2000 NLM Identifier: NCT02486653. Available at: https://www.clinicaltrials.gov/ct2/show/study/NCT02486653. Accessed November 1, 2015.
[33] Dieter AA, Amundsen CL, Edenfield AL, et al. Oral antibiotics to prevent postoperative urinary tract infection: a randomized controlled trial. Obstet Gynecol 2014;123(1):96–103.
[34] Marschall J, Carpenter CR, Fowler S, et al. Antibiotic prophylaxis for urinary tract infections after removal of urinary catheter: meta-analysis. BMJ 2013;346:f3147.
[35] Hartley S, Valley S, Kuhn L, et al. Inappropriate testing for urinary tract infection in hospitalized patients: an opportunity for improvement. Infect Control Hosp Epidemiol 2013;34(11):1204–7.
[36] Drekonja DM, Zarmbinski B, Johnson JR. Preoperative urine cultures at a veterans affairs medical center. JAMA Intern Med 2013;173(1):71–2.
[37] Nicolle LE, Bradley S, Colgan R, et al. Infectious Diseases Society of America guidelines for the diagnosis and treatment of asymptomatic bacteriuria in adults. Clin Infect Dis 2005;40(5):643–54.
[38] Cope M, Cevallos ME, Cadle RM, et al. Inappropriate treatment of catheter-associated asymptomatic bacteriuria in a tertiary care hospital. Clin Infect Dis 2009;48(9):1182–8.
[39] Schuller K, Probst J, Hardin J, et al. Initial impact of Medicare's nonpayment policy on catheter-associated urinary tract infections by hospital characteristics. Health Policy 2014;115(2–3):165–71.
[40] Peasah SK, McKay NL, Harman JS, et al. Medicare non-payment of hospital-acquired infections: infection rates three years post implementation. Medicare Medicaid Res Rev 2013;3(3):E1–13.
[41] Owen RM, Perez SD, Bornstein WA, et al. Impact of surgical care improvement project inf-9 on postoperative urinary tract infections: do exemptions interfere with quality patient care? Arch Surg 2012;147(10):946–53.
[42] Purvis S, Gion T, Kennedy G, et al. Catheter-associated urinary tract infection: a successful prevention effort employing a multipronged initiative at an academic medical center. J Nurs Care Qual 2014;29(2):141–8.
[43] Weaver SJ, Lubomksi LH, Wilson RF, et al. Promoting a culture of safety as a patient safety strategy: a systematic review. Ann Intern Med 2013;158(5 Pt 2):369–74.
[44] Pronovost P, Needham D, Berenholtz S, et al. An intervention to decrease catheter-related bloodstream infections in the ICU. N Engl J Med 2006;355(26):2725–32.
[45] Weaver SJ, Weeks K, Pham JC, et al. On the CUSP: Stop BSI: evaluating the relationship between central line-associated bloodstream infection rate and patient safety climate profile. Am J Infect Control 2014;42(10 Suppl):S203–8.
[46] Haynes AB, Weiser TG, Berry WR, et al. Changes in safety attitude and relationship to decreased postoperative morbidity and mortality following implementation of a checklist-based surgical safety intervention. BMJ Qual Saf 2011;20(1):102–7.

Advances in Surgery 50 (2016) 93–103

ADVANCES IN SURGERY

The Aging Surgeon

Mark R. Katlic, MD, MMM[a,*],
JoAnn Coleman, DNP, ACNP-BC[b]

[a]Department of Surgery, Sinai Center for Geriatric Surgery, Sinai Hospital, Northwest Hospital, 2401 West Belvedere Avenue, Baltimore, MD 21215, USA; [b]Department of Surgery, Sinai Center for Geriatric Surgery, Sinai Hospital, 2401 West Belvedere Avenue, Baltimore, MD 21215, USA

Keywords

• Aging surgeon • Aging physician • Physician competency • Physician retirement • Patient safety • Neuropsychology • Late career practitioner

Key points

- Human faculties diminish with age.
- The variability in cognitive function among individuals increases with advancing age; consequently, functional age differs from chronologic age.
- There should be no mandatory retirement age for surgeons; however, there is a need to evaluate functional age.
- All present methods of evaluating aging surgeons are inadequate.
- A structured aging surgeon program must be comprehensive, multidisciplinary, objective, and confidential to balance patient safety and liability risk with the dignity of a committed surgeon and his or her value to society.

INTRODUCTION

> There is no sadder picture than the Professor who has outgrown his usefulness, and, the only one unconscious of the fact, insists with a praiseworthy zeal, upon the performance of duties for which the circumstances of the time have rendered him unfit.
>
> —William Osler, 1892 [1].

Osler's prescient address to students at the University of Minnesota would resonate with most chiefs of surgery and hospital presidents. He went on to say, "Insensibly, in the fifth and sixth decades, there begins to creep over most of us a change, noted physically among other ways in the silvering of

*Corresponding author. *E-mail address*: mkatlic@lifebridgehealth.org

0065-3411/16/$ – see front matter
http://dx.doi.org/10.1016/j.yasu.2016.03.008

the hair and that lessening of elasticity, which impels a man to open rather than to vault a five-barred gate…and with most of us this physical change has its mental equivalent" [1]. A future surgical giant, Ferdinand Sauerbruch, was a teenager at the time of Osler's address. He would later represent incarnate the sad professor to whom Osler referred.

CASE REPORT

Ferdinand Sauerbruch (1875–1951) was one of the world's greatest surgeons. A brilliant diagnostician and exquisite technician, he attracted to his clinic and operating theaters at the Charité Hospital in Berlin a stream of students and patients from across Europe, Russia, and the United Kingdom. Always innovative, he developed a functioning prosthetic arm and later the differential pressure chambers that facilitated thoracic surgery before the widespread use of endotracheal intubation.

In his late 1960s, however, Sauerbruch began to change. Colleagues noted that he "had sudden changes in mood and periods of forgetfulness." He "struck assistants with instruments during operations," operations that were "performed with growing clumsiness, dragging tissues and tearing blood vessels." The faculty and administration of the Charité, cognizant of his international fame and its financial implications, failed to act; individual efforts by his friends suggesting retirement were met with flat refusal. A prominent actor died from bleeding during a simple herniorrhaphy; a child succumbed when Sauerbruch failed to restore gastrointestinal continuity after a stomach resection. He finally relented in 1949, at age 74, when threatened with a humiliating public dismissal [2,3]. Even then, Sauerbruch had little insight. He continued to operate at his home, with disastrous results. His 1953 autobiography is titled *Master Surgeon* [4].

IS THE AGING SURGEON STILL A PROBLEM?

Sixty years after Sauerbruch's dismissal, there is overwhelming anecdotal evidence and some published evidence that the aging surgeon remains a problem.

Hartz and colleagues [5] found that mortality rates of surgeons performing coronary artery bypass grafts increased with increasing years of practice. Older surgeons performing carotid endarterectomy had higher mortality rates than younger surgeons in O'Neill and associates' [6] study. Laparoscopic inguinal herniorrhaphy led to higher hernia recurrence rates when performed by older surgeons compared with younger surgeons [7]. Waljee and coworkers [8] examined the files of 461,000 Medicare patients and reported that older surgeons had higher operative mortality rates for pancreatectomy, coronary artery bypass grafts, and carotid endarterectomy relative to younger surgeons, but the difference was small and limited to surgeons with low procedure volumes. She concluded that "surgeon age is a relatively weak predictor of operative mortality in aggregate and certainly much worse for discriminating performance among individual surgeons."

Those few individual surgeons, however, are the problem, a problem encountered by nearly every chief of surgery, vice-president of medical affairs, and hospital president sometime during his or her tenure [9]. One of us (MRK) sought anecdotes from members of the Society of Surgical Chairs and was told "he fell asleep taking down the internal mammary artery," "had to organize an 'intervention' led by other senior/retired surgeons," and "operating room nurses were in tears in my office, saying 'you must stop him.'" One e-mail communication (Anonymous, personal communication, 2013) touched many common themes:

> I personally had to ask the former chair of surgery 15 years my senior (age 72) to 'step down with dignity today or face a credentialing committee for a wrong side surgery tomorrow.' I had heard that he needed a 'seeing eye resident' and there were multiple grumblings that he and I had discussed—nothing documented or formal. That day I had senior faculty sit by my side during the 'talk.' I would like to end by saying it went well, but it was awful. He was hurt, resentful, angry. He stormed out, packed up his stuff, said (expletive) you. He even refused a retirement party. I clearly mismanaged the situation from the faculty member's perspective. I was clearly late to the game from the institutional risk perspective but I never had any hard evidence. Perhaps I should have been more proactive when I heard rumors of his needs for residents.

This vignette touches on the lack of self-awareness that is common in, although not exclusive to, this small group of problematic senior surgeons. Bieliauskas and colleagues [10], in a study of 359 surgeons over a 6-year period, reported that although self-perceived cognitive changes play a role in the decision to retire, they are not related to objective measures of cognitive change and are not reliable in the decision to retire. A subsequent survey of 995 surgeons by Greenfield's group [11] found that most senior surgeons reported no changes in perceived cognitive abilities with age. A review of this subject in 2006 concluded "the preponderance of evidence suggests that physicians have a limited ability to accurately self-assess" [12].

How large a potential issue is this? Greenfield and Proctor [13] surveyed 659 members of the American Surgical Association and found that 18% of those over age 70 continued to operate, the majority of those maintaining their customary operative workload; 12% had no retirement plan whatsoever. The American College of Surgeons lists 5763 senior fellows over age 70 years, a category defined as 'actively practicing but no longer required to pay dues' (Van Tornhout R, personal communication, 2013). Given that only 25% to 30% of surgeons are fellows at all, the total number of septuagenarian surgeons practicing may approach 20,000.

ARE SURGEONS HUMAN?

As everyone else, surgeons face the inexorable deterioration in cognitive and physical faculties that accompanies increasing age. Neuropsychological studies have shown that–whether owing to innate aptitude from birth, better health, on-going stimulation, self-selection, or other factors–certain groups of people, to which surgeons belong, start out higher or decline slower: higher income, higher socioeconomic class, working versus retired. Nevertheless, all decline with age.

Even elite athletes manifest decreasing maximal oxygen consumption (VO_2 max), forced expiratory volume in 1 second (FEV_1), and glomerular filtration rate, often decreasing at different rates in different individuals. Decrements in sensory function such as vision and hearing are expected by all [14]. Similarly, we all experience varying declines in visual-spatial ability, inductive reasoning, verbal memory, and other areas of cognition [15] (Fig. 1). Mani and associates [16] studied age-related decrements in performance on a continuous performance test, a well-known measure of attention, under "clear" and "noisy" trial conditions; older age was associated with increased numbers of commission and false alarm errors, supporting the concept of age-related inhibition problems, particularly under degraded or noisy conditions.

An elderly physician's vast fund of knowledge and experience is not sufficient to mitigate the inevitable change in cognition. In a review of the negative

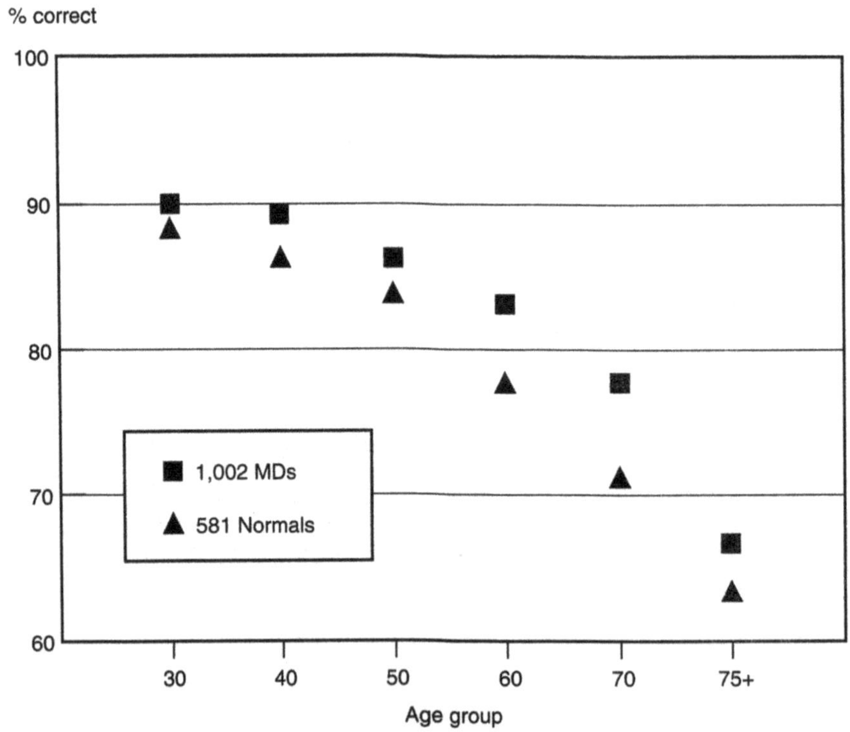

Fig. 1. Human faculties deteriorate with age: age-related differences in MicroCog total score. (*From* Powell DH. Profiles in cognitive aging. Cambridge: Harvard University Press; 1994. Copyright © 1994 by the President and Fellows of Harvard College.)

relationship between physician age and performance, Eva [17] pointed out that crystallized intelligence (eg, accumulated knowledge) was better preserved than fluid intelligence (eg, negotiating a maze or overcoming first impressions by recognizing that alternatives are possible) and that habitual memory was better preserved than controlled analytical memory. The surgeon needs both. Gallagher and colleagues [18] noted that "surgery differs from other specialties in medicine in that the operator must be prepared to make decisions about procedural performance in real time and with incomplete information…must have the technical capability to perform the surgery but they must also have the cognitive resources to decide how to deal with unanticipated events (such as emergencies or recovery from error)."

Greenfield's group [10] studied surgeons specifically, testing visual sustained attention, which addresses stress tolerance; reaction time, which addresses psychomotor abilities; and visual learning and memory, which also address visual-spatial organization. Although surgeons performed better than the general population in psychomotor areas, there was nevertheless "considerable decline with age" in virtually every test.

IS A MANDATORY RETIREMENT AGE THE ANSWER?

Establishing a mandatory retirement age for surgeons would be a straightforward solution, but would be inappropriate and unfair owing to the vast variability in function among older individuals of a given age.

The Age Discrimination in Employment Act of 1967 outlawed forced retirement based on age; this is enforced by the Equal Employment Opportunity Commission, an agency of the Department of Justice. Congress has approved fixed retirement ages for a number of professions that impact public safety: commercial airline pilot (65 years), Federal Bureau of Investigation agent (57 years), National Park Ranger (57 years), air traffic controller (56 years), and lighthouse operator (55 years). Mandatory retirement for surgeons does exist in many countries, for example, England (National Health Service 65 years, private practice 70 years), but–like the Pope and Supreme Court Justices–surgeons in the United States have a lifetime appointment.

Nor should there be a mandatory retirement age for surgeons. There is impressive variability in the rate of cognitive and physical decline, variability that increases with age (Fig. 2). Eva's review [17] of changes in cognitive processing among aging physicians concluded that "one of the more robust findings in ageing research is that the variability across the scores individuals receive tends to increase with age," with many older individuals performing at levels equal to or even above those of their younger counterparts. The majority (61%) of practicing senior surgeons performed within the range of younger surgeons on all 3 tests administered by Drag and coworkers [19]; only 7 of 108 performed significantly below the younger surgeons on more than 1 task. They concluded that, "age alone is not a sufficient predictor of cognitive performance." A number of chairs of surgery lauded surgeons who "are still excellent at age 73" and "continued to operate until 80 and were superb."

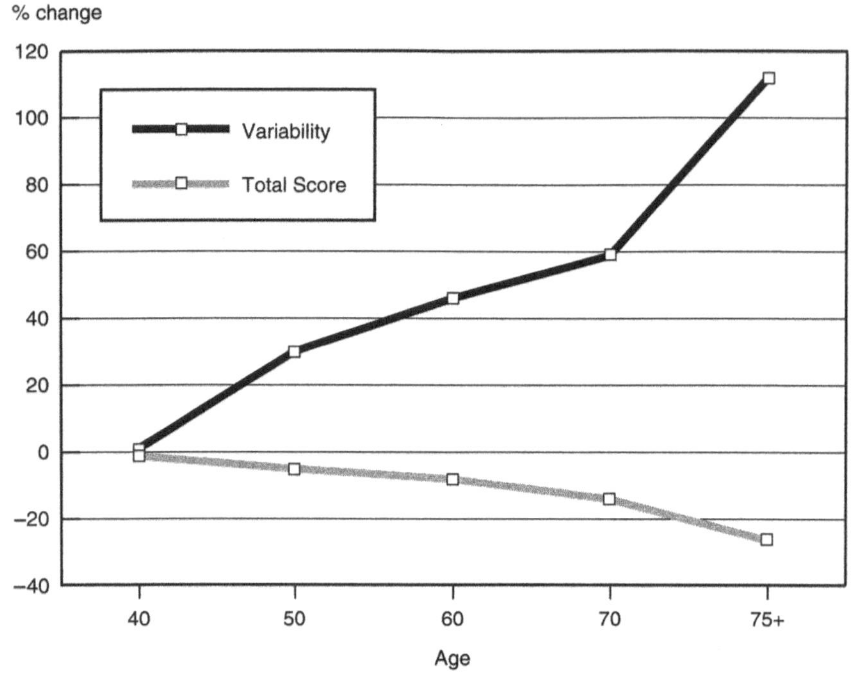

Fig. 2. Variability among individuals increases with age: percentage of change from the age 35 to 44 group in total cognitive score and variability among 1002 physicians. (*From* Powell DH. Profiles in cognitive aging. Cambridge: Harvard University Press; 1994. Copyright © 1994 by the President and Fellows of Harvard College.)

Other arguments against a mandatory retirement age include the fact that treatable causes of poor performance may be found (eg, medication side effect, severe depression, neurologic disease, sleep apnea, vision problems) and the tendency in society as a whole toward ageism, prejudice based purely on chronologic age.

BUT DOES THE SURGICAL PROFESSION POLICE ITSELF?

The public believes that we police ourselves but this is illusory. Initial certification to be a surgeon is difficult but recertification is relatively easy [9]. Ongoing Professional Practice Evaluations, mandatory in all hospitals every 6 months, are hospital specific and highly variable. Our malpractice system is neither constructed nor capable of hobbling bad doctors (cf. *USA Today* investigative report) [20]. We are left with the scrutiny of our peers and, with respect to the aging surgeon, many barriers to this exist.

In a 2005 study, Farber and associates [21] found that physicians would be more likely to report a colleague impaired because of substance abuse compared with one impaired by cognitive decline or psychological impairment. In a later study [22], 17% of physicians reported that in the previous 3 years they had encountered an impaired colleague but one-third of them had taken no action.

Senior surgeons are the most respected members of their community. They have been the teachers and mentors of their younger colleagues, some of whom may now be their chief. These younger colleagues may even become 'enablers' [23,24], assigning senior residents to assist, the best scrub nurse, and the most experienced anesthetist. The senior surgeons have brought fame to their hospital and have been the "rain-makers" for surgical volumes. Few medical staff bylaws contain any provision for dealing with an aging staff physician. Some changes in performance may be hard to document, falling into a gray zone of worrisome but within standard practice. It often takes a patient death or a sentinel event to force action (cf. Sauerbruch and chair of surgery vignettes elsewhere in this article).

We must do better, or others will impose arbitrary rules such as mandatory retirement. We are a profession (from the Latin, "to speak forth") and it is ethically imperative [25]. The American Medical Association Code of Ethics states that "Physicians' responsibilities to colleagues who are impaired by a condition that interferes with their ability to engage safely in professional activities include timely intervention to ensure these colleagues cease practicing and receive appropriate assistance from a physician health program" [26]. Basic ethical principles underlie this, including the nonmaleficence-based duty to colleagues and patients to identify and assist impaired physicians in their recovery [27].

The Joint Commission in Standard MS.06.01.05 [28] requires that medical staff determine a practitioner's "evidence of physical ability to perform the requested privilege" and "documentation regarding an applicant's health status and his or her ability to practice should be confirmed." Adding to the problem, one-third of doctors have no personal physician and the cognitive impairment itself may lead to diminished self-awareness, a phenomenon termed *anosognosia* [29,30].

Ironically, in many states it is more difficult to maintain one's driving privileges than one's surgical privileges [31]. Two states, Illinois and New Hampshire, require a road test at age 75. Ten states require a vision test at a specific age, although the age threshold for this varies from 40 to 80 years. In 5 states, older drivers must renew in person rather than by mail and in 15 states they must renew at more frequent intervals than other drivers. What can we do that balances patient safety and liability risk with the dignity of a committed surgeon and his or her value to society (Fig. 3)?

THE AGING SURGEON PROGRAM

The Aging Surgeon Program is a 2-day comprehensive, multidisciplinary, objective, and confidential evaluation of a surgeon's physical and cognitive function. It is 1 option for striking that balance illustrated. Ironically, this was advocated by the American College of Surgeons 20 years ago. In a 1992 monograph published by the newly formed Committee on the Impaired Physician of the Board of Governors (now the Workforce on Physician Competency

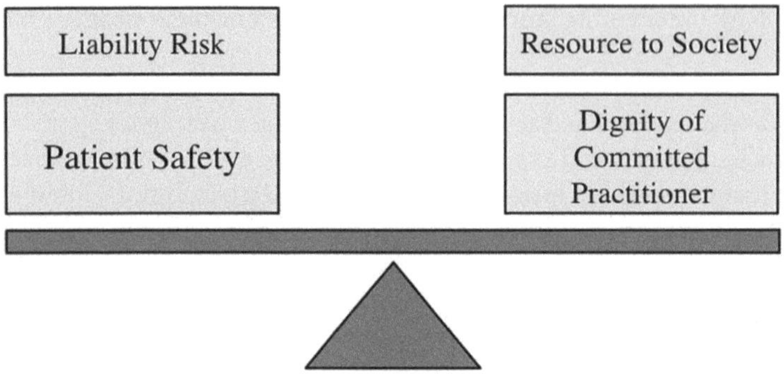

Fig. 3. The aging surgeon: balancing the issues.

and Health), the authors wrote, "Specific mechanisms must be developed to address issues of age-related decline in skills" and "The review procedure must include an assessment of physical, psychological, and intellectual functions" [32]. Greenfield wrote 2 years later, "Both cognitive and functional test results should be evaluated under controlled circumstances so that objective as opposed to subjective criteria for performance can be established" [33]; he reiterated this in 2008 [10]. Trunkey and Botney [34] in 2001 suggested rigorous evaluation. More recently, Leape and Fromson [35] advocate replacing the current ad hoc approach to physician performance with a routine, formal, proactive system that would use validated measures and be objective, fair, and responsive.

Developed over 12 months of literature review, expert consensus, rigorous debate, and reiteration, The Aging Surgeon Program at Sinai Hospital of Baltimore opened on January 1, 2014. The goals of the program (Box 1) are to protect surgeons from arbitrary or unreliable methods of assessing competence or cognitive capacity; identify potentially treatable or reversible disorders that, if treated, could restore or improve functional capacity [36]; aid surgeon in

Box 1: The aging surgeon program goals

- Protect surgeons from arbitrary or unreliable methods of assessing competence or cognitive capacity.
- Identify potentially treatable or reversible disorders that, if treated, could restore or improve functional capacity.
- Aid surgeon in decision of when to retire.
- Protect patients from unsafe surgeons.
- Protect surgeons and hospitals from liability risk.
- Rely on existing structures for using results to make licensing and credentialing decisions.
- Provide objective, comprehensive, and unbiased evaluation.

decision when to retire; protect patients from unsafe surgeons; protect surgeons and hospitals from liability risk; rely on existing structures for using results to make credentialing and privileging decisions; and provide objective, comprehensive, unbiased evaluation.

Our multidisciplinary team includes surgery, geriatric surgery, neurology, neuropsychology, physical medicine and rehabilitation, ophthalmology, internal medicine, legal services, and ethics. The program includes a previsit screen of medical history and appropriate recent radiographs (eg, MRI), then travel to Baltimore. Day 1 begins with general physical and neurologic examinations, physical therapy/occupational therapy evaluation (reaction time, distance judgment, coordination, dynamic visual-spatial acuity, fine-motor function, and more; Fig. 4), then lunch. The afternoon comprises neuropsychology testing (attention, memory, executive functioning, emotional status, and more), then dinner and sleep. Day 2 encompasses a morning of neuropsychology, lunch, physical therapy/occupational therapy, ophthalmology, and an exit interview.

The resultant report is sent as an encrypted locked electronic file to the individual who contracted and paid for the program, likely a chief of surgery, hospital president, or the surgeon himself or herself. The report includes only objective findings; decisions about privileges, retirement, or even lifestyle changes must be made by those who receive the report.

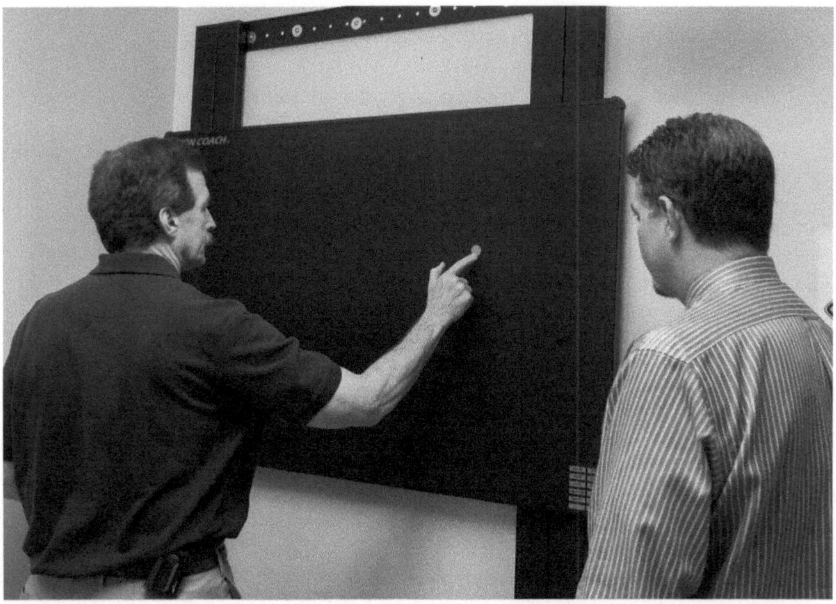

Fig. 4. Author being evaluated for visual-spatial acuity, hand–eye coordination, reaction time, inhibitory control, peripheral and divided attention visual processing, visual–cognitive processing, visual scanning and tracking, visual field deficit, binocularity (eye teaming), and upper body range of motion.

Triggers for the program may include every surgeon age 70 years or older at each hospital recredentialing cycle (typically every 2–3 years), failure of Ongoing Professional Practice Evaluation, failure of focused professional practice evaluation, a sentinel event, worrisome malpractice history, discretion of the chief of surgery, or discretion of the hospital president. Possible hospital actions may include full privileges, no privileges, no operating privileges, assisted by another surgeon (routine; only complex cases), assistant privileges only, focused review of cases (all; certain number), or decreased work hours (eg, no on-call duties).

SUMMARY

Human faculties–even those of surgeons–deteriorate with age; however, there is great variability. Decisions about competency, therefore, should be based on functional age rather than chronologic age. This argues against a mandatory retirement age and argues for an objective evaluation of functional age. Such an assessment would balance the dignity of a committed practitioner and his or her value to society with patient safety and liability risk. One way to do this is presented, namely The Aging Surgeon Program, a comprehensive, multidisciplinary, objective, and confidential evaluation. Both the surgeon and society deserve no less.

References

[1] Osler W. Teacher and student. Aequanamitas. Philadelphia: P. Blackiston's Son & Co., Inc; 1932. p. 23–41.
[2] Thorwald J. The dismissal: the last days of Ferdinand Sauerbruch. 1st American edition. New York: Pantheon Books; 1962.
[3] Cherian SM, Nicks R, Lord RS. Ernst Ferdinand Sauerbruch: rise and fall of the pioneer of thoracic surgery. World J Surg 2001;25(8):1012–20.
[4] Sauerbruch F. Master surgeon. New York: Thomas Y. Crowell Company; 1953.
[5] Hartz AJ, Kuhn EM, Pulido J. Prestige of training programs and experience of bypass surgeons as factors in adjusted patient mortality rates. Med Care 1999;37(1):93–103.
[6] O'Neill L, Lanska DJ, Hartz A. Surgeon characteristics associated with mortality and morbidity following carotid endarterectomy. Neurology 2000;55(6):773–81.
[7] Neumayer LA, Gawande AA, Wang J, et al. Proficiency of surgeons in inguinal hernia repair: effect of experience and age. Ann Surg 2005;242(3):344–8 [discussion: 348–52].
[8] Waljee JF, Greenfield LJ, Dimick JB, et al. Surgeon age and operative mortality in the United States. Ann Surg 2006;244(3):353–62.
[9] Blasier RB. The problem of the aging surgeon: when surgeon age becomes a surgical risk factor. Clin Orthop Relat Res 2009;467(2):402–11.
[10] Bieliauskas LA, Langenecker S, Graver C, et al. Cognitive changes and retirement among senior surgeons (CCRASS): results from the CCRASS Study. J Am Coll Surg 2008;207(1):69–78 [discussion: 9].
[11] Lee HJ, Drag LL, Bieliauskas LA, et al. Results from the cognitive changes and retirement among senior surgeons self-report survey. J Am Coll Surg 2009;209(5):668–71.e2.
[12] Davis DA, Mazmanian PE, Fordis M, et al. Accuracy of physician self-assessment compared with observed measures of competence: a systematic review. JAMA 2006;296(9):1094–102.
[13] Greenfield LJ, Proctor MC. Attitudes toward retirement. A survey of the American Surgical Association. Ann Surg 1994;220(3):382–9 [discussion: 387–90].

[14] Jackson GR, Owsley C. Visual dysfunction, neurodegenerative diseases, and aging. Neurol Clin 2003;21(3):709–28.
[15] Powell DH. Profiles in cognitive aging. London: Harvard University Press; 1994. p. 87.
[16] Mani TM, Bedwell JS, Miller LS. Age-related decrements in performance on a brief continuous performance test. Arch Clin Neuropsychol 2005;20(5):575–86.
[17] Eva KW. The aging physician: changes in cognitive processing and their impact on medical practice. Acad Med 2002;77(Suppl 10):S1–6.
[18] Gallagher AG, Satava RM, O'Sullivan GC. Attentional capacity: an essential aspect of surgeon performance. Ann Surg 2015;261(3):e60–1.
[19] Drag LL, Bieliauskas LA, Langenecker SA, et al. Cognitive functioning, retirement status, and age: results from the Cognitive Changes and Retirement among Senior Surgeons study. J Am Coll Surg 2010;211(3):303–7.
[20] Eisler P, Hansen B. Bad docs often keep practicing medicine. USA Today 2013.
[21] Farber NJ, Gilibert SG, Aboff BM, et al. Physicians' willingness to report impaired colleagues. Soc Sci Med 2005;61(8):1772–5.
[22] DesRoches CM, Rao SR, Fromson JA, et al. Physicians' perceptions, preparedness for reporting, and experiences related to impaired and incompetent colleagues. JAMA 2010;304(2): 187–93.
[23] LoboPrabhu SM, Molinari VA, Hamilton JD, et al. The aging physician with cognitive impairment: approaches to oversight, prevention, and remediation. Am J Geriatr Psychiatry 2009;17(6):445–54.
[24] Burroughs J. Dealing with the aging physician advocacy or betrayal? Physician Exec 2012;38(6):38–41.
[25] Wynia MK. The role of professionalism and self-regulation in detecting impaired or incompetent physicians. JAMA 2010;304(2):210–2.
[26] American Medical Association. American Medical Association. 2004. Available at: www.ama-assn.org/ama/pub/physician-resources/medical-ethics/code-medical-ethics/opinion 9.031. Accessed October 26, 2013.
[27] Bernat J. Ethical issues in neurology. 3rd edition. Philadelphia: Lippincott Williams & Wilkins; 2008. p. 62–3.
[28] The Joint Commission. Standard MS.06.01.05. Comprehensive accreditation manual for hospitals. Oakbrook Terrace (IL): Joint Commission; 2013. p. 27–30.
[29] Ries ML, Jabbar BM, Schmitz TW, et al. Anosognosia in mild cognitive impairment: Relationship to activation of cortical midline structures involved in self-appraisal. J Int Neuropsychol Soc 2007;13(3):450–61.
[30] Zamboni G, Drazich E, McCulloch E, et al. Neuroanatomy of impaired self-awareness in Alzheimer's disease and mild cognitive impairment. Cortex 2013;49(3):668–78.
[31] Fazzalaro JJ. Requirements in other states for elderly drivers renewing drivers' licenses. 2006. Available at: http://www.cga.ct.gov/2006/rpt/2006-R-0457. Accessed April 18, 2016.
[32] Hyde G, Miscall B. Impairment due to aging. The impaired surgeon: diagnosis, treatment, and reentry. Chicago: American College of Surgeons; 1992. p. 5.
[33] Greenfield LJ. Farewell to surgery. J Vasc Surg 1994;19(1):6–14.
[34] Trunkey DD, Botney R. Assessing competency: a tale of two professions. J Am Coll Surg 2001;192(3):385–95.
[35] Leape LL, Fromson JA. Problem doctors: is there a system-level solution? Ann Intern Med 2006;144(2):107–15.
[36] Brannon W. The impaired physician. In: Williams M, editor. Practical ethics in clinical neurology. Philadelphia: Lippincott Williams & Wilkins; 2012. p. 114.

Advances in Surgery 50 (2016) 105–114

ADVANCES IN SURGERY

Maintenance of Certification

Mark A. Malangoni, MD

American Board of Surgery, 1617 John F. Kennedy Boulevard, Suite 860, Philadelphia, PA 19103, USA

Keywords

• Maintenance of certification • Continuous professional development • Board certification • Medical education

Key points

- Maintenance of Certification represents a standard for continuous professional development.
- The American Board of Surgery is responsible for defining the educational and practice standards that allow surgeons to be eligible for certification and maintaining their certification.
- The 4 components of Maintenance of Certification are based on the 6 professional competencies developed by the American Board of Medical Specialties and Accreditation Council on Graduate Medical Education.
- Participation in Maintenance of Certification demonstrates to the public and the profession your ongoing commitment to meet the standards for contemporary practice and to improve care.

BACKGROUND

Board certification in the United States began in 1916 with establishment of the American Board of Ophthalmology. Additional boards were founded over subsequent decades to recognize physicians who had developed specialized skills based in their training or experience. Each board defined the education and practice standards that allowed physicians to be eligible for certification.

The American Board of Surgery (ABS) was founded in 1937 through a joint effort of the American Surgical Association, American Medical Association, American College of Surgeons, and prominent regional surgical societies of that time. Its initial intent was to develop a process that would result in

The author has nothing to disclose.

E-mail address: mmalangoni@absurgery.org

0065-3411/16/$ – see front matter
http://dx.doi.org/10.1016/j.yasu.2016.03.009

certification of individuals who met a defined standard of education, training, knowledge, and clinical judgment in surgery (Box 1).

The impetus for creation of the ABS was "to protect the public and improve the specialty." Assessment of knowledge and judgment through a rigorous examination process differentiated board certification from membership in professional organizations. The ABS was organized in accordance with guidelines of the Advisory Board of Medical Specialties. This organization later became the American Board of Medical Specialties (ABMS), which serves as the oversight body for its member boards and assures the public that its member boards meet common standards for initial certification and maintenance of certification (MOC).

In its mission statement, the ABS emphasizes that its primary purpose is to serve the public (Box 2).

Setting standards for board certification is a privilege of self-regulation that has been granted to the profession of medicine and its specialties by the American public. In return for this trust, the ABS and other boards must commit to serve the best interests of the public through our certification processes and requirements.

Certification by the ABS is based on education, evaluation, and assessment. Appropriate undergraduate medical education, accredited surgical residency training, a broad operative experience, and high ethical standing comprise the essential requirements for certification. As additional specialties have evolved within the ABS, each has developed a certification process using these elements as a framework. The ABS is composed of 7 surgical specialties (Box 3).

Pediatric surgery, vascular surgery, surgical critical care, and complex general surgical oncology have component boards, which are charged to establish the standards for certification and MOC in its discipline. There are several different committees that perform these functions for general surgery. In addition, there are 2 advisory councils within the ABS that represent non–board certified disciplines (transplantation, gastrointestinal surgery) as well as the General Surgery Advisory Council. Through its board of directors, component boards, and advisory councils, the ABS has representation from 39 different surgical societies as well as 3 at large members and one public member.

Box 1: Purposes of the American Board of Surgery

- To conduct examinations of acceptable candidates who seek certification or maintenance of certification by the board
- To issue certificates to all candidates meeting the board's requirements and satisfactorily completing its prescribed examinations
- To improve and broaden the opportunities for graduate education and training of surgeons

Box 2: Mission statement of the American Board of Surgery

The American Board of Surgery serves the public and the specialty of surgery by providing leadership in surgical education and practice, by promoting excellence through rigorous evaluation and examination, and by promoting the highest standards for professionalism, lifelong learning, and the continuous certification of surgeons in practice.

From the American Board of Surgery, Philadelphia, PA. Available at: http://www.absurgery.org/default.jsp?abouthome. Accessed November 13, 2015.

RECERTIFICATION ESTABLISHED

For the first 4 decades of its existence, once ABS certification was achieved, it remained valid for a surgeon's entire professional career. This situation changed in 1976 when the ABS adopted time-limited certification and required its diplomates to recertify by passing a secure written examination every 10 years. This change in requirements was made by the ABS directors in recognition of the rapid evolution of surgical practice. They thought it was necessary for diplomates to demonstrate that they were current with advances in medical knowledge and patient care as assessed by passing a written examination. Forty years later most ABS diplomates in clinical practice have time-limited certification, and these examinations are offered in a computerized format at hundreds of secure testing centers across the United States and worldwide.

In 2000, the ABS adopted a requirement for diplomates to complete 100 credits of continuing medical education (CME), 60 in category 1 and 40 in category 2, during the 2 years before applying for the recertification examination. This requirement was another acknowledgement that medical practice was evolving rapidly and surgeons needed to demonstrate that they were keeping up with new developments in practice through CME.

INTRODUCTION OF MAINTENANCE OF CERTIFICATION

The ABMS introduced its MOC program in 2005. It was based on 6 competencies jointly developed by the Accreditation Council on Graduate Medical Education (ACGME) and the ABMS and adopted by the ABMS member

Box 3: Current specialties of the American Board of Surgery

General surgery
Pediatric surgery
Vascular surgery
Hand surgery
Surgical critical care
Hospice and palliative medicine
Complex general surgical oncology

boards 5 years earlier. These competencies, patient care, medical knowledge, professionalism, interpersonal communication skills, practice-based learning and improvement, and systems-based practice, were thought to represent practice principles that would be applicable across the continuum of the educational spectrum from medical school through residency training and into practice (Box 4).

These competencies, which are the same ones used in the ACGME's Next Accreditation System, are incorporated in the ABMS Program for MOC within a 4-part framework (Box 5).

David Nahrwold, MD, a general surgeon and ABS diplomate, led the MOC effort initially. Nahrwold recognized that for board certification to remain relevant and for the medical profession to continue its privilege of self-regulation, it had to evolve beyond initial certification as the standard for medical practice. Although the ABMS has established standards for MOC that each board must satisfy, individual boards have been allowed to develop its own specific requirements. The ABMS program for MOC is a system of ongoing professional development and practice assessment and improvement. It challenges physicians to focus on the continuous development of their skill set, including

Box 4: Core competencies of the American Board of Medical Specialties and the Accreditation Council on Graduate Medical Education

- *Patient care and procedural skills:* Provide care that is compassionate, appropriate, and effective treatment of health problems and to promote health.
- *Medical knowledge:* Demonstrate knowledge about established and evolving biomedical, clinical, and cognate sciences and their application in patient care.
- *Professionalism:* Demonstrate a commitment to carrying out professional responsibilities, adherence to ethical principles, and sensitivity to diverse patient populations.
- *Interpersonal and communication skills:* Demonstrate skills that result in effective information exchange and teaming with patients, their families, and professional associates (eg, fostering a therapeutic relationship that is ethically sound, uses effective listening skills with nonverbal and verbal communication; working as both a team member and at times as a leader).
- *Practice-based learning and improvement:* Show an ability to investigate and evaluate patient care practices, appraise and assimilate scientific evidence, and improve the practice of medicine.
- *Systems-based practice:* Demonstrate awareness of and responsibility to the larger context and systems of health care. Be able to call on system resources to provide optimal care (eg, coordinating care across sites or serving as the primary case manager when care involves multiple specialties, professions, or sites).

From the American Board of Surgery, Philadelphia, PA. Available at: http://www.abms.org/board-certification/a-trusted-credential/based-on-core-competencies/. Accessed November 9, 2015.

Box 5: The 4 components of the maintenance of certification program

- Part I: professionalism and professional standing
- Part II: lifelong learning and self-assessment
- Part III: assessment of knowledge, judgment, and skills
- Part IV: improvement in medical practice

those skills that enable them to function effectively in interprofessional teams, integrated systems of care, and community settings. The development of the ABMS MOC reinforced the need for board certification to become a more continuous process as the pace of change in medicine had accelerated beyond any seen previously. Boards and their diplomates also had a responsibility to demonstrate an enduring commitment to maintain professional standards, participate in lifelong education, possess basic medical knowledge, and improve practice performance [1].

REQUIREMENTS FOR THE AMERICAN BOARD OF SURGERY MAINTENANCE OF CERTIFICATION PROGRAM

When the ABS inaugurated its MOC program in July 2005, 3 of the 4 required components were already in place; they have been modified only slightly since. Documentation of professional standing has been required since the ABS was formed. A recertification examination (renamed the MOC examination) has been a requirement for the past 40 years, and the requirement to earn CME credits has been in existence for more than a decade.

Recognizing that surgeons practice in a variety of different settings and that everyone's practice has unique features, the MOC program was designed to be practice relevant. The ABS Board of Directors has crafted these requirements to provide enough flexibility for diplomates to satisfy them in a way best suited to their individual practice environment. There was also due consideration given to minimize adding to the burden of requirements for clinical practice.

The ABS MOC program requirements are organized in identical 3-year reporting cycles, with each year running from January 1 to December 31. Diplomates must submit information through the ABS Web site (www.absurgery.org) on how they are meeting MOC requirements for parts I, II, and IV within 2 months after their 3-year cycle ends. A summary of MOC requirements is presented in Table 1.

Professional standing (as known as part I of MOC) is intended to assure the public that diplomates exhibit professionalism in their practice, including acting in the patients' best interests; behaving professionally with patients, families, and colleagues across the health professions; taking appropriate self-care; and representing their board certification and MOC status appropriately. This requirement is satisfied by maintaining a full and unrestricted medical license in at least one state, having a hospital or ambulatory surgery center where

Table 1
Maintenance of certification requirements of the American Board of Surgery

Diplomates must submit information by the end of each 3-y cycle on the following:	
Professionalism and professional standing (part I)	• Diplomates must have a full and unrestricted medical license. • Diplomates must have hospital or surgical center privileges if clinically active. • Diplomates must have recommendations from the chief of surgery and chair of credentialing where most work in performed.
Lifelong learning and self-assessment (part II)	• Diplomates must have 90 category I CME credits relevant to their practice over the 3-y cycle; at least 60 of the 90 credits must include a self-assessment (written or electronic question-and-answer exercise); a score of 75% or higher must be required on the self-assessment activity. • The ABS will waive 60 CME self-assessment credits for passing a certifying or MOC examination given by the ABS or another ABMS board.
Improvement in medical practice (part IV)	• Diplomates must have participation in a local, regional, or national outcomes registry or quality assessment program; if involved in a local activity, diplomates are asked to describe how they are meeting this requirement. No data are collected by the ABS.
Every 10 y, diplomates are required to successfully complete the following:	
Assessment of knowledge, judgment, and skills (part III)	• Diplomates must pass an examination of cognitive knowledge. • Surgeons can apply for an MOC examination starting 3 y before expiration of their certificate. A full examination application is required, including a 12-mo operative. • Diplomates must have a log, reference forms, and documentation of CME activity. Diplomates must be in compliance with MOC to apply. • For surgeons who hold multiple ABS certificates, this is the *only requirement* that must be repeated for each certificate. Once the examination is passed, the surgeon receives a new certificate with an expiration date 10 y from the previous certificate's expiration.

operative privileges are granted, and providing recommendation letters from the chief of surgery and chair of the credentials committee at their major institution. For diplomates who are not clinically active, operative or clinical privileges are not required; however, professional references are still required; the diplomate will be listed as clinically inactive by the ABS.

Lifelong learning/self-assessment (part II of MOC) requires ongoing participation in high-quality, unbiased learning and self-assessment activities that are relevant to the diplomate's specialty and areas of practice within the specialty. The ABS has selected CME credits as satisfying this requirement. Diplomates are required to earn 90 category 1 CME credits during each 3-year cycle (see Table 1). Sixty of the 90 credits must include a self-assessment activity with a minimum passing score of 75% correct. Self-assessment activities provide a means to actively demonstrate comprehension of the material presented, as opposed to only signing in to a course or reading material. CME activities required by state medical licensing boards are considered practice related and can be applied to the CME requirement.

An assessment of cognitive knowledge (part III) is required every 10 years. Diplomates can take the MOC examination up to 3 years before expiration of their certification. These computer-based examinations are administered at local secure testing centers. The use of an external objective assessment demonstrates that the diplomate has remained current in the core subject matter of the specialty. This assessment can drive learning both through preparing for the examination and targeted learning in response to examination results. This requirement is the only MOC requirement that must be repeated for each specialty certification.

Improvement in medical practice (MOC part IV) provides an assessment of the aspect of care provided by diplomates in their individual practices and/or in the larger hospital, health system, or community setting in which they practice. This assessment may include activities that result in improved patient or population health outcomes, improved access to health care, improved patient experience of care, and/or increased value in the health care system. This requirement is fulfilled by active participation in a national patient outcomes registry, state or regional collaborative, or locally based activity. Examples of practice assessment resources are maintained on the ABS Web site (www.absurgery.org) (Box 6). This list is not inclusive.

The ABS participates in the Multi-Specialty MOC Portfolio Approval Program (MSPP) of the ABMS. This program offers a streamlined approach for physicians across multiple disciplines to obtain MOC part IV credit through health care organizations that sponsor and support multiple well-designed quality-improvement efforts.

If there are no hospital-based or individual programs available, the ABS expects that a diplomate will select a focused area of practice for assessment. A brief description of the activity should include the practice area or types of procedures studied; definitions of the measures and goals; an outline of how outcomes were tracked, analyzed, and compared with the goals; and how areas for improvement were identified. A key element of practice performance improvement is to reassess the process after implementing changes based on the results.

RELEVANCE OF AMERICAN BOARD OF SURGERY MAINTENANCE OF CERTIFICATION

Physicians are facing an increasing burden of regulations and requirements for documentation. Likewise, the failure to coordinate these activities and agree on a common set of requirements has resulted in frustration about the duplication of effort with little apparent benefit. There has been criticism that MOC adds to this burden, is not relevant to today's practice of medicine, and does not lead to improvements in the quality of care. Each board has developed its own specific

Box 6: Examples of some acceptable programs for American Board of Surgery part IV credit

- ACS Surgeon Specific Registry (case log system with tracking of 30-day complications)
- Mastery of Breast Surgery (ASBS)
- Metabolic and Bariatric Surgery Accreditation and Quality Improvement Program
- Multi-Specialty MOC Portfolio Approval Program (ABMS)
- National Burn Repository (ABA)
- NCDB
- NCDB Rapid Quality Reporting System
- National Surgical Quality Improvement Program (ACS)
- National Trauma Data Bank
- Organ Procurement and Transplantation Network
- Statewide collaboratives (eg, SCOAP, MSQC, and so forth)
- STS National Database
- Trauma Quality Improvement Program (ACS)
- VA Surgical Quality Improvement Program

Vascular surgery–related programs

- NCDR PVI Registry
- Vascular Quality Initiative

Pediatric surgery–related programs

- ACS Surgeon Specific Registry (case log system with tracking of 30-day complications)
- ELSO Registry
- National Surgical Quality Improvement Program, Pediatric
- Pediatric Trauma Quality Improvement Program

Abbreviations: ABA, American Burn Association; ACS, American College of Surgeons; ASBS, American Society of Breast Surgeons; ELSO, Extracorporeal Life Support Organization; MSQC, Michigan Surgical Quality Collaboration; NCDB, National Cancer Data Base; NCDR, National Cardiovascular Data Registry; PVI, Peripheral Vascular Intervention; SCOAP, Surgical Clinical Outcomes Assessment Program; STS, Society of Thoracic Surgeons; VA, Veterans Affairs.

From the American Board of Surgery, Philadelphia, PA. Available at: http://www.absurgery.org/default.jsp?exam-mocpa. Accessed November 13, 2015.

requirements for MOC based on the principles of the 4-part framework. These requirements will vary in order to be relevant to practitioners within each specialty. Some boards have developed their own products for diplomates to use, whereas others have done this in partnership with their professional organizations or have relied on existing sources.

Achieving and maintaining board certification signifies a physician has met board developed standards of practice. Prystowsky and coauthors [2] have investigated whether ABS certification was associated with better patient outcomes following partial colon resection. Using an administrative state database, they found that surgeons with active ABS certification had significantly lower mortality and risk of complications compared with noncertified surgeons. Their analysis included surgeons who had initial certification as well as those who had recertified. This study is the only study the author is aware of that addresses the effect of having board certification on important patient outcomes. Although this study was performed before the advent of MOC, it demonstrates the value of achieving and maintaining ABS certification.

There is recent evidence that active participation in a clinical outcomes-based registry results in improved quality of care [3,4]. Participation in the American College of Surgeons National Surgical Quality Improvement Program has been associated with improvements in care that accrue with the duration of engagement in the program [4]. State-based quality consortiums have also demonstrated a reduction in adverse outcomes associated with participation in outcomes registries [5–7]. Because there is unlikely to be a prospective randomized trial performed in this area, we need to rely on the results of these and other reports that demonstrate a high level of evidence.

CME is recognized as a common means to maintain an understanding of contemporary medical practice. The rapid developments in clinical care emphasize the importance of staying current. The inclusion of self-assessment as part of the CME requirement fulfills the initial level of clinical competence by demonstration of knowledge acquisition.

The ABS MOC program was designed to create a national standard for professionalism, learning, demonstration of knowledge, and practice improvement throughout a surgeon's career. Now more than 90% of ABS diplomates with time = limited certificates are meeting its requirements. The ABS is committed to having an MOC program that is meaningful and valuable for diplomates as well as our patients while remaining flexible and accommodating of differences in diplomates' practices. There is little doubt that the ABS MOC will continue to evolve and improve.

References

[1] Malangoni MA. The American Board of Surgery Maintenance of Certification program: building on past successes. JAMA Surg 2015;150:697–8.

[2] Prystowsky JB, Bordage G, Feinglass JM. Patient outcomes for segmental colon resection according to surgeon's training, certification, and experience. Surgery 2002;132:663–72.

[3] Stey AM, Russell MM, Ko CY, et al. Clinical registries and quality measurement in surgery: a systematic review. Surg 2015;157:381–95.

[4] Cohen ME, Liu Y, Ko CY, et al. Improved surgical outcomes for ACS NSQIP hospitals over time: evaluation of hospital cohorts with up to 8 years of participation. Ann Surg 2015;263(2):267–73.

[5] Hakkarainen TW, Steele SR, Bastaworous A, et al. Nonsteroidal anti-inflammatory drugs and the risk for anastomotic failure: a report from Washington State's Surgical Care and Outcomes Assessment Program (SCOAP). JAMA Surg 2015;150:223–38.

[6] Guillamondegui OD, Gunter OL, Hines L, et al. Using the National Surgical Quality Improvement Program and the Tennessee Surgical Quality Collaborative to improve surgical outcomes. J Am Coll Surg 2012;214:709–16.
[7] Healy MA, Krell RW, Abdelsattar ZM. Pancreatic resection results in a statewide surgical collaborative. Ann Surg Oncol 2015;22:2468–74.

Advances in Surgery 50 (2016) 115–128

ADVANCES IN SURGERY

Treatment of Locally Advanced Pancreatic Ductal Adenocarcinoma

Andrew P. Loehrer, MD, Christine V. Kinnier, MD, Cristina R. Ferrone, MD*

Department of Surgery, Massachusetts General Hospital, Boston, MA, USA

Keywords

• Neoadjuvant Therapy • Pancreatic cancer • Pancreatic ductal adenocarcinoma

Key points

- Pancreatic cancer is increasingly common, and up to 40% of cases are locally advanced at the time of presentation.
- The incorporation of neoadjuvant chemotherapy and more aggressive surgical resections have provided incremental improvement in survival, but overall prognosis for most patients remains poor.
- Ongoing study of multimodality therapy and prognostic markers are needed to more accurately and appropriately tailor treatment for individual patients.

INTRODUCTION

Pancreatic ductal adenocarcinoma (PDAC) is increasingly common and the fourth leading cause of cancer mortality in the United States, with overall 5-year survival of less than 4% [1]. Surgical resection remains the only potential for cure. Unfortunately, less than 20% of patients present with resectable disease and 45% present with overtly metastatic disease [2]. Increasing attention has been placed on the remaining 40% of patients with locally advanced PDAC (LA-PDAC). Although the overall prognosis for pancreatic cancer remains quite poor, increased use of more effective multimodality therapy has allowed for significantly improved survival for even the most challenging cases of LA-PDAC [3]. With this review, the authors aim to summarize recent

The authors have nothing to disclose.

*Corresponding author. Massachusetts General Hospital, Wang 460, 15 Parkman Street, Boston, MA 02114. *E-mail address*: cferrone@partners.org

0065-3411/16/$ – see front matter
http://dx.doi.org/10.1016/j.yasu.2016.03.010

advances in the management and treatment of patients with LA-PDAC as well as to highlight some promising new directions moving forward.

SIGNIFICANCE OF RESECTABILITY

For patients with LA-PDAC, surgical consideration rests on the ability to obtain negative resection margins. A recent analysis compared survival between wide R0 resections, R0 resections with tumor within 1 mm of margin, and R1 resections. Median survival for patients with wide R0 resections was significantly greater than those with margins of less than 1 mm or R1 resections (35 vs 16 vs 14 months, respectively; $P < .001$) [4]. Yet preoperative determination of resectability has been challenging; therefore, multiple definitions of LA-PDAC or borderline resectable PDAC have been established. Early radiologic definitions deemed tumors locally advanced if tumors abutted the celiac trunk or superior mesenteric artery or involved the portal vein or superior mesenteric vein (SMV) [5]. Because of the heterogeneity of definitions, the University of Texas MD Anderson Cancer Center, Americas Hepato-Pancreato-Biliary Association/Society of Surgical Oncology/Society for Surgery of the Alimentary Tract, and the National Comprehensive Cancer Network have modified these definitions based on vascular involvement [6–9]. At the authors' center, they consider locally advanced tumors as cancers with (1) no distant metastasis, (2) absence of blood flow through the SMV and/or portal vein lumen or venous involvement not amenable to reconstruction, (3) involvement of the common hepatic artery or superior mesenteric artery over greater than 180° of the vessel circumference, (4) any celiac abutment, or (5) aortic or inferior vena cava invasion or encasement. The utility of these traditional definitions is under ongoing evaluation as we determine the accuracy of radiographic imaging following neoadjuvant therapy (discussed later). Examples of computed tomography (CT) images before and after neoadjuvant therapy are seen in Fig. 1. The challenges of identifying truly

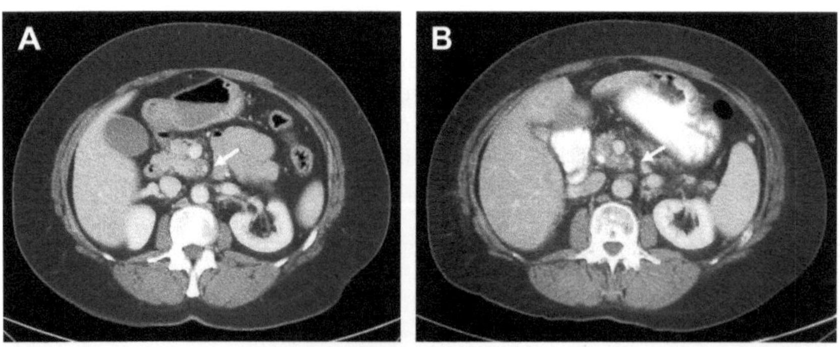

Fig. 1. CT scan of patients with pancreatic adenocarcinoma (*A*) before and (*B*) after neoadjuvant chemotherapy ± chemoradiation. The white arrows are pointing to the superior mesenteric arty.

resectable disease, even after radiographic response to neoadjuvant therapy, are further exemplified by Fig. 2. Each of these patients ultimately underwent an R0 resection. Inclusion of additional factors beyond radiology, including biomarkers, such as carbohydrate antigen 19 to 9 or SMAD4 mutation status, have also been proposed to refine our present classification system and guide more appropriate treatment [7,10].

NEOADJUVANT CHEMOTHERAPY

Until recently, nearly 30% of patients with LA-PDAC had progression of disease or metastasis during early cycles of treatment and only 30% of patients were converted from unresectable to surgical candidates after receipt of chemotherapy and/or chemoradiation (CRT) [11,12]. However, multiple recent studies have provided promising results that these numbers could be shifting with neoadjuvant chemotherapy and/or CRT.

FOLFIRINOX

The ACCORD-11 trial demonstrated an improved survival associated with FOLFIRINOX (oxaliplatin, irinotecan, fluorouracil, and leucovorin) versus gemcitabine in patients with metastatic disease [13]. Since this time, multiple additional groups have looked to the regimen as a potential neoadjuvant therapy for patients with borderline resectable or LA-PDAC. A recent cohort of 188 patients undergoing resection for PDAC compared the results for those with locally advanced/borderline tumors who received neoadjuvant FOLFIRINOX and those who had an operation followed by adjuvant gemcitabine [14]. Despite post-FOLFIRINOX imaging suggesting that 70% of patients had persistent locally advanced/borderline disease, pathology demonstrated a 92% R0 resection rate and significantly lower rates of positive lymph nodes and perineural or lymphatic invasion as compared with those who underwent an operation alone. These findings are consistent with other studies suggesting that radiologic indicators of resectability are unreliable after receipt of neoadjuvant chemotherapy or CRT [15]. Although the study had a

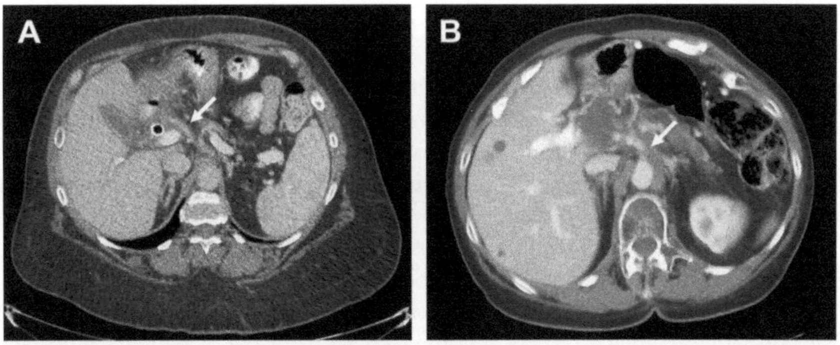

Fig. 2. CT scans of patients at the completion of neoadjuvant therapy and before undergoing R0 resection. Images show unclear involvement of (*A*) hepatic artery and (*B*) celiac trunk (*arrows*).

relatively short median follow-up time of 11 months, the FOLFIRINOX-treated cohort was associated with improved overall survival ($P = .008$). Other groups have demonstrated similarly encouraging results [16,17]. Christians and colleagues [17] showed resection in 83% of patients after neoadjuvant FOLFIRINOX and CRT, with an R0 resection in all 12 patients resected and node positivity in only 17% of patients. It is hoped that long-term follow-up of these patients will elucidate if promising early results in resectability translate into an actual survival benefit with neoadjuvant FOLFIRINOX.

Although FOLFIRINOX has shown promising results in terms of overall survival and conversion of locally advanced tumors to potentially resectable, the regimen is also associated with higher rates of neutropenia (45.0%), febrile neutropenia (5.4%), thrombocytopenia (9.1%), and diarrhea (12.7%) [10]. Therefore, this regimen has mostly been limited to patients with relatively good functional status (Eastern Cooperative Oncology Group performance status 0 or 1). Subsequent analyses of the ACCORD-11 trial noted persistently higher rates of diarrhea in the FOLFIRINOX cohort but a longer time until deterioration of quality of life as compared with patients in the gemcitabine arm [18]. Others have slightly modified the FOLFIRINOX regimen to be more tolerable, including elimination of bolus 5-fluorouracil (5-FU) and adding prophylactic pegfilgrastim [19,20]. Such modified regimens have shown to be safe and effective, with Blazer and colleagues [20] reporting subsequent resection possible in 72% of patients with an R0 resection rate in 86.4%.

Gemcitabine-based therapy

Gemcitabine has been a staple agent in the treatment of PDAC since the CONKO-001 trial. The trial compared adjuvant chemotherapy with gemcitabine with observation alone after an R0 or R1 resection for PDAC. The gemcitabine group had a median survival of 13.4 months compared with 6.9 months in the observation alone group ($P < .001$) [21].

Combination therapy with gemcitabine and nab-paclitaxel has also been investigated for LA-PDAC following the phase 3 randomized trial for patients with metastatic PDAC [22]. The combination was associated with a 2-month longer median overall survival (hazard ratio for death 0.72, 95% confidence interval [CI] [0.62–0.83], $P < .001$) but also higher rates of peripheral neuropathy and myelosuppression than gemcitabine alone. Use of gemcitabine plus nab-paclitaxel in the neoadjuvant setting for LA-PDAC is still limited to case reports, but trials are presently underway [23]. Furthermore, the efficacy of gemcitabine plus nab-paclitaxel compared with FOLFIRINOX is yet to be evaluated on a head-to-head basis.

Barugola and colleagues [24] retrospectively examined the utilization of gemcitabine-based neoadjuvant chemotherapy and subsequent surgical outcomes. Of the 41 patients who received neoadjuvant therapy, nearly 71.0% went on to have an R0 resection compared with 59.7% of patients who went directly to the operating room ($P = .20$). Patients receiving neoadjuvant therapy had lower nodal positivity compared with up-front surgery

(31.7% vs 86.2%, respectively; $P < .001$), comparable rates of postoperative morbidity (41.5% vs 33.7%, respectively; $P = .390$), and a comparable median survival from time of resection (35 months vs 27 months, respectively; $P = .740$). Although this report did not follow all patients receiving neoadjuvant therapy, the study provided encouraging data that patients with locally advanced disease can benefit and see comparable outcomes with those who present with initially resectable disease.

In a single-institutional series, Leone and colleagues [25] evaluated efficacy of neoadjuvant gemcitabine with oxaliplatin (GEMOX) followed by neoadjuvant CRT for patients with LA-PDAC. Nine of 15 patients with borderline resectable disease ultimately proceeded to an R0/R1 resection. The median survival for patients undergoing resection was 31.5 months compared with 12.3 months for unresected patients ($P < .001$). Another multi-institutional phase 2 study of neoadjuvant GEMOX with radiation examined 68 patients with resectable or borderline disease [26]. Forty-three of these patients underwent resection, 84% with an R0 resection; median survival was 34.6 months. Trials comparing gemcitabine with nab-paclitaxal or oxaliplatin to FOLFIRINOX have also yet to be completed.

NEOADJUVANT CHEMORADIATION

Given the significance of having negative surgical margins, neoadjuvant CRT has long been promoted for the treatment of LA-PDAC [27,28]. Evaluation of the Surveillance, Epidemiology, and End Results registry from 1994 to 2003 found that patients receiving neoadjuvant CRT have significantly higher rates of survival relative to no neoadjuvant CRT (hazard ratio, 0.55; 95% CI 0.38–0.79, $P = .001$) and adjuvant radiation therapy (hazard ratio 0.63; 95% CI, 0.45–0.90, $P = .03$) [29]. Furthermore, neoadjuvant CRT is not only associated with improved survival but also a significantly lower cost than surgery-first approaches [30].

However, CRT alone in the absence of neoadjuvant chemotherapy seems to be suboptimal. Arvold and colleagues [31] examined 70 consecutive patients with unresectable or LA-PDAC who received either CRT alone or neoadjuvant gemcitabine-based chemotherapy followed by CRT. Twenty percent of patients in both groups subsequently underwent surgical resection. Patients receiving chemotherapy in addition to CRT had a median survival of 18.7 months versus 12.4 months ($P = .02$) for patients receiving CRT alone. Other studies, although underpowered, suggested that the addition of CRT to gemcitabine therapy conferred a marginal survival benefit with comparable toxicity profiles [32,33]. Correspondingly, CRT usually follows induction chemotherapy, which allows for identification of patients, approximately 30%, with initially undetected metastatic disease [34,35]. The optimal chemotherapeutic regimen and radiation dosages also remain in question. In their systematic review, Gillen and colleagues [12] highlighted that most published studies include radiotherapy doses between 40 Gy and 60 Gy, with most patients receiving 1.8 to 2.0 Gy per fraction.

The histologic response of tumors to neoadjuvant CRT has been shown to be an important prognostic factor in which patients with complete pathologic responses have improved overall survival [36,37]. However, the timing between completion of radiation and surgical resection remains unclear. In a retrospective analysis, Chen and colleagues [38] examined the pathologic response of patients having received different intervals of chemotherapy after completion of neoadjuvant CRT and before surgical resection. Compared with patients who received between 0 and 10 weeks of chemotherapy between radiation and surgery, patients undergoing greater than 20 weeks of chemotherapy between CRT and surgery had a significant increase in rates of R0 resection, progression-free survival, and overall survival.

Few studies have explicitly compared the chemotherapy with use in conjunction with radiotherapy. Takai and colleagues [39] evaluated patients with LA-PADC who received neoadjuvant CRT with either 5-FU and cisplatin or gemcitabine. Eight patients remained unresectable after neoadjuvant chemoradiotherapy, 6 patients (42%) received 5-FU/cisplatin and 2 patients (11%) received gemcitabine. Toxicities of preoperative radiation as well as survival of resected patients were comparable between both 5-FU/cisplatin and gemcitabine cohorts. Another study out of France followed 61 patients treated with 5-FU/cisplatin and radiation, with only 23 patients (38%) demonstrating an objective response allowing reexploration and only 13 patients (21%) undergoing R0/R1 resection [40]. The median survival for those undergoing a resection was 28 months and 20 months for the 10 patients who underwent a palliative procedure. Although 5-FU and gemcitabine have been the most widely used agents, other phase I trials and case series have been presented using additional or alternative chemosensitizers, including capecitabine, bevacizumab, and paclitaxel [41–43]. The optimal combination is under ongoing investigation.

SURGICAL RESECTION AND INTRAOPERATIVE THERAPY

As previously discussed, the traditional extent of disease denoting unresectable disease includes tumor encasement of the superior mesenteric artery, celiac trunk, or hepatic artery. Portal venous involvement becomes unresectable when there is complete occlusion with the development of multiple collaterals, which cannot be reconstructed. Given the significant improvement in survival in patients resected as compared with those left with unresected primary tumors, groups have studied the feasibility of vascular resection and reconstruction. Yekebas and colleagues [44] evaluated 585 patients who underwent a potentially curative pancreatic resection with (N = 136) or without (N = 449) vascular reconstruction. Of those undergoing vascular resection, 128 (94%) of these involved the mesenteric-portal axis and 13 (10%) involved the hepatic artery or superior mesenteric artery. Five patients had both venous and arterial reconstruction. Their results suggested comparable morbidity and mortality in patients undergoing en bloc resection of LA-PDAC relative to those not undergoing vascular resection. Similarly, Tseng and colleagues [45] examined patients undergoing pancreatic resection with (N = 141) and without

(N = 181) vascular resection over a 12-year period at the M.D. Anderson Cancer Center. These resections were also predominantly venous resection and reconstructions, with concomitant hepatic artery resections in 17 of the patients (12%). Patients undergoing vascular reconstruction had comparable major morbidity and mortality rates. Median survival for patients undergoing pancreaticoduodenectomy with vascular resection was not significantly different than patients having resection without reconstruction (23.4 months vs 26.5 months, respectively; $P = .18$). However, acute thrombosis of the portal venous reconstruction following pancreatic resection is not only associated with increased perioperative mortality (22.2% vs 4.6%, $P = .023$) but is also associated with a decreased median survival (7.1 months vs 15.9 months, $P = .011$) even when nonfatal [46].

Although the cumulative literature on feasibility and efficacy of venous reconstruction are promising, outcomes following arterial resection remain in question. A recent meta-analysis found that pancreatectomy with simultaneous arterial resection was associated with increased perioperative mortality (odds ratio [OR] 5.04, 95% CI, 2.69–9.45; $P < .001$) as well as decreased survival at 1 year (OR 0.49, 95% CI, 0.31–0.78; $P = .02$) and at 3 years (OR 0.39, 95% CI, 0.17–0.86; $P = .02$) [47]. Bockhorn and colleagues [48] shared their experience with arterial resection and reconstruction, finding significantly higher rates of major complications, higher mortality, and lower rates of R0 resections. Yet median survival for patients undergoing arterial reconstruction was comparable with those patients who underwent pancreatic resection without concomitant vascular resection and significantly better than patients who underwent palliative bypass alone. Thus, the investigators appropriately caution that marginal benefits in overall survival must be very carefully weighed, on a case-by-case basis, against the considerable perioperative morbidity and mortality associated with arterial vascular reconstruction.

Intraoperative Radiotherapy

Intraoperative radiotherapy (IORT) has been studied extensively over the past few decades. Patients receiving IORT at the authors' institution have usually already received full-dose external beam radiation. IORT is then administered as a single dose of 10 to 25 Gy focally targeted at the surgical margin, residual disease, or unresectable cancer. This modality has great appeal in being able to shield healthy tissue from radiation while potentially reducing the risk of wider external beam radiation toxicity. Previous publications from the Massachusetts General Hospital have found favorable oncologic and survival outcomes in select patients with unresectable pancreatic cancer with 1-year, 2-year, and 3-year overall survival rates of 49%, 16%, and 6% [49,50]. For the 194 patients treated, a Charlson Comorbidity Index of 3 or less, IORT applicator diameter of 8 cm or less, and receipt of chemotherapy were independently predictive of improved overall survival. Data on the use of IORT as an adjunct to surgical resection for LA-PDAC are inconclusive, with most studies suggesting no survival benefit [51–54]. A more recent Japanese study of 210 patients treated with resection and IORT, in conjuction with chemotherapy and/or external beam radiation, resulted in 2-year local control rates of 87.1% and 74.6% following R0 and R1 resections, respectively [55]. There was no clear association between IORT dose (20, 25, or 30 Gy) and local control or overall survival. R0 versus R1 resection and use of adjuvant chemotherapy was associated with an improved overall survival. Another multi-institutional European cohort found a 5-year local control rate in 23.3% of patients with significantly greater local control and survival in patients who also received preoperative radiotherapy (median survival 30 months) versus external beam radiation therapy alone (median survival 22 months, $P<.001$) or IORT alone (median survival 13 months, $P<.001$) [56]. However, these investigators also acknowledge the limitations of the 20-year study period because significant improvements in IORT technology, adjunctive chemotherapy regimens, and improved surgical techniques over this period limit the generalizability of findings in the setting of present-day, multimodality treatment. In general, toxicities related to IORT are limited and include colitis, gastrointestinal bleeding, epigastric discomfort, and ileus [57,58]. Multiple series from select institutions, including a propensity score–matched analysis, have suggested no significant difference in perioperative complications with the use of IORT [59,60].

Intraoperative Electroporation

Newer technologies have also been increasingly applied with hopes of increasing local control at the time of surgery. Irreversible electroporation (IRE) uses short, high-voltage pulses to tissue causing increased cellular membrane permeability and tumor ablation [61]. Recent multi-institutional studies integrating IRE into the multimodality treatment of LA-PDAC have demonstrated improvements in local control and survival with progression-free and median overall survival of 11 months and 22 months, respectively [62,63]. Complication rates in these early experiences seem to be comparable with outcomes following resection and multi-modality therapy in the absence of IRE. How this technique will be most effectively incorporated into newer chemotherapeutic and radiation-based regimens is an area of ongoing investigation.

ADJUVANT THERAPY

Studies from both the United States as well as Italy suggest that both perioperative and overall survival following surgery have improved significantly over the past 25 years [64,65]. Adjuvant chemotherapy has become a mainstay following resection of PDAC, and the role of adjuvant CRT remains to be clearly defined [66–70]. Many found flaws in the adjuvant CRT study designs and analyses, resulting in ongoing trials, such as Radiation Therapy Oncology Group (RTOG) 0848, to evaluate the role of modern CRT regimens following surgical resection [71]. However, no studies to date have examined the efficacy of chemotherapy or CRT in patients with LA-PDAC following neoadjuvant treatment and resection. Much more data on adjuvant after neoadjuvant

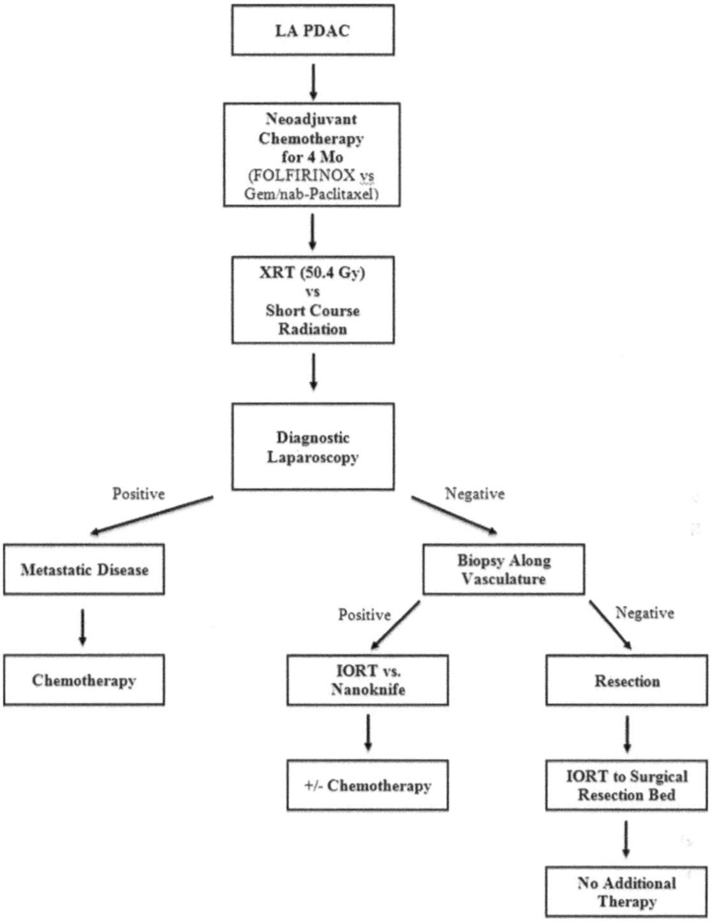

Fig. 3. Management strategy for locally advanced pancreatic cancer used at authors' institution. XRT, external beam radiation therapy.

therapy will surface in the coming years as the utilization of neoadjuvant protocols increases.

FUTURE DIRECTIONS

Advances in imaging technology have improved the diagnosis and staging of patients with pancreatic cancer, and neoadjuvant therapy has demonstrated promising early results; however, the prognosis of patients presenting with LA-PDAC remains poor. Helical CT scanning inadequately assesses the true response to neoadjuvant therapy [14]. Additional imaging modalities are needed to evaluate the true response to treatment, provide more accurate prognostic information, and guide optimal treatment. Furthermore, novel tumor markers or other prognostic factors might also better guide therapeutic options, including determination of who might best benefit from surgical resection. Fluorouracil and gemcitabine-based chemotherapy has been the mainstay in treatment. Newer regimens, including FOLFIRINOX, GEMOX, and gemcitabine with paclitaxel, are still in their infancy. Newer drugs and incorporation of immunotherapy, including ipilimumab or erlotinib, may provide additional benefit, though data for LA-PDAC remains to be seen [72,73].

SUMMARY

Pancreatic cancer is increasingly common, and up to 40% of cases are locally advanced at the time of presentation. The incorporation of neoadjuvant chemotherapy and more aggressive surgical resections has provided incremental improvement in survival, but the overall prognosis for most patients remains poor. Therefore, multimodality strategies in the management of locally advanced pancreatic cancer continue to evolve (Fig. 3). Ongoing study of a newer medical therapy as well as prognostic markers is needed to more accurately and appropriately tailor treatment of individual patients.

References

[1] Jemal A, Siegel R, Ward E, et al. Cancer statistics, 2008. CA Cancer J Clin 2008;58: 71–96.
[2] Vincent A, Herman J, Schulick R, et al. Pancreatic cancer. Lancet 2004;27:1049–57.
[3] Truty MJ, Thomas RM, Katz MH, et al. Multimodality therapy offers a chance for cure in patients with pancreatic adenocarcinoma deemed unresectable at first operative exploration. J Am Coll Surg 2012;215:41–52.
[4] Konstantinidis IT, Warshaw AL, Allen JN, et al. Pancreatic ductal adenocarcinoma: is there a survival difference for R1 resections versus locally advanced unresectable tumors? What is a "true" R0 resection? Ann Surg 2013;257:731–6.
[5] Lu DS, Reber HA, Krasny RM, et al. Local staging of pancreatic cancer: criteria for unresectability of major vessels as revealed by pancreatic-phase thin-section helical CT. AJR Am J Roentgenol 1997;168:1439–43.
[6] Varadhachary GR, Tamm EP, Abrruzzese JL, et al. Borderline resectable pancreatic cancer: definitions, management and role of preoperative therapy. Ann Surg Oncol 2006;13: 1035–46.
[7] Katz MH, Pisters PW, Evans DB, et al. Borderline resectable pancreatic cancer: the importance of this emerging stage of disease. J Am Coll Surg 2008;206:833–46.
[8] Callery MP, Chang KJ, Fishman EK, et al. Pretreatment assessment of resectable and borderline resectable pancreatic cancer: expert consensus statement. Ann Surg Oncol 2009;16: 1727–33.
[9] Katz MH, Marsh R, Herman JM, et al. Borderline resectable pancreatic cancer: need for standardization and methods for optimal clinical trial design. Ann Surg Oncol 2013;20(8):2787–95.
[10] Evans DB, Erickson BA, Ritch P. Borderline resectable pancreatic cancer: definitions and the importance of multimodality therapy. Ann Surg Oncol 2010;17:2803–5.
[11] He J, Page AJ, Weiss M, et al. Management of borderline and locally advanced pancreatic cancer: where do we stand? World J Gastroenterol 2014;20:2255–66.
[12] Gillen S, Schuster T, Meyer zum Büschenfelde C, et al. Preoperative/neoadjuvant therapy in pancreatic cancer: a systematic review and meta-analysis of response and resection percentages. PLoS Med 2010;7:e1000267.

[13] Conroy T, Desseigne F, Ychou M, et al. FOLFIRINOX versus gemcitabine for metastatic pancreatic cancer. N Engl J Med 2011;364:1817–25.
[14] Ferrone CR, Marchegiani G, Hong T, et al. Radiological and surgical implications of neoadjuvant treatment with FOLFIRINOX for locally advanced and borderline resectable pancreatic cancer. Ann Surg 2015;261:12–7.
[15] Katz MH, Fleming JB, Bhosale P, et al. Response of borderline resectable pancreatic cancer to neoadjuvant therapy is not reflected by radiographic indicators. Cancer 2012;118: 5749–56.
[16] Peddi PF, Lubner S, McWilliams R, et al. Multi-institutional experience with FOLFIRINOX in pancreatic adenocarcinoma. JOP 2012;13:497–501.
[17] Christians KK, Tsai S, Mahmoud A, et al. Neoadjuvant FOLFIRINOX for borderline resectable pancreas cancer: a new treatment paradigm? Oncologist 2014;19:266–74.
[18] Gourgou-Bourgad S, Bascoul-Molevi C, Desseigne F, et al. Impact of FOLFIRINOX compared with gemicitabine on quality of life in patients with metastatic pancreatic cancer: results from the PRODIGE 4/ACCORD 11 randomized trial. J Clin Oncol 2012;31:23–9.
[19] Mahaseth H, Brutcher E, Kauh J, et al. Modified FOLFIRINOX regimen with improved safety and maintained efficacy in pancreatic adenocarcinoma. Pancreas 2013;42: 1311–5.
[20] Blazer M, Wu C, Goldberg RM, et al. Neoadjuvant modified (m) FOLFIRINOX for locally advanced unresectable (LAPC) and borderline resectable (BRPC) adenocarcinoma of the pancreas. Ann Surg Oncol 2015;22:1153–9.
[21] Oettle H, Post S, Neuhaus P, et al. Adjuvant chemotherapy with gemcitabine vs observation in patients undergoing curative-intent resection of pancreatic cancer: a randomized control trial. JAMA 2007;297:267–77.
[22] Von Hoff DD, Ervin T, Arena FP, et al. Increased survival in pancreatic cancer with na-paclitaxel plus gemcitabine. N Engl J Med 2013;369:1691–703.
[23] Olowokure O, Torregroza-Sanchez MP, Bedoya-Apraez ID. Gemcitabine plus nab-paclitaxel with chemoradiation in locally advanced pancreatic cancer. J Gastrointest Oncol 2013;4:E16–8.
[24] Barugola G, Partelli S, Crippa S, et al. Outcomes after resection of locally advanced or borderline resectable pancreatic cancer after neoadjuvant therapy. Am J Surg 2012;203:132–9.
[25] Leone F, Gatti M, Massucco P, et al. Induction gemcitabine and oxaliplatin therapy followed by a twice-weekly infusion of gemcitabine and concurrent external-beam radiation for neoadjuvant treatment of locally advanced pancreatic cancer: a single institutional experience. Cancer 2013;119:277–84.
[26] Kim EJ, Ben-Josef E, Herman JM, et al. A multi-institutional phase 2 study of neoadjuvant gemcitabine and oxaliplatin with radiation therapy in patients with pancreatic cancer. Cancer 2013;119:2692–700.
[27] A multi-institutional comparative trial of radiation therapy alone and in combination with 5-fluorouracil for locally unresectable pancreatic carcinoma. The Gastrointestinal Tumor Study Group. Ann Surg 1979;189:205–8.
[28] Treatment of locally unresectable carcinoma of the pancreas: comparison of combined-modality therapy (chemotherapy plus radiotherapy) to chemotherapy alone. Gastrointestinal Tumor Study Group. J Natl Cancer Inst 1988;80:751–5.
[29] Stessin AM, Meyer JE, Sherr DL. Neoadjuvant radiation is associated with improved survival in patients with resectable pancreatic cancer: an analysis of data from the Surveillance, Epidemiology, and End Results (SEER) registry. Int J Radiat Oncol Biol Phys 2008;72: 1128–33.
[30] Abbott DE, Tzeng CWD, Merkow RP, et al. The cost-effectiveness of neoadjuvant chemoradiation is superior to a surgery-first approach in the treatment of pancratic head adenocarcinoma. Ann Surg Oncol 2013;20:S500–8.

[31] Arvold ND, Ryan DP, Niemerko A, et al. Long-term outcomes of neoadjuvant chemotherapy before chemoradiation for locally advanced pancreatic cancer. Cancer 2012;118: 3026–35.
[32] Cardenes HR, Moore AM, Johnson CS, et al. A phase II study of gemcitabine in combination with radiation therapy in patients with localized unresectable pancreatic cancer: a Hoosier Oncology Group study. Am J Clin Oncol 2011;34:460–5.
[33] Loehrer PJ, Feng Y, Cardenes Wagner L, et al. Gemcitabine alone versus gemcitabine plus radiotherapy in patients with locally advanced pancreatic cancer: an Eastern Cooperative Oncology Group trial. J Clin Oncol 2011;29:4105–12.
[34] Krishnan S, Rana V, Janjan NA, et al. Induction chemotherapy selects patients with locally advanced, unresectable pancreatic cancer for optimal benefit from consolidative chemoradiation therapy. Cancer 2007;110:47–55.
[35] Huguet F, André T, Hammel P, et al. Impact of chemoradiotherapy after disease control with chemotherapy in locally advanced pancreatic adenocarcinoma in GERCOR phase II and III studies. J Clin Oncol 2007;25:326–31.
[36] White RR, Xie HB, Gottfried MR, et al. Significance of histological response to preoperative chemoradiotherapy for pancreatic cancer. Ann Surg Oncol 2005;12:214–21.
[37] Chatterjee D, Katz MH, Rashid A, et al. Histologic grading of the extent of residual carcinoma following neoadjuvant chemoradiation in pancreatic ductal adenocarcinoma: a predictor of patient outcome. Cancer 2012;118:3182–90.
[38] Chen KT, Devarajam K, Milestone BN, et al. Neoadjuvant chemoradiation and duration of chemotherapy before surgical resection for pancreatic cancer: does time interval between radiotherapy and surgery matter? Ann Surg Oncol 2014;21:662–9.
[39] Takai S, Satoi S, Yanagimoto H, et al. Neoadjuvant chemoradiation in patients with potentially resectable pancreatic cancer. Pancreas 2008;36:e26–32.
[40] Cunha AS, Rault A, Laurent C, et al. Surgical resection after radiochemotherapy in patients with unresectable adenocarcinoma of the pancreas. J Am Coll Surg 2005;201:359–65.
[41] Stokes JB, Nolan NJ, Stelow EB, et al. Preoperative capecitabine and concurrent radiation for borderline resectable pancreatic cancer. Ann Surg Oncol 2011;18:619–27.
[42] Crane CH, Ellis LM, Abbruzzesse JL, et al. Phase I trial evaluating the safety of bevacizumab with concurrent radiotherapy and capecitabine in locally advanced pancreatic cancer. J Clin Oncol 2006;24:1145–51.
[43] Pisters PW, Wolff RA, Janjan NA, et al. Preoperative paclitaxel and concurrent rapid-fractionation radiation for resectable pancreatic adenocarcinoma: toxicities, histologic response rates, and event-free outcome. J Clin Oncol 2002;20:2537–44.
[44] Yekebas EF, Bogoevski D, Cataldegirmen G, et al. En bloc vascular resection for locally advanced pancreatic malignancies infiltrating major blood vessels: perioperative outcome and long-term survival in 136 patients. Ann Surg 2008;247:300–9.
[45] Tseng JF, Raut CP, Lee JE, et al. Pancreaticoduodenectomy with vascular resection: margin status and survival duration. J Gastrointest Surg 2004;8:935–50.
[46] Gawlas I, Epelboym I, Winner Dinorcia J, et al. Short-term but not long-term loss of patency of venous reconstruction during pancreatic resection is associated with decreased survival. J Gastrointest Surg 2014;18:75–82.
[47] Mohllberg N, Rhbari NN, Koch M, et al. Arterial resection during pancreatectomy for pancreatic cancer: a systematic review and meta-analysis. Ann Surg 2011;254: 882–93.
[48] Bockhorn M, Burdelski C, Bogoevski D, et al. Arterial en bloc resection for pancreatic carcinoma. Br J Surg 2011;98:86–92.
[49] Willett CG, Fernandez-del Castillo C, Shih HA, et al. Long-term results of intraoperative electron beam irradiation (IOERT) for patients with unresectable pancreatic cancer. Ann Surg 2005;241:295–9.
[50] Cai S, Hong TS, Goldberg SI, et al. Updated long-term outcomes and prognostic factors for patients with unresectable locally advanced pancreatic cancer treated with intraoperative

radiotherapy at the Massachusetts General Hospital, 1978-2010. Cancer 2013;119: 4196–204.
[51] Ruano-Ravina A, Ortega RA. Guedea. Intaroperative radiotherapy in pancreatic cancer: a systematic review. Radiother Oncol 2008;87:318–25.
[52] Roldan GE, Gunderson LL, Nagorney DM, et al. Exernal beam versus intraoperative and external beam irradiation for locally advanced pancreatic cancer. Cancer 1988;61: 1110–6.
[53] Zerbi A, Fossati V, Parolini D, et al. Intraoperative radiation therapy adjuvant to resection in the treatment of pancreatic cancer. Cancer 1994;73:2930–5.
[54] Alfieri S, Morganti A, Di Giorgio A, et al. Improved survival and local control after intraoperative radiation therapy and postoperative radiotherapy: a multivariate analysis of 46 patients undergoing surgery for pancreatic head cancer. Arch Surg 2001;136: 343–7.
[55] Ogawa K, Karasaw K, Ito Y, et al. Intraoperative radiotherapy for resected pancreatic cancer: a multi-institutional retrospective analysis of 210 patients. Int J Radiat Oncol Biol Phys 2010;77:734–42.
[56] Valentini V, Calvo F, Reni M, et al. Intra-operative radiotherapy (IORT) in pancreatic cancer: joint analysis of the ISIORT-Europe experience. Radiother Oncol 2009;91:54–9.
[57] Sindelar WF, Kinsella TJ. Normal tissue tolerance to intraoperative radiotherapy. Surg Oncol Clin N Am 2003;12:925–42.
[58] O'connor JK, Suase WT, Hazard LJ, et al. Survival after attempted surgical resection and intraoperative radiation therapy for pancreatic and peiampullary adenocarcinoma. Int J Radiat Oncol Biol Phys 2005;63:1060–6.
[59] Farrell TJ, Barbot DJ, Rosato FE. Pancreatic resection combined with intraoperative radiation therapy for pancreatic cancer. Ann Surg 1997;226:66–9.
[60] Showalter TN, Rao AS, Anne PR, et al. Does intraoperative radiation therapy improve local tumor control in patients undergoing pancreaticoduodenectomy for pancreatic adenocarcinoma? A propensity score analysis. Ann Surg Oncol 2009;16:2116–22.
[61] Al-Sakere B, André F, Bernat C, et al. Tumor ablation with irreversible electroporation. PLoS One 2007;2:e1135.
[62] Martin RCG, McFarland K, Ellis S, et al. Irreversible electroporation in locally advanced pancreatic cancer: potential improved overall survival. Ann Surg Oncol 2013;20:S443–9.
[63] Kwon D, McFarland K, Velanovich V, et al. Borderline and locally advanced pancreatic adenocarcionoma margin accentuation with intraoperative irreversible electroporation. Surgery 2014;156:910–22.
[64] Mayo SC, Gilson MM, Herman JM, et al. Management of patients with pancreatic adenocarcinoma: national trends in patient selection, operative management, and use of adjuvant therapy. J Am Coll Surg 2012;214:33–45.
[65] Barugola G, Partelli S, Crippa S, et al. Time trends in the treatment and prognosis of resectable pancreatic cancer in a large tertiary referral centre. HPB (Oxford) 2013;15: 958–64.
[66] Kalser MH, Ellenberg SS. Pancreatic cancer. Adjuvant combine radiation and chemotherapy following curative resection. Arch Surg 1985;120:899–903.
[67] Yeo CJ, Abrams RA, Grochow LB, et al. Pancreaticoduodenectomy for pancreatic adenocarcinoma: postoperative adjuvant chemoradiation improves survival. Ann Surg 1997;225: 621–36.
[68] Neoptolemos JP, Dunn JA, Stocken DD, et al. Adjuvant chemoradiotherapy and chemotherapy in resectable apncreatic cancer: a randomised controlled trial. Lancet 2001;358:1576–85.
[69] Neoptolemos JP, Stocken DD, Friess H, et al. A randomized trial of chemoradiotherapy and chemotherapy after resection of pancreatic cancer. N Engl J Med 2004;350: 1200–10.

[70] Stocken DD, Büchler MW, Dervenis C, et al. Meta-analysis of randomised adjuvant therapy trials for pancreatic cancer. Br J Cancer 2005;92:1372–81.
[71] Chuong MD, Boggs DH, Patel KN, et al. Adjuvant chemoradiation for pancreatic cancer: what does the evidence tell us? J Gastrointest Oncol 2014;5:166–77.
[72] Royal RE, Levy C, Turner K, et al. Phase 2 trial of single agent ipilimumab (Anti-CTLA-4) for locally advanced or metastatic pancreatic adenocarcinoma. J Immunother 2010;33: 828–33.
[73] Gemcitabine hydrochloride with or without erlotinib hydrochloride followed by the same chemotherapy regimen with or without radiation therapy and capecitabine or fluorouracil in treating patients with pancreatic cancer that has been removed by surgery. Available at: https://clinicaltrials.gov/ct2/show/NCT01013649. Accessed April 15, 2015.

Advances in Surgery 50 (2016) 129–141

ADVANCES IN SURGERY

Prevention of Perioperative Anastomotic Healing Complications

Anastomotic Stricture and Anastomotic Leak

Kristina L. Guyton, MD, Neil H. Hyman, MD, John C. Alverdy, MD*

Department of Surgery, The University of Chicago Medicine, University of Chicago, 5841 South Maryland Avenue, MC 5095, Chicago, IL 60637, USA

Keywords

• Anastomotic complications • Anastomotic healing • Anastomotic stricture • Anastomotic leak • Diverting ileostomy • Leak test • Mechanical bowel preparation

Key points

- Anastomotic leak and anastomotic stricture remain persistent and poorly understood phenomena in gastrointestinal surgery.
- Inconsistent definitions and reporting of anastomotic complications lead to difficulty in comparing the results obtained in different studies and the impact of interventions.
- Few interventions have led to a significant decrease in the incidence of anastomotic complications.
- Consistent definitions and improved understanding of the pathophysiology of anastomotic healing complications will lead to interventions that target underlying causes of the complications themselves.

ANASTOMOTIC COMPLICATIONS: A SPECTRUM OF CLINICAL PRESENTATIONS

Anastomotic complications encompass a wide variety of clinical manifestations, ranging from bleeding and stricture to leakage and perforation. Patients may exhibit a broad spectrum of symptoms that can present acutely, in a delayed

The authors have nothing to disclose.

*Corresponding author. *E-mail address*: jalverdy@surgery.bsd.uchicago.edu

0065-3411/16/$ – see front matter
http://dx.doi.org/10.1016/j.yasu.2016.03.011

fashion, or chronically. Anastomotic leakage may present acutely as septic shock or with much less severe symptoms, such as vague discomfort or ileus [1]. Emerging technology has allowed many of the most feared complications of anastomotic surgery, including bleeding and leakage, to be detected early and often to be treated without surgery [2,3]. For example, frequently anastomotic bleeding can be treated with endoscopic clipping or cauterization when the anastomotic site is within the reach of the endoscope [2]. Yet anastomotic complications can be severe and can lead to disability and occasionally death [4]. To understand how to prevent anastomotic complications, an evidence-based approach grounded on an understanding of the pathophysiology and on clinical trials that demonstrate efficacy is needed. This review focuses on two complications: anastomotic stricture and anastomotic leak. Although there is much dogma passed on from generation to generation regarding how to prevent anastomotic complications, the fact remains that, even among high-volume surgeons working in high-volume centers, anastomotic strictures and leaks continue to occur, often with devastating or disabling consequences.

BEYOND TENSION AND ISCHEMIA: PHYSICS IS IMPORTANT, BUT BIOLOGY IS A MAJOR FACTOR IN ANASTOMOTIC HEALING

The classic question asked during morbidity and mortality conferences on anastomotic healing complication is, "Was the anastomosis ischemic or under tension?" No surgeon would willingly leave the operating room with a grossly ischemic anastomosis or with an anastomosis under tension. Yet anastomotic leaks still occur after technically well-constructed anastomoses. This prompts the question of the technique used. Since the turn of the century, surgeons have evaluated multiple technical aspects of anastomotic surgery: everting versus inverting, suture types, 1-layer versus 2-layer techniques, and hand sewing versus stapling [5]. Collectively, these studies have failed to demonstrate significant differences in effectiveness [6]. Most surgeons would agree that the specific technique used, assuming the methods adhere to good surgical principles, is rarely the determinant of optimum healing. Even well-perfused, well-constructed anastomoses under no tension can develop a leak or stricture. Despite surgeons' belief in their own predictive capacities, clinical studies demonstrate that surgeons cannot predict which anastomoses will leak [7]. In the aggregate, studies reveal that although meticulous attention to the tenets of good surgical practice is important and should be rigorously adhered to, some factors that significantly impact anastomotic healing are not fully understood.

Over the past several decades, a primary focus on using engineering principles to reduce complications has driven device improvement and compound development (eg, glues or seam bindings) to promote healing. However, most of these studies are decoupled from the biologic factors that underlie the pathophysiology. Despite iterative improvements in technology, application of these innovations has had little impact on anastomotic stricture and leak rates. Focusing research on the pathobiology of anastomotic complications at the cellular and molecular levels will lead to new insights and solutions for these problematic healing complications.

CURRENT UNDERSTANDING: WE HAVE PROBABILISTIC MEASUREMENTS AND WE NOW NEED DETERMINISTIC ANALYSES

Fortunately for patients and physicians, both anastomotic stricture and anastomotic leak are relatively low incidence events. Because of this, it is difficult to study anastomotic complications and to evaluate preventive measures and their clinical efficacy. A plethora of studies have examined the incidence and risk factors for both stricture and leak; however, few studies explore the biologic underpinnings of these phenomena. Additional retrospective studies and speculative conclusions will not bring us closer to understanding and eliminating these postoperative healing complications because the studies merely demonstrate associations, not the causal mechanism. More basic investigative work using next-generation technology and molecular analysis is needed.

Anastomotic stricture

Retrospective analyses examining anastomotic stricture often focus on the incidence, symptomatic presentation, and subsequent management of the complication itself. There is little understanding of the normal process of intestinal healing and how it becomes altered to lead to stricture formation. This lack of knowledge leaves the clinician wondering why, when the same technique is used, one patient's anastomosis strictures but that of another patient heals without incident. There have been numerous proposed reasons for why anastomoses constrict: ischemia, tension, subacute obstruction, circular staplers, narrow diameter staplers, and the occurrence of an anastomotic leak [8]. Few studies have shed light on why anastomotic strictures occur; they have neglected to include factors outside of the technique and conduct of the operation. The intestinal tract is a complex organ made up of epithelial cells, immune cells, stromal cells, and microbial organisms whose number exceeds the total quantity of human cells. A more holistic understanding of the entire host–microbe interaction throughout the course of surgery and healing is essential to elucidate the pathobiology of both anastomotic leak and stricture. One major obstacle has been the lack of access to observe, sample, and analyze an anastomosis as it heals. If we are to advance our understanding of anastomotic healing, future studies need to be designed that can directly examine and sample anastomotic tissues in humans as they heal.

Anastomotic leak

Clinical studies evaluating causes of anastomotic leak have relied on retrospective analyses that determine associated risk factors. Such studies yield recurring themes generalizable to most complications after surgery, such as poor nutritional status, comorbid diseases, smoking, immunosuppression, advanced tumor grade, hypotension, and blood loss/transfusion [6,9,10]. Studies of the two anatomic regions with the highest anastomotic leak occurrence–the esophagus and rectum–often identify anatomic and physiologic risk factors for leak such as tension, ischemia, and location of the anastomosis [11,12]. However, even in the most carefully conducted multivariate analyses, identified risk factors fall short of explaining why the majority (>75%) of patients with identified risk factors do not leak. Anastomotic leakage is generally a low frequency event, with approximately 10% to 15% incidence in the esophagus and rectum and 5% to 10% elsewhere [1,13]. The rate of leak has remained largely unchanged over the past 25 years. Risk factor analyses may indicate the probability of leak but do not allow us to determine how a given factor contributes to leak pathogenesis. In many cases, even the risk factor calculations fall short of identifying the degree of contribution to leak. For example, if smoking, blood loss, and a low rectal anastomosis all significantly contribute to leak, there is little explanation as to why the majority of low rectal anastomoses in smokers subjected to major blood loss do not leak. Adherence to this theoretic framework has led to the perpetual generation of retrospective analyses both confirming and invalidating various risk factors associated with anastomotic leak. Retrospective reviews have neither advanced our understanding of the pathophysiology nor decreased the overall incidence. Although numerous potential risk factors may contribute to a leak, the mechanisms by which they contribute and the pathogenesis of an anastomotic leak remain poorly understood and need to be studied properly. Even within preclinical models, potential innovations and methods of preventing anastomotic leak are not being evaluated effectively [14,15]. Although interventional studies may provide clinically meaningful and statistically significant evidence for potential mechanisms of anastomotic leak, the conclusions of many of these studies are weakened by the lack of a precise definition of an anastomotic leak.

THE CHALLENGE OF DEFINING ANASTOMOTIC HEALING COMPLICATIONS

Anastomotic stricture

The significance of anastomotic stricture varies highly based on the anatomic location of the stricture and the degree of luminal obstruction. Although high-grade strictures are immediately recognized owing to patient symptoms, low-grade strictures may go completely unidentified. The clinical presentations are also varied in the timing of symptom development after surgery. Early onset obstruction is often attributed to technical error or tissue edema; delayed onset obstruction and stricture formation is felt to be related to chronic inflammation. One of the identified risk factors for stricture includes anastomotic leak, but how this situation differs from a stricture that forms outside of the setting of a leak is unknown [16]. Again, because there are no studies that have defined the natural history of anastomotic healing in real time by directly examining anastomotic tissues over the course of healing (ie, endoscopy, fluid sampling), much of the pathogenesis of stricture formation remains speculative. In addition, because stricture formation is addressed only when there are gross symptoms of obstruction, the technical and physiologic factors that govern its occurrence and outcome remain unknown. Finally, most endoscopic studies in which the anastomosis can be reached and dilated have not attempted to classify strictures in a defined way that might advance our understanding of their pathogenesis and their response to treatment.

Anastomotic leak

Conceptually, anastomotic leak is a single entity: the breakdown or insufficiency of the anastomotic line resulting in spillage of intestinal contents outside of the bowel lumen. However, this physical event may have a variety of anatomic consequences that range from a contained abscess that spontaneously resolves to free spillage into the peritoneal cavity. The clinical manifestations mimic this wide variation: no symptoms, ileus, pain, fever, or fatal sepsis [1]. Given the increasing utilization of low colorectal anastomoses, there is an increased focus on the incidence and pathophysiology of anastomotic leak in this area. Depending on the study and the definition of anastomotic leak used, the observed incidence of colorectal leak varies from almost zero to one-third of low colorectal anastomoses [1,17]. Some studies define leak as extravasation of rectally administered contrast identified on radiographic imaging, whereas others include perianastomotic abscesses identified on CT scan, and still others only include patients who exhibit specific symptoms. Literature reviews have found more than 40 definitions for anastomotic leak in 107 publications [18]. Inconsistencies in definitions of leak among these studies lead to further challenges in comparing and analyzing the results and in reaching meaningful conclusions [19]. Several methods of classification have been proposed to eliminate the variation in definitions, some based on imaging findings and others based on required intervention (Table 1) [1]. To adequately monitor and evaluate preventive interventions, we need to develop a consistent method of defining and classifying anastomotic complications.

SPECIFIC INTERVENTIONS TO PREVENT ANASTOMOTIC HEALING COMPLICATIONS

Anastomotic stricture

In recent years, randomized controlled studies that compare anastomotic technique directly have been abandoned largely, given the perception that the

Table 1
Proposed classification for postoperative anastomotic disruption

Class	Imaging finding
1	Free pelvic or presacral fluid on CT with no extravasation of contrast medium
2A	Postoperative *perianastomotic abscess* with no extravasation of contrast medium
2B	Postoperative *remote intraabdominal abscess* with no extravasation of contrast medium
3	Presacral extravasation of contrast medium
4	Free extravasation of contrast medium

From Caulfield H, Hyman NH. Anastomotic leak after low anterior resection: a spectrum of clinical entities. JAMA Surg 2013;148(2):181; with permission.

technique itself (hand sewing, circular vs linear stapler, 1 layer vs 2 layer) is not a likely factor involved in leak, assuming that good surgical principles are followed. The one exception to this generalization has been the stricture rate with staplers. Circular staplers are reported to have higher stricture rates compared with linear stapling [20,21]. Why this occurs has not yet been addressed in any scientific way. Although there have been multiple speculations using physics and mathematics to explain this observation, little biology has been applied in experimentation. With circular stapling, a granulation 'membrane' often develops that is soft and easy to dilate endoscopically. The smaller the circular diameter of the stapler, the greater the likelihood becomes that this granulation membrane will cause symptoms. As such, it is generally practiced that, to the degree that the bowel lumen allows, larger circular staplers are used, resulting in a lower risk of symptomatic stricture. It is not known why linear staplers do not form strictures at similar rates as circular staplers. The pathophysiology of stricture formation has been assumed to be local inflammation that results in collagen overproduction and poor bowel wall remodeling. Although multiple engineering-based explanations have been offered, there is no credible evidence that these factors are indeed causative mechanistically [22]. Again, a more holistic understanding of stricture formation will require detailed, dynamic studies of anastomotic healing via direct examination with tissue sampling and analysis. To date there has been little enthusiasm for such an approach, because it is perceived to be excessively risky.

Anastomotic leak: hand sewn versus stapling, intraoperative evaluation, and diverting ileostomy

In construction of gastrointestinal anastomoses, it is very important to adhere to the tenets of good surgical practice: optimizing the patient preoperatively, avoiding tension, and ensuring adequate blood supply to the healing anastomosis. Yet even the most conscientious and technically proficient surgeons occasionally experience the complication of an anastomotic leak and its occurrence is most often not anticipated [7]. There is a longstanding debate regarding the superiority of stapled versus hand-sewn anastomoses. For ileocolic anastomoses, a recent Cochrane review suggests that nondiverted stapled anastomoses have a lower anastomotic leak rate as compared with hand sewn anastomoses [23]. However, in difficult to access regions of intestinal tract, such as the esophagus and the rectum, there remains significant debate. For colorectal anastomoses, there is not enough evidence to determine the superiority of one method over another [24]. In the construction of esophageal anastomoses, the numerous methods used to create the connection–stapled, hand sewn, cervical, intrathoracic, end-to-end, side-to-side–have made it difficult to determine superiority of one technique over another; however, there has been a recent trend toward a side-to-side linearly stapled technique [25,26].

Intraoperative evaluation, known as a "leak test," is commonly performed after creation of esophageal, gastric, and rectal anastomoses, where the anastomosis is proximal or distal enough in the bowel to be accessible by endoscopy.

The anastomosis is examined for staple line bleeding or gross abnormalities, and the integrity of the anastomosis is tested by examining for bubbles escaping from the insufflated lumen as the bowel is submerged in liquid. Studies have demonstrated that intraoperative endoscopic assessment of the anastomotic line is safe, feasible, and able to identify gross bleeding and abnormalities. Recent studies suggest that this method may reduce anastomotic complications and no studies have shown any harm in performing the procedure [27–29].

In colorectal anastomoses, many surgeons choose to perform a diverting ileostomy. Although it is known that this procedure and its subsequent reversal carry the independent risks of morbidity and add costs, the impact that diversion has on prevention of anastomotic leak remains unclear [30–32]. The theory behind fecal diversion is that it eliminates the anastomotic stress of bowel wall dilation during healing and that any leakage that occurs has less severe consequences by avoiding large volume fecal spillage. The question that remains is this: does fecal diversion have any impact on prevention of anastomotic leak, or does it simply minimize the severity of the leak? A metaanalysis of randomized controlled trials examining this issue concluded that defunctioning stomas decrease the leak rate as defined by clinical symptoms such as peritonitis, pelvic abscess, rectovaginal fistula, or fecal discharge from a drain; radiologically demonstrated leakage without these clinical sequelae was not included in the analysis [33]. This study and similar studies are plagued by the recurrent issue of lack of a standardized definition of anastomotic leak. If a diverting stoma serves to decrease the severity of leak, many clinically evident leaks may then be categorized only as radiologically detectible leaks, leading to the false conclusion that fecal diversion decreases the anastomotic leak rate.

THE BIOLOGY OF ANASTOMOTIC HEALING

A great deal is known about healing of the external skin after injury, but much less is known about intestinal healing. This is owing to the easy accessibility of the skin as it heals as opposed to the intestinal mucosa. The gastrointestinal tract wall is composed of the surrounding serosa, the smooth muscle-containing muscularis propria, the collagen-containing submucosa providing tensile strength, and the epithelial mucosa and mucous layer that provide the interface with and barrier to the luminal contents. Most important, the intestinal mucosa heals in close contact with the intestinal microbiota, the densest biomass in the body. The process of intestinal healing is characterized by the three phases of inflammation, proliferation, and remodeling. The greatest risk to the anastomosis is thought to occur during the inflammatory phase when collagen proteolytic activity is greatest. After 48 hours, the strength in esophageal anastomoses decreases by almost 40%, whereas colonic anastomoses lose 70% of their initial strength. These strengths increase gradually as fibroblasts and smooth muscle cells synthesize new collagen while the wound is remodeled [34,35]. Disorders of this process may contribute to the development of anastomotic stricture and anastomotic leak. It is known that local inflammation impairs wound healing by prolonging the inflammatory phase and increasing tissue proteases [35]. There is some evidence in rats that a general tissue protease inhibitor has a beneficial effect during uncomplicated anastomotic healing, yet a detrimental effect after colonic obstruction [36]. The process of creating an anastomosis significantly alters the local microbiota at the site of the anastomosis [37]. There is new evidence that the presence of specific bacterial families and low microbial diversity correlates with anastomotic leakage [38]. Although the details remain to be discovered, the bacterial contribution to healing and to the development of anastomotic complications is likely to be significant.

MICROBES: THE COMMON DENOMINATOR OF ANASTOMOTIC COMPLICATIONS?

A role for intestinal microbiota in anastomotic healing has been known for more than 60 years. Much of the evidence for this role has been gathered indirectly, in studies where antibiotics are administered and leak rates are examined in both animals and humans. In the aggregate, these studies provide indisputable evidence that microbes are a contributing factor in the occurrence and outcome of leak. In one of the first studies, Isadore Cohn performed a colon anastomosis in dogs and devascularized the anastomotic segment until it seemed to be grossly ischemic. The dogs were then administered either antibiotics or saline directly onto the anastomotic site by placing a feeding tube just proximal to the anastomosis. Dogs assigned to antibiotics demonstrated normal healing and reversal of the ischemia, whereas dogs administered saline developed leaks and peritonitis [39]. Since then, numerous animal and clinical studies have shown that oral nonabsorbable antibiotics decrease but do not eliminate anastomotic leak rates [40]. These studies provide evidence that microbes play a significant role in anastomotic leak. Yet surgeons do not consistently apply oral, nonabsorbable antibiotics as a prophylactic measure to prevent infectious complications [41]. Potentially, the lack of molecular detail and causative inference needed to implicate the role of microbes in these anastomotic leak studies is the reason that surgeons continue to dismiss microbes as important causative agents.

Our laboratory has been studying anastomotic leak at the molecular level and has provided exciting details that continue to implicate the role of microbes as initiating and causative agents in leak. We have isolated microbial organisms (*Pseudomonas aeruginosa, Enterococcus faecalis*) that, when reintroduced into animals, can cause leak independent of the anastomotic technique itself. The mechanism is a result of the abilities of these bacteria to produce the collagen-degrading enzyme collagenase. Bacteria produce a collagenase that can breakdown intestinal tissues at seven orders of magnitude higher than intestinal tissue collagenase; these bacterial collagenases are therefore much more likely to alter the dynamics of healing than the host tissue enzymes alone [42,43]. We have also shown that these microbial-derived collagenases trigger intestinal tissues to produce matrix metalloproteinase 9, which has an important tissue destructive capacity. Surprisingly, both our studies and the studies of other laboratories have shown that, despite the best efforts to deliver intestinal antisepsis before surgery (purgatives, oral antibiotics, intravenous antibiotics), these collagenase-producing organisms persist at anastomotic sites [44].

Because many pathogenic bacteria remain on anastomotic tissues during the healing process, it remains unclear under which circumstances certain bacteria become 'triggered' to cause a leak. Our studies demonstrate that the role of the normal intestinal microbiome is very important in containing the virulence of these pathogens. When the normal intestinal microbiome refaunates after surgery, it can provide colonization resistance against these blooming pathogens. However, if the normal microbiome cannot repopulate itself after surgery, high-collagenase pathogens with the capacity to adhere to and colonize the anastomotic tissue may then complicate anastomotic healing. Clinical trials are under development to test this hypothesis in a manner that would inform more effective preventative measures than the current approach of undirected antibiotic elimination of all potential pathogens. It should be kept in mind that the current approach to intestinal antisepsis is based on 50-year-old culture data that are not only outdated, but, owing to being culture based, miss many important aspects of the intestinal microbiome such as microbial community structure, phenotype, proteome, and metabolome [45]. A new understanding of the role of the intestinal microbiome in health and disease is likely to have a major influence on how we prepare for bowel anastomoses in future patients.

PREPARING THE BOWEL FOR ANASTOMOTIC SURGERY: HOW WE GOT IT RIGHT, WHY WE STILL HAVE IT WRONG

Our understanding of preparation of the bowel before surgery has evolved over time. In the first one-half of the 20th century, when surgeons recognized that microbes played a role in anastomotic leak and surgical site infection, patients were admitted preoperatively for bowel preparations to decrease the fecal load and eliminate bacteria from the intestinal lumen. Postoperative infection rates decreased from nearly 40% to 20% [46]. Increasingly, the intent was to sterilize the bowel lumen before surgery. This was achieved with oral, nonabsorbable antibiotics and mechanical cleansing, using large-volume osmotic agents, motility agents, and enemas. In the 1990s, with the increasing use of intravenous antibiotics at the beginning of surgery and the shift to outpatient bowel preparations, the oral antibiotic component of the bowel preparation and the need for purgative cleansing were considered unnecessary and often omitted [47,48]. The "bowel preparation," defined as purgative cleansing agents and oral antibiotics, came under attack and many studies demonstrated that it was not needed to prevent infectious related complications. However, resurgence in bowel preparation use has developed owing to persistent infectious complications after colorectal procedures. In addition, patient concerns regarding discomfort and the efficacy of the bowel preparation have been reevaluated recently. Observational and randomized clinical trials have demonstrated that, compared with no bowel preparation, mechanical bowel preparation alone provides no benefit in key infectious outcomes [47]. However, when mechanical bowel preparation is combined with oral and intravenous antibiotic prophylaxis in colorectal surgery, there is a 44% reduction in surgical site infection [40].

Throughout the history of intestinal surgery, surgical prophylaxis has been reflective of the understanding of the intestinal microbiome. In the mid-20th century, the intention was to eliminate all intestinal bacteria before surgery. The integral role that our intestinal microbiome plays in promoting our health and the potential detriments of an imbalanced microbiome were not yet appreciated. Given studies demonstrating improvement in surgical site infection after colorectal surgery–with the use of oral and intravenous antibiotics and mechanical bowel preparation–it is becoming increasingly clear that intestinal bacteria play an important role in infectious complications. We know that mechanical bowel preparation and antibiotic use dramatically alter the intestinal microbiome [49,50]. Yet how to specifically eliminate the 'bad actors' in our microbiome while at the same time preserving our health-promoting microbiota remains a challenge. Surgical prophylaxis has had to evolve with the growing understanding of the anatomic variation of the intestinal microbiome; surgery on the jejunum requires different preparation and prophylaxis from surgery on the sigmoid colon. Increasingly, surgical practice reflects the biologic composition of the various intestinal bacterial ecosystems: no bowel preparation or oral antibiotics for the lower microbial load environment of the small bowel, but mechanical bowel preparation and oral antibiotics for the high microbial load environments of left-sided colon and rectum [41]. The existing body of evidence upon which we are basing our practices is unfortunately weak. There is now an opportunity to understand more completely the impact of present practices and to refine approaches using genetic analysis of the intestinal microbiome at specific regional and spatial niches (ie, anastomotic tissue sites). Such studies will help to elucidate the complex biological processes present on and within anastomotic tissues. This will in turn inform the path forward to a more pathophysiologically based intestinal antisepsis method of containing the harmfulness of certain microbes while preserving the health benefits of others.

SUMMARY: HOW DO WE MOVE FORWARD IN THE PREVENTION OF ANASTOMOTIC HEALING COMPLICATIONS?

The creation of an anastomosis requires meticulous attention to detail, both technically and biologically. Anastomotic healing complications are not as simple as too much or not enough collagen, not as simple as patient risk factors, and not as simple as bad bacterial actors. The development of an anastomotic stricture or leak is a result of the complex interactions of genetics, the microbiome, operative technique, a patient's antecedent health, prior patient exposures, the subsequent hospital course, and exposures ranging from infectious agents to antibiotics. Further research evaluating the relationship and impact these many factors have on the progression of anastomotic healing is needed. To develop a higher resolution pathophysiologic understanding, we need methods to directly and serially examine anastomoses and extract meaningful information. With a further understanding of the dynamic factors that impact healing at the anastomotic site, we will be able to develop more informed and scientifically based interventions and preventive measures. Technological advances are now available to execute these studies in real time and to develop a more complete understanding of the impact of the intestinal ecosystem on anastomotic healing.

References

[1] Caulfield H, Hyman NH. Anastomotic leak after low anterior resection: a spectrum of clinical entities. JAMA Surg 2013;148(2):177–82.
[2] Amr MA, Alzghari MJ, Polites SF, et al. Endoscopy in the early postoperative setting after primary gastrointestinal anastomosis. J Gastrointest Surg 2014;18(11):1911–6.
[3] Lou Z, Zhang W, Yu E, et al. Colonoscopy is the first choice for early postoperative rectal anastomotic bleeding. World J Surg Oncol 2014;12:376.
[4] Konishi T, Watanabe T, Kishimoto J, et al. Risk factors for anastomotic leakage after surgery for colorectal cancer: results of prospective surveillance. J Am Coll Surg 2006;202(3): 439–44.
[5] Chen C. The art of bowel anastomosis. Scand J Surg 2012;101(4):238–40.
[6] Nandakumar G, Stein SL, Michelassi F. Anastomoses of the lower gastrointestinal tract. Nat Rev Gastroenterol Hepatol 2009;6(12):709–16.
[7] Karliczek A, Harlaar NJ, Zeebregts CJ, et al. Surgeons lack predictive accuracy for anastomotic leakage in gastrointestinal surgery. Int J Colorectal Dis 2009;24(5):569–76.
[8] Hashemi M, Novell JR, Lewis AA. Side-to-side stapled anastomosis may delay recurrence in Crohn's disease. Dis Colon Rectum 1998;41(10):1293–6.
[9] Fujita F, Torashima Y, Kuroki T, et al. Risk factors and predictive factors for anastomotic leakage after resection for colorectal cancer: reappraisal of the literature. Surg Today 2014;44(9):1595–602.
[10] Kang CY, Halabi WJ, Chaudhry OO, et al. Risk factors for anastomotic leakage after anterior resection for rectal cancer. JAMA Surg 2013;148(1):65–71.
[11] Morse BC, Simpson JP, Jones YR, et al. Determination of independent predictive factors for anastomotic leak: analysis of 682 intestinal anastomoses. Am J Surg 2013;206(6):950–6.
[12] Markar SR, Arya S, Karthikesalingam A, et al. Technical factors that affect anastomotic integrity following esophagectomy: systematic review and meta-analysis. Ann Surg Oncol 2013;20(13):4274–81.
[13] Turrentine FE, Denlinger CE, Simpson VB, et al. Morbidity, mortality, cost, and survival estimates of gastrointestinal anastomotic leaks. J Am Coll Surg 2015;220(2):195–206.
[14] Oines MN, Krarup PM, Jorgensen LN, et al. Pharmacological interventions for improved colonic anastomotic healing: a meta-analysis. World J Gastroenterol 2014;20(35): 12637–48.
[15] Yauw ST, Wever KE, Hoesseini A, et al. Systematic review of experimental studies on intestinal anastomosis. Br J Surg 2015;102(7):726–34.
[16] Baird R, Laberge J-M, Lévesque D. Anastomotic stricture after esophageal atresia repair: a critical review of recent literature. Eur J Pediatr Surg 2013;23(3):204–13.
[17] Hyman N, Manchester TL, Osler T, et al. Anastomotic leaks after intestinal anastomosis: it's later than you think. Ann Surg 2007;245(2):254–8.
[18] Bruce J, Russell EM, Mollison J, et al. The measurement and monitoring of surgical adverse events. Health Technol Assess 2001;5(22):1–194.
[19] Whistance RN, Forsythe RO, McNair AG, et al. A systematic review of outcome reporting in colorectal cancer surgery. Colorectal Dis 2013;15(10):e548–60.

[20] Castro PM, Ribeiro FP, Rocha Ade F, et al. Hand-sewn versus stapler esophagogastric anastomosis after esophageal resection: systematic review and meta-analysis. Arq Bras Cir Dig 2014;27(3):216–21.

[21] Wang W-P, Gao Q, Wang K-N, et al. A prospective randomized controlled trial of semi-mechanical versus hand-sewn or circular stapled esophagogastrostomy for prevention of anastomotic stricture. World J Surg 2013;37(5):1043–50.

[22] Rice TW. Anastomotic stricture complicating esophagectomy. Thorac Surg Clin 2006;16(1):63–73.

[23] Choy PY, Bissett IP, Docherty JG, et al. Stapled versus handsewn methods for ileocolic anastomoses. Cochrane Database Syst Rev 2011;(9):CD004320.

[24] Neutzling CB, Lustosa SA, Proenca IM, et al. Stapled versus handsewn methods for colorectal anastomosis surgery. Cochrane Database Syst Rev 2012;(2):CD003144.

[25] Allaix ME, Herbella FA, Patti MG. Hybrid trans-thoracic esophagectomy with side-to-side stapled intra-thoracic esophagogastric anastomosis for esophageal cancer. J Gastrointest Surg 2013;17(11):1972–9.

[26] Harustiak T, Pazdro A, Snajdauf M, et al. Anastomotic leak and stricture after hand-sewn versus linear-stapled intrathoracic oesophagogastric anastomosis: single-centre analysis of 415 oesophagectomies. Eur J Cardiothorac Surg 2015; http://dx.doi.org/10.1093/ejcts/ezv395.

[27] Kamal T, Pai A, Velchuru VR, et al. Should anastomotic assessment with flexible sigmoidoscopy be routine following laparoscopic restorative left colorectal resection? Colorectal Dis 2015;17(2):160–4.

[28] Li VK, Wexner SD, Pulido N, et al. Use of routine intraoperative endoscopy in elective laparoscopic colorectal surgery: can it further avoid anastomotic failure? Surg Endosc 2009;23(11):2459–65.

[29] Kanaji S, Ohyama M, Yasuda T, et al. Can the intraoperative leak test prevent postoperative leakage of esophagojejunal anastomosis after total gastrectomy? Surg Today 2015; http://dx.doi.org/10.1007/s00595-015-1243-y.

[30] Leahy J, Schoetz D, Marcello P, et al. What is the risk of clinical anastomotic leak in the diverted colorectal anastomosis? J Gastrointest Surg 2014;18(10):1812–6.

[31] Åkesson O, Syk I, Lindmark G, et al. Morbidity related to defunctioning loop ileostomy in low anterior resection. Int J Colorectal Dis 2012;27(12):1619–23.

[32] Liang MK, Li LT, Avellaneda A, et al. Outcomes and predictors of incisional surgical site infection in stoma reversal. JAMA Surg 2013;148(2):183–9.

[33] Tan WS, Tang CL, Shi L, et al. Meta-analysis of defunctioning stomas in low anterior resection for rectal cancer. Br J Surg 2009;96(5):462–72.

[34] Thornton FJ, Barbul A. Healing in the gastrointestinal tract. Surg Clin North Am 1997;77(3):549–73.

[35] Thompson SK, Chang EY, Jobe BA. Clinical review: healing in gastrointestinal anastomoses, Part I. Microsurgery 2006;26(3):131–6.

[36] Rehn M, Krarup P-M, Christensen LH, et al. GM6001 Increases anastomotic leakage following colonic obstruction possibly by impeding epithelialization. Surg Infect (Larchmt) 2015;16(6):702–8.

[37] Shogan BD, Smith DP, Christley S, et al. Intestinal anastomotic injury alters spatially defined microbiome composition and function. Microbiome 2014;2:35.

[38] van Praagh JB, de Goffau MC, Bakker IS, et al. Intestinal microbiota and anastomotic leakage of stapled colorectal anastomoses: a pilot study. Surg Endosc 2015; http://dx.doi.org/10.1007/s00464-015-4508-z.

[39] Cohn I Jr, Rives JD. Antibiotic protection of colon anastomoses. Ann Surg 1955;141(5):707–17.

[40] Nelson RL, Gladman E, Barbateskovic M. Antimicrobial prophylaxis for colorectal surgery. Cochrane Database Syst Rev 2014;(5):CD001181.

[41] Moghadamyeghaneh Z, Hanna MH, Carmichael JC, et al. Nationwide analysis of outcomes of bowel preparation in colon surgery. J Am Coll Surg 2015;220(5):912–20.

[42] Shogan BD, Belogortseva N, Luong PM, et al. Collagen degradation and MMP9 activation by Enterococcus faecalis contribute to intestinal anastomotic leak. Sci Transl Med 2015;7(286):286ra68.
[43] Olivas AD, Shogan BD, Valuckaite V, et al. Intestinal tissues induce an SNP mutation in Pseudomonas aeruginosa that enhances its virulence: possible role in anastomotic leak. PLoS One 2012;7(8):e44326.
[44] Ohigashi S, Sudo K, Kobayashi D, et al. Significant changes in the intestinal environment after surgery in patients with colorectal cancer. J Gastrointest Surg 2013;17(9):1657–64.
[45] Bartlett JG, Condon RE, Gorbach SL, et al. Veterans administration cooperative study on bowel preparation for elective colorectal operations: impact of oral antibiotic regimen on colonic flora, wound irrigation cultures and bacteriology of septic complications. Ann Surg 1978;188(2):249–54.
[46] Baum ML, Anish DS, Chalmers TC, et al. A survey of clinical trials of antibiotic prophylaxis in colon surgery: evidence against further use of no-treatment controls. N Engl J Med 1981;305(14):795–9.
[47] Güenaga KF, Matos D, Wille-Jørgensen P. Mechanical bowel preparation for elective colorectal surgery. Cochrane Database Syst Rev 2011;(9):CD001544.
[48] Bratzler DW, Houck PM, Richards C, et al. Use of antimicrobial prophylaxis for major surgery: baseline results from the National Surgical Infection Prevention Project. Arch Surg 2005;140(2):174–82.
[49] Harrell L, Wang Y, Antonopoulos D, et al. Standard colonic lavage alters the natural state of mucosal-associated microbiota in the human colon. PLoS One 2012;7(2):e32545.
[50] Ferrer M, Martins dos Santos VAP, Ott SJ, et al. Gut microbiota disturbance during antibiotic therapy: a multi-omic approach. Gut Microbes 2014;5(1):64–70.

Advances in Surgery 50 (2016) 143–155

ADVANCES IN SURGERY

Is Health Services Research Important for Surgeons?

Kristen A. Ban, MD[a,b], Karl Y. Bilimoria, MD, MS[a,c,d,*]

[a]Division of Research and Optimal Patient Care, American College of Surgeons, 633 North St. Clair Street, 22nd Floor, Chicago, IL 60611, USA; [b]Department of Surgery, Loyola University Medical Center, 2160 South 1st Avenue, Maywood, IL 60153, USA; [c]Surgical Outcomes and Quality Improvement Center, Department of Surgery, Feinberg School of Medicine, Northwestern University, 633 North St. Clair Street, 20th Floor, Chicago, IL 60611, USA; [d]Center for Healthcare Studies, Feinberg School of Medicine, Northwestern University, 633 North St. Clair Street, 20th Floor, Chicago, IL 60611, USA

Keywords

• Health services research • Surgical outcomes research • Health care outcomes • Quality improvement

Key points

- Health services research (HSR), also known as surgical outcomes research, is an important and expanding field that examines health care delivery and outcomes in the real world.
- Traditional measures of quality care in HSR include health system structures, processes, and outcomes.
- A variety of research domains exist within HSR to evaluate health care delivery at the patient, hospital, and policy levels.
- Important domains in HSR include comparative effectiveness research, quality improvement, patient safety, and cost-effectiveness analyses.
- With increasing emphasis placed on the provision of economic, high-quality care, surgeons will be well positioned as leaders in their health systems if they are familiar with HSR techniques.

INTRODUCTION

Health services research (HSR) has expanded dramatically in the recent decades, particularly in surgery. Clinicians have access to increasing volumes of data via large national datasets as well as their own institutional records

Disclosure Statement: The authors have nothing to disclose.

*Corresponding author. Surgical Outcomes and Quality Improvement Center, Department of Surgery, Feinberg School of Medicine, Northwestern University, 633 North St. Clair Street, 20th Floor, Chicago, IL 60611. *E-mail address*: k-bilimoria@northwestern.edu

0065-3411/16/$ – see front matter
http://dx.doi.org/10.1016/j.yasu.2016.03.012

via electronic medical record (EMR) systems. These data lend themselves to the analysis of health care delivery and outcomes in the real world, which is the cornerstone of HSR as the authors describe in this article. Further, there is increasing external pressure on surgeons by government and regulatory agencies to provide high-quality, economic care. HSR will allow surgeons to evaluate the care they currently provide, to identify areas for improvement, and, ultimately, to prove that the care they provide is high quality. At the end of the day, all surgeons are invested in providing the best care possible to their individual patients; HSR is a practical, applied field with the same goal.

SIGNIFICANCE OF HEALTH SERVICES RESEARCH FOR SURGEONS

Defining health services research

The goal of medical research is to improve patient care. Numerous fields of study exist within medical research, and each field is uniquely suited to address certain research questions. Basic science research aims to elucidate the underlying biological mechanisms of health and disease. Clinical research aims to determine the best treatment of a given disease by comparing therapies. HSR examines patients in a broader context that includes the physician, the hospital, and the health care system at large.

One of the most widely accepted definitions of HSR was published by the Agency for Healthcare Research and Quality (AHRQ) in 2002:

> Health services research examines how people get access to health care, how much care costs, and what happens to patients as a result of this care. The main goals of health services research are to identify the most effective ways to organize, manage, finance, and deliver high quality care, reduce medical errors, and improve patient safety [1].

HSR within surgery is also referred to as *surgical outcomes research.* This field of study has expanded dramatically in recent years. In the United States, major changes in health policy have occurred at the federal level. Priorities are shifting to value outcomes and patient perception of care; surgeons will be compensated based on their ability or failure to deliver high-quality, economic care. HSR is uniquely suited to evaluate existing care models and to guide future changes and improvements to the health care delivery system.

A framework for health sciences research: structure, process, and outcomes

Donabedian [2] provided the framework for HSR in 1966 in a landmark publication that defined a scheme to measure the quality of care. This framework is composed of 3 elements: structures, processes, and outcomes, as seen in Fig. 1.

Structure

Medical care as experienced by patients is the sum of numerous components organized into a larger health care delivery system. *Structural measures* of a health care system include both the concrete resources in that system, like staff and

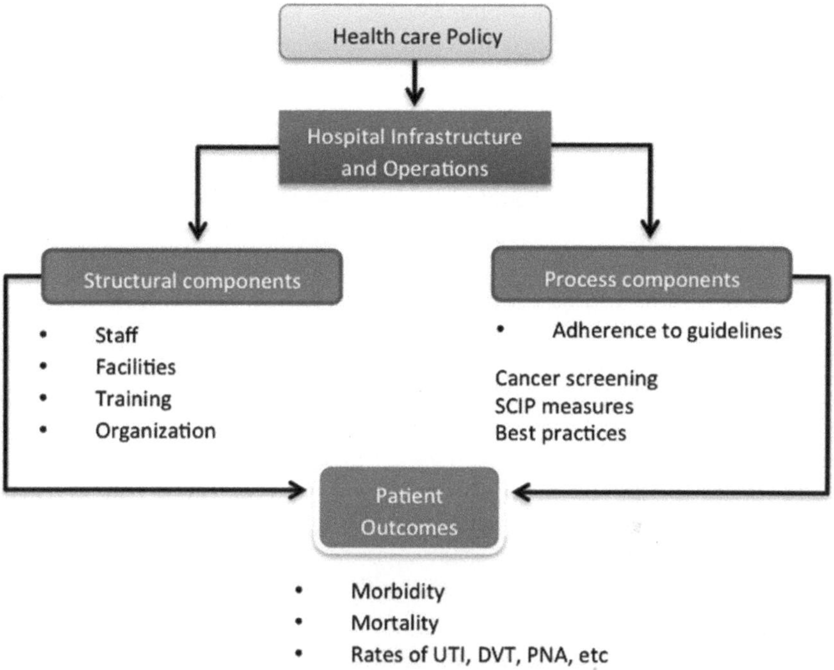

Fig. 1. Donabedian framework for HSR: structure, process, and outcomes. DVT, deep vein thrombosis; PNA, pneumonia; SCIP, Surgical Care Improvement Project; UTI, urinary tract infection.

facilities, as well as the training background and organization of those resources. Examples of structural measures include the number of beds in a hospital, whether a hospital uses an EMR system, nurse to patient ratios, or the proportion of surgeons in a given hospital who are fellowship trained.

Structural components of the health care system are overall assumed to be equal; various accreditation agencies exist to ensure that all physicians broadly possess the same knowledge base and skill set and that all hospitals generally meet the same standards of safety and organization, but variations can and do exist between different hospitals. Significant HSR has examined structural components of health systems and how these components affect outcomes.

Multiple studies have demonstrated worse outcomes as the patient to nurse ratio increases. Aiken and colleagues [3] found that in surgical patients, increased patient to nurse ratios were associated with higher 30-day mortality and increased odds of failure to rescue. The volume-outcome relationship is another well-known example in this domain. Multiple studies have demonstrated that, particularly for highly complex or highly morbid surgeries, high-volume hospitals achieve better outcomes. Kelly and Hellinger [4] were the first to publish this effect in a surgical population, and numerous subsequent studies have validated their findings. Studies linking fellowship training with improved outcomes in complex surgery is an example of research into how physician training impacts outcomes. Porter and colleagues [5] first published that fellowship-trained colorectal surgeons (and surgeons performing a high volume and large total number of colorectal operations) had improved local recurrence and survival for rectal cancer compared with non–fellowship-trained colleagues.

All of the aforementioned studies demonstrated that structural components of a health system impact patient care and outcomes. Further, the findings described earlier broadly affect patient care in the real world. The results of these studies were used to support changes to nursing staffing ratios as well as calls to regionalize care for specific, highly complex surgical oncology patients in centers with both volume and specialty-trained physicians. Unfortunately, some structure measures are difficult to change. For example, some communities and hospitals are unable to support multiple specialized, fellowship-trained surgeons. An individual patient with cancer may not have the resources or desire to travel to a tertiary referral center for a complex cancer operation despite knowing that outcomes are better at high-volume hospitals. These factors should not be ignored, as they contribute to the feasibility of enacting changes within hospitals and health care systems.

Process

Process measures reflect how care is delivered and consist of individual practices or bundles of practices that are applicable to large numbers of patients. Examples of process measures include administration of venous thromboembolism (VTE) prophylaxis, surgical site marking, and compliance with cancer screening guidelines. Process measures are now widely tracked and reported as part of the Surgical Care Improvement Project, which is mandated by the Joint Commission. Among the process measures tracked for surgical patients are administration of prophylactic antibiotics within 1 hour before incision, administration of beta-blocker therapy for patients on a beta-blocker at home, and timely removal of Foley catheters by postoperative day 1 if no surgical contraindications to doing so exist.

The evidence to support routine tracking and adherence to these measures is now widely accepted, but HSR was essential to document that clinicians were failing to adhere to recommended guidelines and to demonstrate that patient outcomes were better when adherence improved. In 1994, Keane and colleagues [6] demonstrated that only 33% of critically ill medical intensive care unit (MICU) patients were receiving VTE prophylaxis despite 87% of patients in the MICU qualifying as high risk for a thromboembolic event. Numerous studies have demonstrated that compliance with VTE prophylaxis guidelines can be improved with smart order sets in EMR systems and that patients experience fewer thromboembolic events when adherence improves [7]. Similar research has supported process measures to reduce catheter-associated urinary tract infections (CAUTIs). These measures include early Foley catheter removal and improved adherence to hand hygiene with Foley catheter insertion. Kachare and colleagues [8] were able to demonstrate an 85% reduction in the total number of CAUTIs over a 1-year period with improved adherence to these measures.

Processes are popular measures to track because they intuitively affect patient care, and many have now been demonstrated to be effective in improving patient outcomes in the literature. Many process measures can be improved regardless of the structural components of a given hospital or health system, making them an attractive means of comparing care delivered within different systems. These measures have proven popular targets for quality improvement (QI) initiatives because they are easily measured and have consequences for patient care and hospital finances. Process measures are now heavily emphasized by organizations like the Joint Commission; but it is important to note that a given measure, for example, VTE prophylaxis administration, must still consider the unique situation of an individual patient. For example, patients with a contraindication to receiving VTE prophylaxis, like a trauma patient with an intracranial bleed, should not receive this intervention. Care must be taken to document these exceptions and account for them because hospital and physician reimbursement will increasingly be linked to compliance with these measures.

Outcomes

Outcomes measures reflect the overall success of a patient's treatment within the health system. In surgery, outcomes measures, including morbidity and mortality, are commonly tracked. Numerous other measures are now commonly included in health services analyses, including length of stay (LOS), readmission rates, and functional status. Outcomes measures can also be more subjective, including patient satisfaction. Within cancer, important outcomes measures include disease-free and overall survival.

Because outcomes measures represent the bottom line in patient care, they are an obvious means of comparing care delivered in different systems and by different physicians. Comparing outcomes measures like mortality among various surgeons in one hospital or from one surgeon against the national average for his or her peers can reveal important deficiencies or highlight an individual who is providing exceptional care. Complex and important databases have been built using outcomes data in an effort to help physicians and hospitals identify areas for improvement. The national Veterans Affairs Surgical Quality Improvement Program (VASQIP), born in the Veterans Affairs (VA) system, aggregates hospital-specific outcomes data across a wide range of procedures and specialties. After the success of VASQIP in achieving improved outcomes at the VA, the American College of Surgeons launched the National Surgical Quality Improvement Program (NSQIP) to help hospitals understand their performance on key outcomes compared with similar hospitals with similar patients. A key component of the NSQIP program is the frequent feedback hospitals receive regarding their performance. Data are reported within 30 days of a patient's admission, and hospitals receive information and models on their performance regularly throughout the year. The tools available via NSQIP continue to evolve and now include on-demand analyses that help clinicians track their outcomes and progress with greater frequency.

One challenge in interpreting outcomes measure data is that an outcome represents the totality of the structures and processes that comprise a health care system. If a given surgeon has suboptimal outcomes, such as morbidity or mortality, what is the underlying cause? Is it poor operative technique by that surgeon? Is it a lack of appropriate or cutting-edge equipment? Is it a shortage of nursing staff on the floor? The causes of a poor outcome are far more complex to tease apart than measuring the outcome itself. Initiatives to improve outcomes can require cumbersome, multidisciplinary action plans. Often, numerous interventions are attempted simultaneously, making it difficult to know which individual changes contributed most to an outcome improvement. Nonetheless, outcomes reflect the totality of patient care and are ultimately the most important measures to improve.

Disciplines within health services research and research modalities

From a practical perspective, HSR can be conducted in 3 different conceptual domains as outlined by Greenberg and colleagues [9], first, at the patient/disease management level, second, at the hospital level, and third, at the health policy level. These domains are interrelated and together comprise the US health care system. A variety of intellectual fields and research modalities exist within each of the aforementioned domains (Fig. 2), all of which are outlined later.

Patient/disease-management level

Evidence to support disease management at the individual patient level has traditionally been provided by clinical research, including randomized clinical trials. These studies can demonstrate safety and efficacy but are designed to minimize all external variables and, thus, occur in a relative vacuum.

HSR at the patient level examines these same interventions applied in real life to a wider range of patients. This discipline, called *comparative effectiveness research*, is defined by the Institute of Medicine as:

> The generation and synthesis of evidence that compares the benefits and harms of alternative methods to prevent, diagnose, treat, and monitor a clinical condition or to improve delivery of care. [10]

The goal of this research is to compare existing health care interventions to determine which work best for a given set of patients. Although not a new field of study, the relevance and potential of this field to answer important clinical questions was highlighted recently: The Patient Protection and Affordable Care Act of 2010 created the Patient-Centered Outcomes Research Institute (PCORI) with a mandate to fund and promote comparative effectiveness research, among other goals. To date, PCORI has awarded more than $300 million in federal grants to support comparative effectiveness research projects.

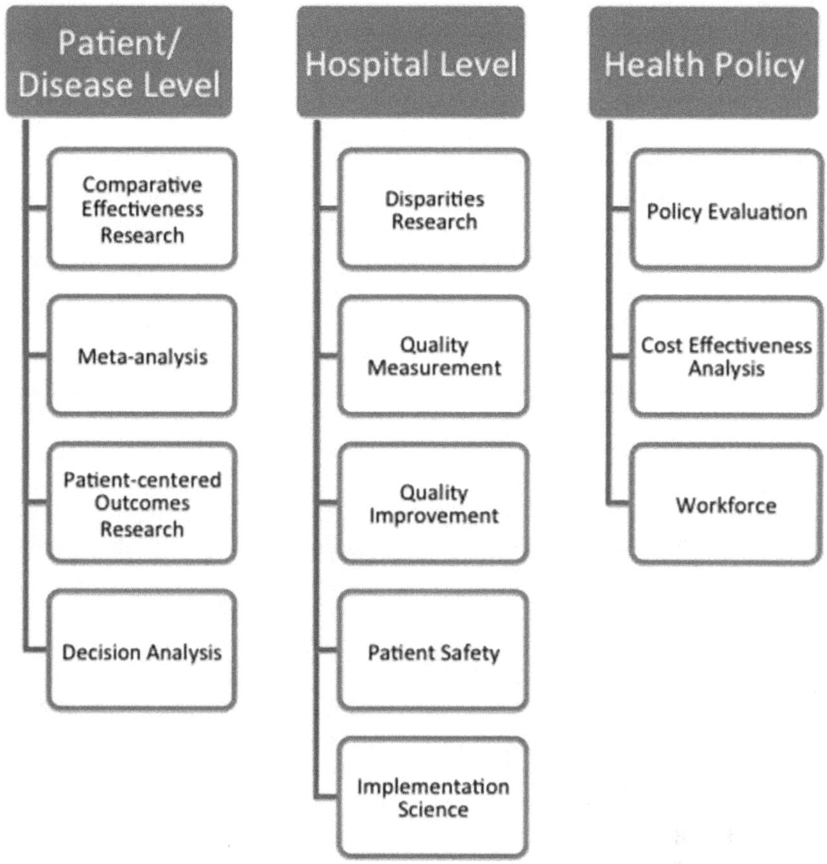

Fig. 2. Domains of HSR.

Comparative effectiveness research can be carried out using retrospective or prospective data collection and a variety of study designs. Retrospective data are usually obtained from large population databases including patient registries, such as Surveillance, Epidemiology, and End Results Program, from clinical databases like NSQIP, or from health insurance or Medicare claims data. Retrospective comparative effectiveness research studies must account for various confounders because they are not randomized and controlled as prospective clinical trials are. This effort is accomplished by approximating randomization to the greatest extent possible and by using statistical tools to correct for confounding variables. These tools include multivariable regression models, propensity scores, and instrumental variables.

Data can also be collected prospectively, and various study designs exist depending on whether or not randomization occurs. Nonrandomized studies are termed *prospective observational cohort studies.* In these studies, patients are grouped according to a given treatment modality or based on shared characteristics. A study in which randomization occurs is termed a *pragmatic clinical trial*, so-called because the study more accurately reflects real-world conditions and includes a broader range of patients. If randomization takes place at the level of the provider or institution (as opposed to among patients or treatment modalities), a study is termed a *cluster randomized trial*.

One example of a prospective cohort study was the Keystone ICU project, which was initiated to examine whether a series of evidence-based interventions could reduce catheter-related bloodstream infections. All hospitals in Michigan with adult intensive care units (ICUs) were invited to participate, so the study was performed on a large scale under real-world conditions. The intervention was education and surveillance regarding a series of evidence-based practices associated with central line insertion and maintenance. Catheter-related bloodstream infections were reduced from a mean rate of 7.7 per 1000 catheter-days to 1.4 at 16 to 18 months after intervention implementation [11]. In addition to benefiting patients, the reduction in infection rates could also be linked to cost savings for the health system at large. By demonstrating a substantial and sustained reduction in infection rates, the Keystone ICU study changed ICU practices on a large scale.

Synthesis of existing data represents another component of patient-level HSR. *Meta-analyses* can combine data from multiple independent, previously conducted trials to better evaluate a given intervention or provide more statistical power to the conclusions drawn by prior, smaller studies. Meta-analyses rely on rigorous statistical methods to combine data from multiple studies, which may be conducted under variable conditions on dissimilar patient cohorts. A meta-analysis is conducted by performing a thorough systematic review of the literature to identify studies for inclusion. Next, the data and results of these studies are evaluated for the presence of heterogeneity. Sensitivity analysis is used to determine if the main findings change based on how data were selected and aggregated in each of the studies. Although complex to perform, meta-analyses can allow researchers to answer a clinical question that would not be feasible to test with a clinical trial.

Patient-centered outcomes research examines how an individual patient experiences health care. Variables measured by this research include quality of life, patient satisfaction, and shared decision-making. This field is rapidly expanding, in part because health care has shifted to place greater importance on patient satisfaction and in part because hospitals increasingly view patients as health care consumers who have a choice in where to seek care. In the 2001 publication *Crossing the Quality Chasm: A New Health System for the 21st Century*, the Institute of Medicine highlighted patient-centered care as one of 6 key components of a high-quality health care system [12]. Many of these outcomes rely on information solicited from patients themselves, usually in the form of a survey or questionnaire; however, alternative means of data collection include structured interviews and focus groups. One challenge in this area of research is the creation of validated scoring rubrics that allow patients to be accurately and reliably compared with each other as well as to themselves over time.

Health-related quality of life (HRQOL) is the primary outcome examined in patient-centered outcomes research. Numerous validated tools exist to measure HRQOL either in general or as it relates to a specific disease. Tools to measure general HRQOL include the Healthy Days Measures, developed by the Centers for Disease Control and Prevention, and the 36-Item Short Form Health Survey (SF-36), which was developed commercially by QualityMetric. With both tools, patients are prompted to answer a series of questions. The Healthy Days Measures calculates a summary index of unhealthy days, which can be physical, mental, or both, whereas the SF-36 generates validated physical and mental health scores. Numerous disease-specific HRQOL measures have been developed for a variety of diseases, including cancer and diabetes. In addition to utilization of preexisting HRQOL measures, methods have been described for the development and validation of new tools.

Numerous other patient-centered outcomes exist, including patient satisfaction, patient preference, decision regret, and shared decision-making. Decision regret is a particularly interesting outcome as we move towards greater patient involvement in the decision-making process. Decision regret has proven challenging to measure, in part because the degree of regret described by a patient frequently changes with time. Shared decision-making is a related concept that describes the current paradigm for medical decisions. Ideally, patients and their providers develop a plan based on both scientific evidence and an individual patient's values, preferences, and priorities. The degree of patient involvement in shared decision-making is the primary outcome that can be measured, and several validated tools exist to this end.

Hospital level

HSR at the hospital level is a dynamic and active field. Clinical and comparative effectiveness research can support what interventions or therapies a given patient should receive, but patients receive care within a hospital or health system. A growing body of research demonstrates a concerning lag between when a given therapy or intervention is supported by the literature and when it is adopted and put into widespread practice. Further, care varies widely among different patient populations, between hospitals, and between regions. These realities demonstrate the importance of a system in the delivery of high-quality care. HSR at the hospital level can elucidate barriers to the implementation of evidence-based practices and can demonstrate how care delivery systems within a hospital can be improved based on cost, safety, and efficiency.

Research by Ghaferi and colleagues [13] in 2009 explored the concept of failure to rescue and the importance of the hospital on patient outcomes. This study demonstrated a similar incidence of postoperative complications between hospitals with the highest and lowest mortality rates for a subset of surgeries. Patient outcomes were driven by the availability and sophistication of hospital resources to mitigate complications rather than variations in individual surgeons' complication rates.

Until recently, most HSR at the hospital/systems level focused on describing differences. *Disparities research* is a field devoted to describing and understanding differences in access to and utilization of care based on socioeconomic or racial differences. Research in this field has demonstrated that differences in delivery of care and outcomes do exist based on race and socioeconomic factors.

Lautner and colleagues [14] recently demonstrated that patients with early stage breast cancer who would normally qualify for breast-conserving therapy were more likely to undergo mastectomy instead if they lacked insurance, were in a lower socioeconomic group, lived far from their hospital, or were located in the South. The investigators suggest that the inability to obtain regular transportation to radiation therapy, required after breast-conserving surgery, is likely a major barrier to patients who might otherwise elect a less radical intervention. Regional differences can highlight both what treatments are advocated by local physicians and also what resources are available in a given area. Areas with a paucity of radiation oncologists may be unable to meet the community needs for radiation therapy following breast-conserving therapy.

Notably, disparities research can highlight the intersection between how care is delivered in a given hospital and the surrounding patient community served in that hospital. Many of the inequalities uncovered by disparities research would require intervention beyond the physician or hospital level. Nonetheless, describing what differences are present is a key first step to addressing them.

As discussed previously, federal initiatives driven by the Patient Protection and Affordable Care Act of 2010 as well as Medicare/Medicaid now emphasize the provision of high-quality patient care. Hospitals must demonstrate that they provide high-quality care in order to receive compensation. But how is high-quality care defined? *Quality measurement* is a field that compares the performance of hospitals and providers against recognized quality standards. Quality can be measured at 3 primary levels, consistent with Donabedian's scheme described earlier. Quality measures apply at the structure level, the process level, and the outcome level. An updated version of this framework also evaluates patient experience measures.

Once quality has been defined, hospitals and health care systems can embark on QI initiatives. These projects often focus on a specific measure of quality. Barriers to improving the chosen measure are identified, and interventions are undertaken to address these barriers. Many hospitals adopt QI methodology developed in industry, such as Lean, Six Sigma, define measure analyze improve control, or others. These programs emphasize a core series of steps and multidisciplinary teams of involved individuals and incorporate an auditing process to assess implementation. Many QI projects set tangible goals so that progress can be easily tracked. A key component of QI is buy-in from the hospital culture and all parties involved in the proposed intervention.

A collaborative in the state of Illinois, the Illinois Surgical Quality Improvement Collaborative (ISQIC), was formed to provide hospitals with support and formal mentorship for QI initiatives and to embark on a collaborative statewide QI project. ISQIC is modeled off prior statewide collaboratives in Michigan, Tennessee, and Florida that promoted networking between hospitals to share experiences, best practices, successes, and challenges in an effort to spur QI. ISQIC hospitals are all enrolled in NSQIP and, thus, report data on demographics, comorbidities, and detailed postoperative outcomes. Key components of ISQIC include identification of key individuals within a given hospital to promote QI initiatives called surgeon champions, mentors for hospitals new to NSQIP with experience leading QI initiatives, formal education in QI methodology, and financial support to improve infrastructure.

QI and its associated methodology is becoming an increasing priority to hospital administrators and regulatory bodies. Surgeons with expertise in QI are well positioned to be leaders within their hospitals on such initiatives. Key components to success in undertaking QI endeavors include formal education in QI methodology, mentorship from experienced QI leaders or via a collaborative, and buy-in from hospital administration and relevant stakeholders.

Patient safety research is a field that aims to define and explore the root causes of errors in the medical field. The importance of this field was highlighted by the infamous *To Err Is Human* report, released by the Institute of Medicine in 1999, that estimated almost 100,000 deaths annually related to medical errors [15]. Subsequent studies have estimated double to triple this number [16]. It is clear that medical errors represent a financial burden on the medical system and, more importantly, are responsible for adverse patient outcomes. As a field characterized by invasive, high-risk procedures that rely on both advanced technology and numerous specialized providers, surgery offers numerous opportunities for improvements in patient safety.

Patient safety research led to the development of the World Health Organization's Safe Surgery Checklist, a series of mandatory steps to be completed before and after every surgery. The goals of the checklist are to reduce errors in the operating room and to improve communication between team members. In a study published in *the New England Journal of Medicine* in 2009, Haynes and colleagues [17] demonstrated that the use of this checklist improved morbidity and mortality in a diverse group of hospitals across the world.

Implementation science is a field that often overlaps with patient safety and QI. Research in this area studies how to promote the widespread adoption of new practices in a given health care system. These practices are usually evidence based and can be identified as areas for improvement via QI or patient safety initiatives. Implementation science also examines the obstacles facing implementation of new research, explores new approaches to health care programming, and examines the impact of a given intervention within a health care system. A key component of implementation science is the construction of formal models to guide implementation efforts and an emphasis on achieving results that are reproducible across a wide range of hospitals and systems.

Health policy level

Numerous high-level factors influence medical care, namely, health care policy and regulation, payer organizations, such as insurance companies and Medicare, professional organizations that publish guidelines, and the health care workforce at large. Although all of these components have the potential to exert enormous influence on how care is provided, very little research focuses on how changes at this upper level affect care. It is largely assumed that policies enacted at the highest level of the system must be based on solid evidence and research; however, this is not always the case. Additionally, every intervention can have unintended consequences.

Evaluation of health care policy can help elucidate whether legislation enacted at the local or federal level achieves the intended goal or whether it results in unintended consequences. Interestingly, health policy changes can sometimes precede robust, validated research to support the measures that are enacted. One challenge facing this field is the constant addition of new policies. The effects of a new policy can also be delayed, resulting in a lag between when a policy is enacted and when a change can be measured.

A recent study by Rajaram and colleagues [18] examined the implications of the new Centers for Medicare and Medicaid Services (CMS) Hospital-Acquired Condition Reduction Program, which reduced payments to the lowest-performing hospitals. Paradoxically, hospitals penalized under this program were found to have higher rates of quality accreditation, offered more advanced services, were major teaching institutions, and performed better on other process and outcome measures than hospitals that were not penalized. This important study illuminated potential problems with the criteria used by CMS to determine reimbursement.

Cost-effectiveness research is an important field in HSR that evaluates the financial implications of a specific treatment or practice in the health care system. Many studies have examined how these various practices affect LOS, which can be easily linked to cost. Enhanced recovery protocols represent a promising development in gastrointestinal surgery. These protocols can be labor intensive to enact, but studies have demonstrated that they result in a decreased LOS. Surgeons can leverage the results of these HSR studies to convince hospital administrations that the costs associated with implementing enhanced recovery protocols will ultimately pay dividends to the health care system in addition to improving patient outcomes.

SUMMARY

HSR has expanded dramatically in recent years, particularly in surgery. As a procedural specialty that relies on complex, highly trained teams of providers, surgery is an ideal medium to examine structure and process components of health systems. Further, patient outcomes and cost can feasibly be measured. At the regulatory and federal levels, priorities are changing to prioritize value, outcomes, and patient perception of care. HSR is uniquely suited to evaluate existing care models and to guide future improvements. Surgeons will remain leaders in their health care systems if they understand and are actively involved in these research efforts as well as QI initiatives.

References

[1] Agency for Healthcare Research and Quality. What is health services research? Rockville, MD: Agency for Healthcare Research and Quality; 2002.
[2] Donabedian A. Evaluating the quality of medical care. Milbank Mem Fund Q 1966;44(3 Suppl):166–206.
[3] Aiken LH, Clarke SP, Sloane DM, et al. Hospital nurse staffing and patient mortality, nurse burnout, and job dissatisfaction. JAMA 2002;288(16):1987–93.
[4] Kelly JV, Hellinger FJ. Physician and hospital factors associated with mortality of surgical patients. Med Care 1986;24(9):785–800.
[5] Porter GA, Soskolne CL, Yakimets WW, et al. Surgeon-related factors and outcome in rectal cancer. Ann Surg 1998;227(2):157–67.
[6] Keane MG, Ingenito EP, Goldhaber SZ. Utilization of venous thromboembolism prophylaxis in the medical intensive care unit. Chest 1994;106(1):13–4.
[7] Zeidan AM, Streiff MB, Lau BD, et al. Impact of a venous thromboembolism prophylaxis "smart order set": improved compliance, fewer events. Am J Hematol 2013;88(7):545–9.
[8] Kachare SD, Sanders C, Myatt K, et al. Toward eliminating catheter-associated urinary tract infections in an academic health center. J Surg Res 2014;192(2):280–5.
[9] Chen HK, Kao LS, editors. Success in academic surgery. London: Springer-Verlag London Limited; 2012.
[10] Council NR. Initial national priorities for comparative effectiveness research. Washington, DC: The National Academies Press; 2009.
[11] Pronovost P, Needham D, Berenholtz S, et al. An intervention to decrease catheter-related bloodstream infections in the ICU. N Engl J Med 2006;355(26):2725–32.
[12] Institute of Medicine (IOM). Crossing the quality chasm: a new health system for the 21st century. Washington, DC: National Academy Press; 2001.
[13] Ghaferi AA, Birkmeyer JD, Dimick JB. Complications, failure to rescue, and mortality with major inpatient surgery in Medicare patients. Ann Surg 2009;250(6):1029–34.
[14] Lautner M, Lin H, Shen Y, et al. Disparities in the use of breast-conserving therapy among patients with early-stage breast cancer. JAMA Surg 2015;150(8):778–86.
[15] Institute of Medicine (IOM). To err is human: building a safer health system. In: Kohn LT, Corrigan JM, Dinaldson MS, editors. Washington, DC: National Academy Press; 2000. p. 1.
[16] James JT. A new, evidence-based estimate of patient harms associated with hospital care. J Patient Saf 2013;9(3):122–8.
[17] Haynes AB, Weiser TG, Berry WR, et al, Safe Surgery Saves Lives Study Group. A surgical safety checklist to reduce morbidity and mortality in a global population. N Engl J Med 2009;360(5):491–9.
[18] Rajaram R, Chung JW, Kinnier CV, et al. Hospital characteristics associated with penalties in the Centers for Medicare & Medicaid Services Hospital-Acquired Condition Reduction Program. JAMA 2015;314(4):375–83.

Advances in Surgery 50 (2016) 157–171

ADVANCES IN SURGERY

Robotic Colorectal Surgery

Advance or Expense?

Rahila Essani, MD[1], Roberto Bergamaschi, MD, PhD, FRCS*

Division of Colon & Rectal Surgery, State University of New York, Nichols Road, Stony Brook, NY 11794-819, USA

Keywords

• Robotic colorectal surgery • Colorectal surgery • Laparoscopic colorectal surgery • Hand-sewn ileocolic anastomoses • Rectal cancer • Circumferential resection margin • Quality of total mesolectal excision

Key points

- Robotic colorectal surgery offers most of the advantages of laparoscopy with additional increased features, particularly in colorectal surgery.
- The current disadvantages of robotic colorectal surgery include high cost, large size, complex setup, limited range of surgical field, and the lack of haptic interface.
- The cost may make up for the clinical advantages it provides in terms of improved circumferential resection margin in rectal cancer surgery as well as the ability to facilitate intracorporeal hand-sewn bowel anastomosing.

INTRODUCTION

The introduction of robotic surgery has been slow, and the use of robots to assist in performing surgical tasks has been developing over the past 20 years. Colorectal surgery in the era of laparoscopy presents a few unique challenges, such as difficulty of operating in the confines of a narrow bony pelvis, particularly in obese men with radiated low rectal cancer.

Furthermore, performing intracorporeal ileocolic anastomosis laparoscopically is technically difficult and has never been broadly implemented with

The authors have nothing to disclose.

[1]Present address: 116 Vista Lane, Georgetown, TX 78633.

*Corresponding author. Division of Colon & Rectal Surgery, State University of New York, Health Science Center T18, Suite 046B, Stony Brook, NY 11794-8191. *E-mail address:* rcmbergamaschi@gmail.com

0065-3411/16/$ – see front matter
http://dx.doi.org/10.1016/j.yasu.2016.04.001

the exception of a few centers. Similarly, the urologic community has embraced robotic surgery to circumvent the difficulties of laparoscopic hand-sewn urethra-vesical anastomosis. Robots are defined as "a machine capable of automatically carrying out a complex series of movements, especially one which is programmable" (Oxford Dictionary). Thomas Sheridan, the "Father of automation and robotics" from the Massachusetts Institute of Technology used automation and robotics interchangeably: "Automation includes all those things that computers and machines can do to perform tasks for people faster, more accurately, and more efficiently (in terms of time, resources, and human labor) than if they were done directly by people." Robots have been used in many industries such as manufacturing cars, planes, and computers for many decades. Robots do not tire and operate at a level of precision and accuracy with dedicated motions scalable in speed and force unreachable for human beings [1]. Although this technology is not new to the operating room, there are several factors that differentiate the adoption process of current robots and their use from the other surgical technologies. Currently, there is only one dominant company that produces and sells a surgical robot. Both purchasing and operation of these robots is expensive, making the robotic platform unaffordable for most hospitals. The cost of the robot is around $1.65 to $2 million; disposable robotic instruments cost $2000 each as well as the yearly maintenance cost $150,000 [2]. Furthermore, the various vessel sealers and staplers used widely in laparoscopic surgery are incompatible with the current robot platform, leading to the need to either invest in these instruments or have an assistant by the patient's side to perform this task. In addition, because of the depreciation over 5 years with 150 procedures a year, the robotic system is 2.7 times more expensive [3]. It has been highlighted that caution needs to be taken when interpreting costs because it may differ significantly between hospitals [4]. Different health care systems between countries will also have an impact on costs. However, maximizing the use of the robot by different surgical subspecialties within the hospital might increase savings to the overall running costs. A bias of all of the cost studies is that all cost assumptions were largely based on operating time and depreciation of the robotic system calculation [4]. Despite the increase in cost, robotic systems offer most advantages of laparoscopic surgery with additional features particularly useful in colorectal surgery.

OPERATING IN CONFINES OF NARROW BONY PELVIS

Robotic rectal surgery has potential advantages over laparoscopic rectal surgery: increased degree of freedom (DOF) of the operating instruments, surgeon motion filter for tremor-free surgery, high-definition 3-dimensional (3D) images, and surgeon-controlled camera on a stable platform. One important limitation of laparoscopic surgery is the loss of 2 of the 6 movements of the surgeon's hands. In fact, there are concerns that laparoscopic proctectomy may decrease the width of the radial margin as a result of restricting movements of the surgeon's hand when performing proctectomy for cancer in a narrow pelvis. Robotic surgery, however, allows the surgeon to retain all 6 movements by using wristed instruments (Fig. 1). The value of these 6 movements becomes evident in procedures performed within a confined space, such as the pelvis. Another aspect of both laparoscopic and robotic techniques that should be borne in mind is the changes in tactile sensation [5]. However, tactile feedback is only reduced in laparoscopic surgery, whereas it is completely abolished in robotic surgery. Accordingly, concerns persist about the impact that robotic proctectomy may have on the quality of total mesorectal excision (TME) due to its complete loss of tactile feedback [6].

There are various different techniques of robotic-assisted surgery for rectal cancer, such as the conventional hybrid, which includes laparoscopic mobilization of the splenic flexure as the first step [7]. Unlike the conventional hybrid, the reverse hybrid is a modified procedure where robotic proctectomy is performed as the first operative step [8]. Other robotic-assisted surgery for rectal cancer has also been described, including hand-assisted laparoscopy with robotic proctectomy [8], robotic transanal minimally invasive surgery (TAMIS) [9] (Fig. 2), as well as natural orifice specimen extraction with hand-sewn anastomosis [10].

IMPACT OF CONING ON CIRCUMFERENTIAL RESECTION MARGIN IN RECTAL CANCER

Circumferential resection margin (CRM) has been shown to be an independent predictor of local recurrence in rectal cancer surgery. There are currently two definitions in the literature for uninvolved CRM: greater than 1 mm and greater than 2 mm [11]. In 2002, it was reported that local recurrence and liver metastases were significantly decreased in nonradiated patients provided that CRM was greater than 2 mm rather than less than 2 mm. Two concerns with laparoscopic low anterior and abdominoperineal resection are adequate CRM and a cylinder without a waist, respectively [12]. The potential benefit of robotic proctectomy is its ability to achieve an increased rate of uninvolved CRM [6,13–15], the result of the robot's wristed instrument's ability to overcome the fulcrum effect, which is a major limitation of laparoscopic surgery. In fact, the trocars placed through the abdominal wall do not allow movements other than spinning the straight laparoscopic instrument around the abdominal wall fulcrum. It is intuitive that the range of such movement is limited in the confined space of a narrow pelvis. Data from preoperative MRI pelvimetry suggest that the interspinous distance can be a predictive factor for involved CRM [15]. Therefore, robotic proctectomy holds the potential benefit of increasing the feasibility of robotic proctectomy in subgroups of patients with unfavorable anatomy [16], thereby decreasing conversion to laparotomy [17–19]. In fact, a recent large administrative database indicated that robotic proctectomy is most commonly performed in male patients [20].

A disadvantage of robotic proctectomy is its possible negative impact on the quality of TME due to the absence of tactile feedback. Although there is limited literature dedicated to assessing the quality of TME in robotic proctectomy

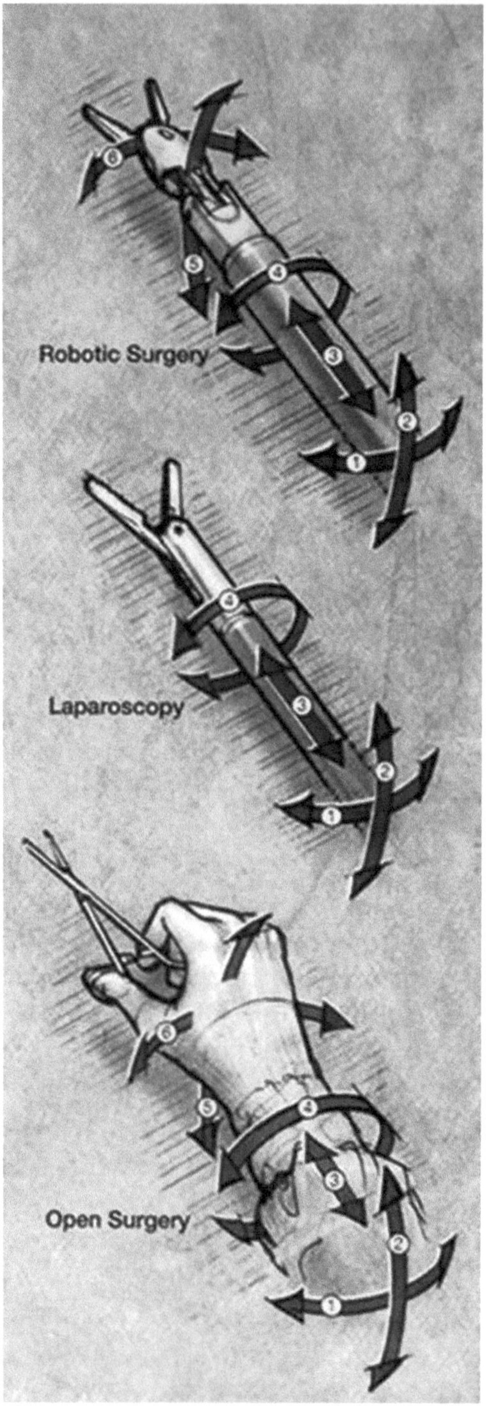

Fig. 1. Robotic surgery allows the surgeon to retain all 6 movements by using wristed instruments.

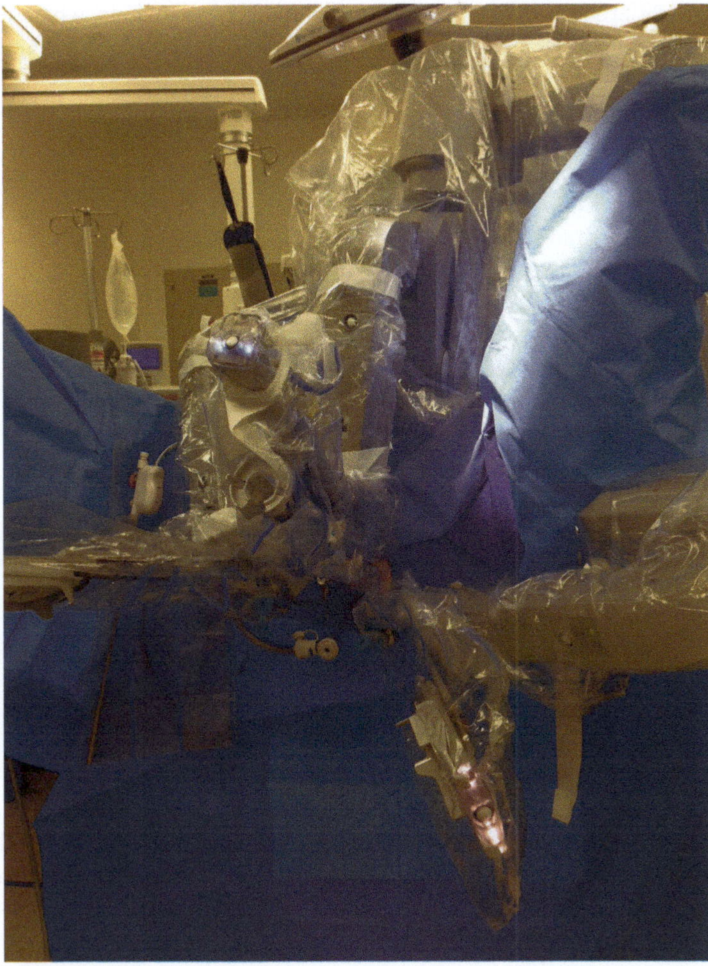

Fig. 2. Robotic TAMIS for rectal cancer.

[6,15,21,22], MRI pelvimetry data suggest that interspinous distance and obstetric conjugate are predictive factors for TME quality [15]. It is still controversial whether high body mass index (BMI) is a predictive factor for decreased TME quality [23,24].

No differences in rates of intraoperative complications were found in a meta-analysis and a systematic review comparing robotic to laparoscopic surgery for rectal cancer [25,26]. Despite a lack of studies on the impact of high BMI on complication rates of robotic-assisted surgery for rectal cancer, the laparoscopic surgery literature reported higher conversion to laparotomy [24], and longer operating time [27]. A recent systematic review and a large administrative database concurred with 3 previous systematic reviews in that there are no significant differences in rates of postoperative complications when robotic-assisted proctectomy is compared with its laparoscopic counterpart [17,18,20,25,26]. However, another recent large administrative database has indicated that robotic-assisted proctectomy performed by low-volume surgeons may actually result in increased rates of postoperative complications when compared with the rates associated with high-volume expert surgeons performing the same operation [28].

The results of 2 randomized trials [29,30] comparing laparoscopic to conventional rectal cancer surgery were published in 2015. These 2 trials differ on the CRM data with the COLOR II [29] reporting lower CRM positivity in the laparoscopic arm as opposed to ACOSOG trial [30], which describes higher CRM positivity in the laparoscopic arm. Regardless, a return to conventional surgery for rectal cancer seems highly unlikely based on the above-mentioned controversy, which may actually indirectly open the way to robotic surgery for rectal cancer.

SUTURING AND KNOT-TYING

Suturing, one of the main tasks in advanced laparoscopic surgery, substantially differs from its open counterpart. The narrower the operative field is, the more relevant the technical drawbacks become. Laparoscopic instruments are usually limited to 4 (5 with instrument actuation) DOF, including pitch, jaw rotation, extraction/insertion, plus the actuation of the instrument. They lack extension and flexion of the wrist. In addition, translational movements are restricted by a pivot point: the trocar position. This restriction results in a fulcrum effect, which may be compared with the picture orientation in a pinhole camera. In addition, most of the laparoscopic instrument is outside the abdomen, which, because of the leverage effect, leads to a considerable and variable motion scaling effect [31], and 2-dimensional systems challenge the surgeon's 3D imagination. The lack of shadows, stereovision, and movement parallax challenge the surgeon to precisely estimate spatial distance, position, and movements and deteriorates his eye-hand coordination [32]. Moreover, the posture of the surgeon can be extremely unergonomic because of placement requirements of the trocars. Also, the discrepancy between the position of the video monitor and the working field usually results in a twisted posture of the surgeon [33]. All of these factors require a higher muscle effort compared with the open surgical procedure [34,35] and may lead to increased wrist and joint forces, resulting in painful injuries, respectively, with long-term sequelae such as disc prolapse or knee arthropathia [31,33–35]. The surgeon also has to train hand-eye coordination with respect to the transfer between video view and instrument movement, resulting in a considerable mental workload [36].

Robotic systems provide corresponding solutions as 3D view, intuitive motion, additional DOF, tremor filtration, and longer instruments that provide full 7 DOF due to an extension/flexion and tilt action of the tip [37–39]. In general, robotic surgical systems have the ability to compensate the most important drawbacks of laparoscopy. Performance studies have shown that the needle can be grabbed and handled more easily due to the above-mentioned advantages of the robotic system. The additional DOF also allow the intuitive motion and manipulation of the needle. These benefits increase the dexterity and accuracy of grabbing the needle at the right position, and DOF allow the tip of needle to be passed easily passed through the tissue, which is particularly important when performing rectopexy. The robotic system also allows easy tying, like in hand-sewn anastomoses, due to the endowrist instrument tip. However, because of the lack of haptic feedback and the power of the instrument, it is possible to bend the needle, and there is an increased risk of damaging threads, especially when performed by inexperienced users.

For colorectal dissection, the enhanced suturing capabilities have been reported by several investigators but also the longer operative times [40] and the need to dock/de-dock the robot several times during the operation, when changing abdominal quadrants; therefore, many robotic-assisted colon resections are hybrid procedures. Procedures such as minimally invasive rectopexy and intracorporeal ileocolic anastomosis benefit from robotic facilitation of suturing with intracorporeal knot tying [41]. Preservation and improvement of function in pelvic floor disorder surgery require meticulous dissection and preservation of the autonomic nerve supply by careful dissection. Robotic assistance can be advantageous particularly in the narrow pelvic space because of the high-definition 3D stereoscopic and magnified vision, instruments with multiple DOF, improved ergonomics, motion scaling, and tremor-free movements [42,43]. Compared with laparoscopy, robotic surgery could provide enhanced dexterity with decreased risk of nerve damage, safer and more precise movements in the pelvis, easier intracorporeal suturing, and less conversions [44].

HAND-SEWN ILEOCOLIC ANASTOMOSES

The potential benefit of robotic assistance in right colectomy consists of the increased feasibility of hand-sewn intracorporeal anastomosis (Fig. 3) [45,46], which is particularly advantageous in patients with high BMI with a very thick abdominal wall. Intracorporeal ileocolic anastomoses have the following advantages as compared with the totally stapled counterpart:

1. There is no need for mobilization of the transverse colon to reach the abdominal wall, allowing anastomosing through a limited laparotomy as in the laparoscopic-assisted technique.
2. Anastomosing away from the abdominal wall could reduce rates of superficial and/or deep surgical site infection (SSI).
3. Because the abdominal cavity is not manipulated by the surgeon's hands, the formation of adhesions and rates of adhesive small bowel obstruction could be reduced.
4. A 50% reduction of the extraction site incision length could lead to clinical benefits, such as less pain and lower rates of superficial and/or deep SSIs.
5. Laparoscopic visualization during the creation of the anastomosis could reduce unrecognized twisting of the terminal ileum mesentery [47].

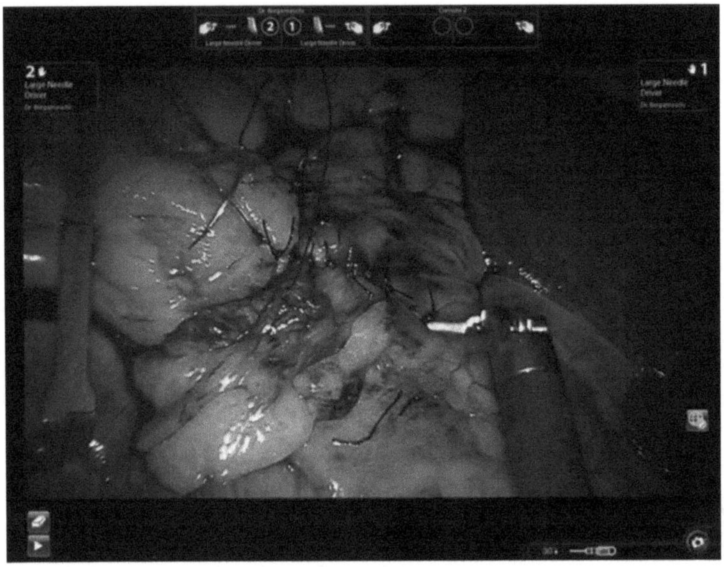

Fig. 3. Increased feasibility of hand-sewn intracorporeal anastomosis with robotic-assistance in right colectomy.

Moreover, the totally stapled intracorporeal ileocolic anastomoses [48] have the following potential disadvantages:

1. Compared with their hand-sewn inverted counterpart, everted anastomoses may increase the risk of complications.
2. They require use of a 60-mm-long cartridge for side-to-side anastomosing because stapling enterocolotomy inevitably excises tissue and thereby reduces the final size of the anastomosis.
3. They most likely require an additional port if performed on the transverse colon.
4. They do not obviate intracorporeal suturing because stay stitches are required to ensure safe stapler application on the enterocolotomy.
5. They may require multiple firings depending on the size of the enterocolotomy or whether the previous stapled line is being excised.
6. They may lead to higher direct cost because of the requirement of additional cartridges.

Another application of intracorporeal suturing is in patients with ileocolic resection for terminal ileitis. The principle of Crohn disease treatment is preserving small bowel length by strictureplasty, which has been shown to have good outcomes in terms of complications and recurrence [49]. However, laparoscopic strictureplasty is technically challenging even in the hands of advanced laparoscopic surgeons [50] unless the suturing is performed extracorporeally. Because of the dexterity and ease of the 360° motion of the robot, it is technically easier to perform a robotic-assisted strictureplasty [51]. In conclusion, these advantages can be further used for cases where intracorporeal anastomosis would be important, such as in patients with a high BMI, or in thickened fore-shortened mesentery in Crohn disease, whereby extracorporeal anastomosis would be difficult after laparoscopic mobilization.

RECTOPEXY

Described operations for rectal prolapse are myriad and include well-recognized eponymous associations. The literature on this rather uncommon condition has stimulated a disproportionate number of diverse operations, which include those directed at narrowing the anal orifice, obliteration of the pouch of Douglas, restoration of the pelvic floor, bowel resection by any number of routes, and suspension by various means (such as suture, mesh). The dilemma of whether suspending the rectum plays a role in containing prolapse recurrence was solved by a randomized controlled trial [52] showing that rectopexy decreases recurrence when randomized to no rectopexy. Previously, some surgeons would argue that scarring after mobilization would work as good as a rectopexy. There is limited literature on robotic rectopexy for rectal prolapse. Several studies reported significantly longer operative times for robotic rectopexy as compared with laparoscopic rectopexy [42,53,54]. Mean operative time ranged from 152 to 221 minutes as compared with a range of 113 to 163 minutes, respectively. However, other studies reported no such differences [55,56]. It is highly unlikely the functional results of robotic rectopexy are any different from the laparoscopic counterpart [57]. Although earlier reports showed similar functional outcomes [42,58], more recent studies claim significantly improved obstructed defecation scores, improved digitation, and straining following robotic rectopexy [54]. In terms of recurrence rates after surgery, one study reported significantly higher rates 2 years after robotic rectopexy [58]. Nonetheless, all papers shared the limitations of small sample size and short-term follow-up.

In recent years, one also encounters publications that use the adjective ventral to indicate that a mesh was sutured to the posterior vaginal wall (and anterior rectal wall), yet was suspended posteriorly to the sacrum [59]. The erosion of the synthetic mesh resulting in perforation of the posterior vaginal wall is a devastating complication. This complication is unacceptable because the literature offers data suggesting that the addition of a mesh does not decrease recurrence rates when compared with suture rectopexy [60]. Furthermore, mesh fixation to the promontory with metal tacks [42,56] is not an acceptable substitute for suturing and most likely reflects inadequate training in minimally invasive suturing.

TRANSANAL MINIMALLY INVASIVE SURGERY

Traditionally, benign neoplasia and early-stage rectal cancers located in the rectum were managed with transanal excision (TAE) using a conventional (Parks) retractor. This approach has important limitations, because exposure and visibility within the rectal lumen curtail the surgeon's ability to perform high-quality oncologic excisions. Furthermore, lesions in the proximal two-thirds of the rectum cannot be approached transanally with Parks TAE, leaving major transabdominal resections as the only alternative for these patients. Robotic TAMIS surgery is one of the developments that has arisen from the natural evolution of transanal endoscopic microsurgery. The benefit of robotic TAMIS is in overcoming the technical limitations of TAMIS using lap instruments involving improved dexterity in cases of difficult manipulation and suturing (Fig. 4). All the above features are ideal for working in a confined space, where conflict between instruments and optics is otherwise common and can hamper operative flow and accuracy [61]. The literature on robotic TAMIS is limited, representing cadaver studies [62] and case reports without comparisons [55,63].

TRANSANAL TOTAL MESORECTAL EXCISION

A transanal approach to rectal cancer is not novel as it precedes the era of laparotomy [64]. Obese male patients with tumors of the distal third of the rectum constitute a well-known challenge to low anterior resection with TME. The meticulous dissection that can be achieved from below while adhering to the concept of an oncologically sound TME seems to have benefits in comparison with a pure minimally invasive approach from above; therefore, transanal total mesorectal excision (taTME) was the natural next step forward. Although endoluminal TAMIS fueled the initial development, it is currently the extraluminal approaches for TAMIS, in particular taTME that is the catalyst for ongoing innovation.

The challenge posed by low rectal cancer is to be distinguished from the subject of tumors located near the dentate line, where transanal intersphincteric resection (ISR) and coloanal anastomosis may be indicated. One of the concerns is, unlike ISR, transanal TME entails a rectal transection inside the pelvis and thereby mandates serious scrutiny due to the potentially increased risk of

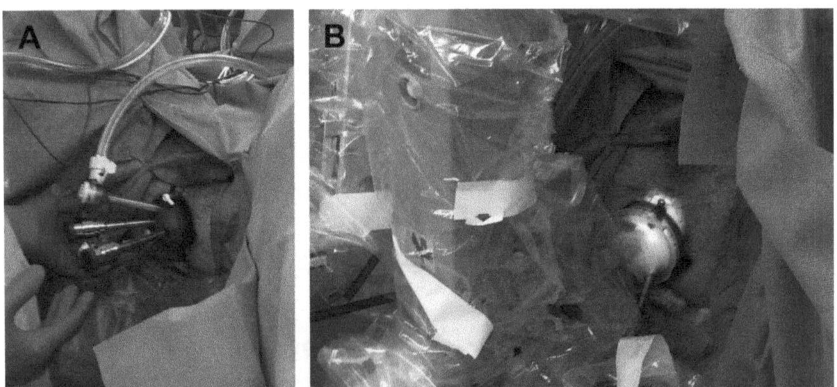

Fig. 4. Robotic TAMIS is overcoming the technical limitations of TAMIS using lap instruments involving improved dexterity in cases of difficult manipulation and suturing. (*A*) Single-port device with robotic ports. (*B*) Si robot docked.

local recurrence [65]. Nonetheless, it has been recently claimed that transanal TME offers at least 3 "oncological advantages" [66]:

1. Longer distal resection margin [67],
2. Decreased rate of involved CRM [68],
3. Improved quality of TME [69].

A recent study claimed longer distal resection margin following transanal TME (2.8 ± 1.8 vs 1.7 ± 1.3 cm; $P<.01$). This result was likely obtained by performing unnecessary low rectal transection with coloanal anastomoses on patients with cancer of the mid rectum. As is understood, a 1.7-cm distal margin would have been adequate even in the case of nonsolid tumors with poor differentiation.

It seems appropriate to distinguish genuine concern for involved CRM and incomplete TME quality in obese men undergoing transabdominal TME for low rectal cancer from the extrapolation of transanal TME to all patients with resectable rectal cancer. The former should abide by the established rules of innovation [69], which include neither nonvalidated metrics [70] nor the bias of historical control studies [71]. Conversely, unwarranted transanal TME might at best inflict a repaired rectal perforation and an unnecessary coloanal anastomosis on patients with resectable cancer of the higher rectum.

SUMMARY

Robotic colorectal surgery offers most of the advantages of laparoscopy with additional increased features particularly in colorectal surgery and is the result of the robotic instruments' ability to intracorporeally simulate the human wrist motion. The current disadvantages of robotic colorectal surgery include high cost, large size, complex setup, limited range of surgical field, and the lack of haptic interface. Nonetheless, the cost may make up for the clinical advantages it provides in terms of improved CRM in rectal cancer surgery as well as the ability to facilitate intracorporeal hand-sewn bowel anastomosing.

References

[1] Szold A, Bergamaschi R, Broeders I, et al, European Association of Endoscopic Surgeons. European Association of Endoscopic Surgeons (EAES) consensus statement on the use of robotics in general surgery. Surg Endosc 2015;29(2):253–88.

[2] Baik SH, Kwon HY, Kim JS, et al. Robotic versus laparoscopic low anterior resection of rectal cancer: short-term outcome of a prospective comparative study. Ann Surg Oncol 2009;16:1480–7.

[3] Link RE, Bhayani SB, Kavoussi LR. A prospective comparison of robotic and laparoscopic pyeloplasty. Ann Surg 2006;243:486–91.

[4] Lotan Y, Cadeddu JA, Gettman MT. The new economics of radical prostatectomy: cost comparison of open, laparoscopic and robot assisted techniques. J Urol 2004;172(4 Pt 1):1431–5.

[5] Bhlat OS, Haluck RS, Murray WB, et al. Tactile feedback is present during minimally invasive surgery. J Am Coll Surg 1999;189:349–55.

[6] Barnajian M, Pettet D, Kazi E, et al. Quality of total mesorectal excision and depth of circumferential resection margin in rectal cancer: a matched comparison of first 20 robotic cases. Colorectal Dis 2014;16(8):603–9.

[7] Pigazzi A, Ellenhorn JD, Ballantyne GH, et al. Robotic-assisted laparoscopic low anterior resection with total mesorectal excision for rectal cancer. Surg Endosc 2006;20(10): 1521–5.
[8] Zawadzki M, Velchuru VR, Albalawi SA, et al. Is hybrid robotic laparoscopic assistance the ideal approach for restorative rectal cancer dissection? Colorectal Dis 2013;15(8): 1026–32.
[9] Hellan M, Stein H, Pigazzi A. Totally robotic low anterior resection with total mesorectal excision and splenic flexure mobilization. Surg Endosc 2009;23(2):447–51.
[10] Pan HF, Ruan H, Zhao K, et al. Totally robotic surgery for rectal cancer with transanal specimen extraction and robot-sewn anastomosis technique. Zhonghua Wei Chang Wai Ke Za Zhi 2012;15(8):807–9.
[11] Nagtegaal ID, Marijnen CA, Kranenbarg EK, et al, Pathology Review Committee, Cooperative Clinical Investigators. Circumferential margin involvement is still an important predictor of local recurrence in rectal carcinoma: not one millimeter but two millimeters is the limit. Am J Surg Pathol 2002;26:350–7.
[12] West NP, Finan PJ, Anderin C, et al. Evidence of the oncologic superiority of cylindrical abdominoperineal excision for low rectal cancer. J Clin Oncol 2008;26(21):3517–22.
[13] D'Annibale A, Pernazza G, Monsellato I, et al. Total mesorectal excision: a comparison of oncological and functional outcomes between robotic and laparoscopic surgery for rectal cancer. Surg Endosc 2013;27(6):1887–95.
[14] Kang J, Yoon KJ, Min BS, et al. The impact of robotic surgery for mid and low rectal cancer: a case-matched analysis of a 3-arm comparison—open, laparoscopic, and robotic surgery. Ann Surg 2013;257(1):95–101.
[15] Baik SH, Kim NK, Lee KY, et al. Factors influencing pathologic results after total mesorectal excision for rectal cancer: analysis of consecutive 100 cases. Ann Surg Oncol 2008;15(3): 751–8.
[16] Weissman JS, Zinner M. Comparative effectiveness research on robotic surgery. JAMA 2013;309(7):721–2.
[17] Trastulli S, Farinella E, Cirocchi R, et al. Robotic resection compared with laparoscopic rectal resection for cancer: systematic review and meta-analysis of short-term outcome. Colorectal Dis 2012;14(4):e134–56.
[18] Memon S, Heriot AG, Murphy DG, et al. Robotic versus laparoscopic proctectomy for rectal cancer: a meta-analysis. Ann Surg Oncol 2012;19(7):2095–101.
[19] Ortiz-Oshiro E, Sánchez-Egido I, Moreno-Sierra J, et al. Robotic assistance may reduce conversion to open in rectal carcinoma laparoscopic surgery: systematic review and meta-analysis. Int J Med Robot 2012;8(3):360–70.
[20] Halabi WJ, Kang CY, Jafari MD, et al. Robotic-assisted colorectal surgery in the United States: a nationwide analysis of trends and outcomes. World J Surg 2013;37(12): 2782–90.
[21] Fernandez R, Anaya DA, Li LT, et al. Laparoscopic versus robotic rectal resection for rectal cancer in a veteran population. Am J Surg 2013;206(4):509–17.
[22] Karahasanoglu T, Hamzaoglu I, Baca B, et al. Robotic surgery for rectal cancer: initial experience from 30 consecutive patients. J Gastrointest Surg 2012;16(2):401–7.
[23] Leonard D, Penninckx F, Fieuws S, et al, PROCARE, a multidisciplinary Belgian Project on Cancer of the Rectum. Factors predicting the quality of total mesorectal excision for rectal cancer. Ann Surg 2010;252(6):982–8.
[24] Denost Q, Quintane L, Buscail E, et al. Short- and long-term impact of body mass index on laparoscopic rectal cancer surgery. Colorectal Dis 2013;15(4):463–9.
[25] Lin S, Jiang HG, Chen ZH, et al. Meta-analysis of robotic and laparoscopic surgery for treatment of rectal cancer. World J Gastroenterol 2011;17(47):5214–20.
[26] Kim CW, Kim CH, Baik SH. Outcomes of robotic-assisted colorectal surgery compared with laparoscopic and open surgery: a systematic review. J Gastrointest Surg 2014;18(4): 816–30.

[27] Chern H, Chou J, Donkor C, et al. Effects of obesity in rectal cancer surgery. J Am Coll Surg 2010;211(1):55–60.
[28] Keller DS, Hashemi L, Lu M, et al. Short-term outcomes for robotic colorectal surgery by provider volume. J Am Coll Surg 2013;217(6):1063–9.
[29] Bonjer HJ, Deijen CL, Abis GA, et al. A randomized trial of laparoscopic versus open surgery for rectal cancer. N Engl J Med 2015;372(14):1324–32.
[30] Fleshman J, Branda M, Sargent DJ, et al. Effect of laparoscopic-assisted resection vs open resection of stage II or III rectal cancer on pathologic outcomes: the ACOSOG Z6051 randomized clinical trial. JAMA 2015;314(13):1346–55.
[31] Frede T, Stock C, Renner C, et al. Geometry of laparoscopic suturing and knotting techniques. J Endourol 1999;13:191–8.
[32] Breedveld P, Stassen HG, Meijer DW, et al. Observation in laparoscopic surgery: overview of impeding effects and supporting aids. J Laparoendosc Adv Surg Tech A 2000;10: 231–41.
[33] Berguer R, Smith WD, Chung YH. Performing laparoscopic surgery is significantly more stressful for the surgeon than open surgery. Surg Endosc 2001;15:1204–7.
[34] Berguer R. Surgical technology and the ergonomics of laparoscopic instruments. Surg Endosc 1998;12:458–62.
[35] Johnson SL. Ergonomic hand tool design. Hand Clin 1993;9:299–311.
[36] Carswell CM, Clarke D, Seales WB. Assessing mental workload during laparoscopic surgery. Surg Innov 2005;12:80–90.
[37] Rassweiler J, Safi KC, Subotic S, et al. Robotics and telesurgery–an update on their position in laparoscopic radical prostatectomy. Minim Invasive Ther Allied Technol 2005;14: 109–22.
[38] Gutt CN, Oniu T, Mehrabi A, et al. Robot-assisted abdominal surgery. Br J Surg 2004;91: 1390–7.
[39] Hanly EJ, Talamini MA. Robotic abdominal surgery. Am J Surg 2004;188(4A Suppl): 19S–26S.
[40] Weber PA, Merola S, Wasielewski A, et al. Telerobotic-assisted laparoscopic right and sigmoid colectomies for benign disease. Dis Colon Rectum 2002;45:1689–94 [discussion: 1695–6].
[41] Buchs NC, Pugin F, Ris F, et al. Early experience with robotic rectopexy. Int J Med Robot 2013;9(4):61–5.
[42] Heemskerk J, de Hoog DE, van Gemert WG, et al. Robot-assisted vs. conventional laparoscopic rectopexy for rectal prolapse: a comparative study on costs and time. Dis Colon Rectum 2007;50(11):1825–30.
[43] Maeso S, Reza M, Mayol JA, et al. Efficacy of the Da Vinci Surgical System in abdominal surgery compared with that of laparoscopy, a systematic review and meta-analysis. Ann Surg 2010;252:254–62.
[44] Ayav A, Bresler L, Hubert J, et al. Robotic-assisted pelvic organ prolapse surgery. Surg Endosc 2005;19:1200–3.
[45] D'Annibale A, Pernazza G, Morpurgo E, et al. Robotic right colon resection: evaluation of first 50 consecutive cases for malignant disease. Ann Surg Oncol 2010;17(11):2856–62.
[46] Morpurgo E, Contardo T, Molaro R, et al. Robotic-assisted intracorporeal anastomosis versus extracorporeal anastomosis in laparoscopic right hemicolectomy for cancer: a case control study. J Laparoendosc Adv Surg Tech A 2013;23(5):414–7.
[47] Stein SA, Bergamaschi R. Extracorporeal versus intracorporeal ileocolic anastomosis. Tech Coloproctol 2013;17(Suppl 1):S35–9.
[48] Ho YH. Laparoscopic right hemicolectomy with intra-corporeal anastomosis. Tech Coloproctol 2010;14:359–63.
[49] Yamamoto T, Fazio VW, Tekkis PP. Safety and efficacy of strictureplasty for Crohn's disease: a systematic review and meta- analysis. Dis Colon Rectum 2007;50:1968–86.

[50] Sonoda T, Lee S, Whelan RL, et al. Robotically assisted small intestinal strictureplasty in dogs: a survival study involving 16 Heineke–Mikulicz strictureplasties. Surg Endosc 2007;21:2220–3.
[51] Tou S, Pavesi E, Nasser A, et al. Robotic-assisted strictureplasty for Crohn's disease. Tech Coloproctol 2015;19(4):253–4.
[52] Karas JR, Uranues S, Altomare DF, et al, Rectal Prolapse Recurrence Study Group. No rectopexy versus rectopexy following rectal mobilization for full-thickness rectal prolapse: a randomized controlled trial. Dis Colon Rectum 2011;54:29–34.
[53] Wong MT, Meurette G, Rigaud J, et al. Robotic versus laparoscopic rectopexy for complex rectocele: a prospective comparison of short-term outcomes. Dis Colon Rectum 2011;54(3): 342–6.
[54] Mantoo S, Podevin J, Regenet N, et al. Is robotic-assisted ventral mesh rectopexy superior to laparoscopic ventral mesh rectopexy in the management of obstructed defaecation? Colorectal Dis 2013;15(8):469–75.
[55] Buchs NC, Pugin F, Volonte F, et al. Robotic transanal endoscopic microsurgery: technical details for the lateral approach. Dis Colon Rectum 2013;56(10):1194–8.
[56] Mäkelä-Kaikkonen J, Rautio T, Klintrup K, et al. Robotic-assisted and laparoscopic ventral rectopexy in the treatment of rectal prolapse: a matched-pairs study of operative details and complications. Tech Coloproctol 2014;18(2):151–5.
[57] Cadeddu F, Sileri P, Grande M, et al. Focus on abdominal rectopexy for full-thickness rectal prolapse: meta-analysis of literature. Tech Coloproctol 2012;16(1):37–53.
[58] de Hoog DE, Heemskerk J, Nieman FH, et al. Recurrence and functional results after open versus conventional laparoscopic versus robot-assisted laparoscopic rectopexy for rectal prolapse: a case-control study. Int J Colorectal Dis 2009;24(10):1201–6.
[59] D'Hoore A, Cadoni R, Penninckx F. Long-term outcome of laparoscopic ventral rectopexy for total rectal prolapse. Br J Surg 2004;91:1500–5.
[60] Raftopoulos Y, Senagore AJ, Di Giuro G, et al, Rectal Prolapse Recurrence Study Group. Recurrence rates after abdominal surgery for complete rectal prolapse: a multicenter pooled analysis of 643 individual patient data. Dis Colon Rectum 2005;48:1200–6.
[61] Atallah S, Parra-Davila E, DeBeche-Adams T, et al. Excision of a rectal neoplasm using robotic transanal surgery (RTS): a description of the technique. Tech Coloproctol 2012;16: 389–92.
[62] Gomez Ruiz M, Martin Parra I, Calleja Iglesias A, et al. Pre-clinical cadaveric study of transanal robotic proctectomy with total mesorectal excision combined with laparoscopic assistance. Int J Med Robot 2015;11(2):188–93.
[63] Atallah S, Nassif G, Polavarapu H, et al. Robotic-assisted transanal surgery for total mesorectal excision (RATS-TME): a description of a novel surgical approach with video demonstration. Tech Coloproctol 2013;17(4):441–7.
[64] Volkmann R. Concerning rectal cancer and the removal of the rectum. Dis Colon Rectum 1986;29:679–85.
[65] Warren OJ, Solomon MJ. The drive toward transanal total mesorectal excision–science or rhetoric? Dis Colon Rectum 2015;58:909–10.
[66] Rullier E. Transanal mesorectal excision: the new challenge in rectal cancer. Dis Colon Rectum 2015;58:621–2.
[67] Fernández-Hevia M, Delgado S, Castells A, et al. Transanal total mesorectal excision in rectal cancer: short-term outcomes in comparison with laparoscopic surgery. Ann Surg 2015;261:221–7.
[68] Denost Q, Adam JP, Rullier A, et al. Perineal transanal approach: a new standard for laparoscopic sphincter-saving resection in low rectal cancer, a randomized trial. Ann Surg 2014;260:993–9.
[69] Velthuis S, Nieuwenhuis DH, Ruijter TEG, et al. Transanal versus traditional laparoscopic total mesorectal excision for rectal carcinoma. Surg Endosc 2014;28:3494–9.

[70] Wexner SD, Berho M. Transanal TAMIS total mesorectal excision (TME)—a work in progress. Tech Coloproctol 2014;18:423–5.
[71] Abraham NS, Durairaj R, Young JM, et al. How does an historic control study of a surgical procedure compare with the "gold standard"? Dis Colon Rectum 2006;49:1141–8.

Advances in Surgery 50 (2016) 173–186
ADVANCES IN SURGERY

Ventilator Management

A Systematic Approach to Choosing and Using New Modes

Theresa Elizabeth Robertson, MD
Department of Surgery, University of Mississippi, 2500 North State Street, Jackson, MS 39216, USA

Keywords
• Ventilator • Mechanical ventilation • Hypoxia • Dyssynchrony • ARDS

Key points

- Modern ventilators have many new modes but most go unused.
- Research has demonstrated that low tidal volumes in acute respiratory distress syndrome and early liberation for all patients are life-saving; other mode choices are made for short-term benefits.
- Guidelines have been shown to improve patient outcomes for ventilators and these should be implemented as a first step in ventilator mode selection.

INTRODUCTION

Modern ventilator management presents a dizzying array of choices in ventilators, modes, and advanced features. The new clinician is assaulted with a list of acronyms that sound impressively similar but can mean the difference between a calm, well-oxygenated patient and an agitated, hypoxic one struggling to breathe. New ventilators are developed with advanced microprocessors and artificial intelligence to reduce the workload of the physician and patient, but with very little data to back them up. What the data do show is that the sooner we rid the patient of the ventilator, the better they will do, and this is our ultimate and daily goal.

The new ventilator modes are often developed by industry and then assigned proprietary names on each ventilator. Some ventilators offer the same modes as other vents, some are unique. All ventilators have the basic modes of ventilation, which are discussed. We then address some common

Disclosure Statement: The author has nothing to disclose.

E-mail address: terobertson@umc.edu

0065-3411/16/$ – see front matter
http://dx.doi.org/10.1016/j.yasu.2016.03.013

advanced modes of ventilation and then some less available types. We also discuss adjuncts to mechanical ventilation, such as extracorporeal membrane oxygenation. It is best to know what ventilators and resources your institution has to be able to plan a strategy for your patients' recoveries.

SIGNIFICANCE

The overwhelming number of unique modes of ventilation available is demonstrated in Table 1 taken from the article by Mireles-Cabodevila and colleagues [1] showing 47 unique mode names on only 4 different ventilators. These names are given by the ventilator manufacturer and do not necessarily represent differences in independent or dependent variables on the machine or differences in appropriate clinical scenarios. For example, the airway pressure release ventilation mode on the Dräger Evita XL (Draeger Medical, Telford, PA) has the same features as the Bi-Vent mode on the Maquet Servo-i (Maquet Getinge Group, Wayne, NJ). To discuss different types of ventilation between ventilators, Chatburn [2] developed a classification of ventilator modes. This separated modes first by pressure or volume as the control variable and then subclassifies them by the breath sequence type: continuous mandatory ventilation (CMV), intermittent mandatory ventilation (IMV), or continuous spontaneous ventilation (CSV). From there, the modes are further subdivided by breath-targeting scheme: set-point, dual, adaptive, optimal, biovariable, or intelligent. Table 2 demonstrates this and is taken from the article by Mireles-Cabodevila and colleagues [1] to demonstrate how the modes from Table 1 fit into an organized classification scheme.

Breath-targeting schemes are one of the key targets for innovation in mechanical ventilation. Early in the development of positive pressure ventilation, you could choose a set-point for your volume or pressure and the machine would hit it. New microprocessors and artificial intelligence allow for heuristics and auto feedback to adjust the vent between, and even within, breaths. Dual targeting switches between pressure control and volume control within a single breath to reach preset volume and pressure targets. Adaptive targeting changes the target between breaths based on the performance of the prior breaths. Optimal targeting bases targets on mathematical models from prior breaths. Intelligent targeting systems are the most complex and based on artificial intelligence modeling of prior breaths.

These breath-targeting schemes vary from completely clinician dependent to completely model dependent and there are problems with both ends of the spectrum. Data show that low tidal volume ventilation is clearly better for acute respiratory distress syndrome (ARDS) [3], but that this is not currently uniformly applied by practitioners [4]. Computerized systems would seem to solve this human problem; however, mathematical models and artificial intelligence systems are easily confused by the patient not behaving according to how the model predicts. The computer then provides inappropriate ventilator support.

We have a taxonomy for ventilation modes and a large variety of these modes to choose from. But, the only high-quality significant data we have to guide our choice is the ARDSNet study in 2000 demonstrating that lower tidal volumes are beneficial in ARDS [3]. We also know that early liberation from ventilation is vital and that should be our ultimate and daily goal [5]. There are a variety of studies demonstrating increased synchrony with the vent, decreased minutes on the vent, and improved prediction for extubation success [6–8], but there is little evidence that these short-term outcomes have a long-term impact for our patients [9]. We do know that to achieve low tidal volumes in ARDS and early extubation, protocols or guidelines driven by nonphysicians are successful [10].

Current usage of ventilator modes in modern intensive care units consists mostly of volume control–CMV, volume control IMV, pressure control–CMV, and pressure control IMV [11–13]. Most patients are not being ventilated with a new advanced ventilator mode and there has not been a clear frontrunner among the systems.

Initial approach

The first step in a systematic approach to new ventilator modes is to prepare a guideline or protocol to be applied automatically to every ventilated patient by a non–physician-level provider. The development of this bundle should include input from a multidisciplinary group with consideration given to local equipment, preferences, disease patterns, and resources. The guideline should include proven best practices for ventilator management, including head of bed elevation, oral care, light sedation, daily awakening trials, and daily assessment for and performance of spontaneous breathing trials [10]. The choice of which ventilator mode to use is based on the one your practitioners are most comfortable with and which is the most comfortable for your patients. Many find this to be a CSV with backup ventilation modes for apnea, although others find that mandatory ventilation is well tolerated.

It is with the unusual, sick, or difficult patient, then, that the physician or affiliate provider is called to the bedside to evaluate the ventilator. When troubleshooting the ventilator and the patient, I find it helpful to diagnose the problems, prioritize the problems, and then choose among the management strategies available. The most common issues in acute ventilator management are hypoxia, high pressures, and dyssynchrony. Acute and chronic liberation from the ventilator is also a frequent problem faced in the critically ill.

Hypoxia

When one approaches a patient with severe hypoxia, the patient has already been placed on 100% Fio_2 and bagged. The ARDSNet trial shows us we should provide low tidal volume ventilation in an open lung strategy to avoid volutrauma and atelectrauma [3,14]. Given this, we may want to use a mode that targets preset volumes. With the new modes, this is possible in a volume or pressure control method according to the simplified taxonomy. For example, the pressure control–CMV with and adaptive breath-targeting scheme is called pressure regulated volume control (PRVC) on the Maquet Servo-i. This mode has a set-point for pressure and a target volume and uses the minimum amount

Table 1
Unique modes from 4 ventilator types

Manufacturer	Model	Manufacturer's mode name
Covidien	PB 840	BiLevel
Covidien	PB 840	Pressure Control Assist Control
Covidien	PB 840	Pressure Control Synchronized Intermittent Mandatory Ventilation
Covidien	PB 840	Pressure Support
Covidien	PB 840	Proportional Assist Ventilation Plus
Covidien	PB 840	Spontaneous
Covidien	PB 840	Tube Compensation
Covidien	PB 840	Volume Control Synchronized Intermittent Mandatory Ventilation
Covidien	PB 840	Volume Control Assist/Control
Covidien	PB 840	Volume Control Plus Assist/Control
Covidien	PB 840	Volume Control Plus Synchronized Intermittent Mandatory Ventilation
Covidien	PB 840	Volume Ventilation Plus Synchronized Intermittent Mandatory Ventilation
Dräger	Evita XL	Airway Pressure Release Ventilation
Dräger	Evita XL	Automatic Tube Compensation
Dräger	Evita XL	Continuous Mandatory Ventilation
Dräger	Evita XL	Continuous Mandatory Ventilation with AutoFlow
Dräger	Evita XL	Continuous Mandatory Ventilation with Pressure-Limited Ventilation
Dräger	Evita XL	Continuous Positive Airway Pressure/Pressure Support
Dräger	Evita XL	Mandatory Minute Volume Ventilation
Dräger	Evita XL	Mandatory Minute Volume with AutoFlow
Dräger	Evita XL	Mandatory Minute Volume with Pressure-Limited Ventilation
Dräger	Evita XL	Pressure-Controlled Ventilation Plus Assisted
Dräger	Evita XL	Pressure-Controlled Ventilation Plus Pressure Support
Dräger	Evita XL	SmartCare/PS

Dräger	Evita XL	Synchronized Intermittent Mandatory Ventilation
Dräger	Evita XL	Synchronized Intermittent Mandatory Ventilation with AutoFlow
Dräger	Evita XL	Synchronized Intermittent Mandatory Ventilation with Pressure-Limited Ventilation
Hamilton	G5	Adaptive Pressure Ventilation Controlled Mandatory Ventilation
Hamilton	G5	Adaptive Pressure Ventilation Synchronized Intermittent Mandatory Ventilation
Hamilton	G5	Adaptive Support Ventilation
Hamilton	G5	Duo Positive Airway Pressure
Hamilton	G5	Noninvasive Ventilation
Hamilton	G5	Pressure-Controlled Mandatory Ventilation
Hamilton	G5	Pressure Synchronized Intermittent Mandatory Ventilation
Hamilton	G5	Synchronized Controlled Mandatory Ventilation
Maquet	Servo-i	Automode (Pressure Control to Pressure Support)
Maquet	Servo-i	Automode (Pressure-Regulated Volume Control to Volume Support)
Maquet	Servo-i	Automode (Control to Volume Support)
Maquet	Servo-i	Bi-Vent
Maquet	Servo-i	Neurally Adjusted Ventilatory Assist
Maquet	Servo-i	Pressure Control
Maquet	Servo-i	Pressure-Regulated Volume Control
Maquet	Servo-i	Synchronizes Intermittent Mandatory Ventilation (Pressure Control)
Maquet	Servo-i	Synchronized Intermittent Mandatory Ventilation (Pressure-Regulated Volume Control)
Maquet	Servo-i	Synchronized Intermittent Mandatory Ventilation (Volume Control)
Maquet	Servo-i	Volume Control
Maquet	Servo-i	Volume Support

From Mireles-Cabodevila E, Hatipoğlu U, Chatburn RL. A rational framework for selecting modes of ventilation. Respir Care 2013;58(2):350; with permission.

Table 2
A simplified taxonomy for ventilator mode classification

Order[a] Control volume	Family Breath sequence	Genus primary breath-targeting scheme	Species secondary breath-targeting scheme	Example mode names	Abbreviation	Variety[b] operational differences
Volume	CMV	Set-point	NA	Volume Control Assist/Control	$VC\text{-}CMV_S$	—
		Dual	NA	Continuous Mandatory Ventilation with Pressure Limited	$VC\text{-}CMV_D$	—
	IMV	Set-point	Set-point	Volume Control Synchronized Intermittent Mandatory Ventilation	$VC\text{-}IMV_{S,S}$	—
		Dual	Set-point	Synchronized Intermittent Mandatory Ventilation (Volume Control Servo-i ventilator)	$VC\text{-}IMV_{D,S}$	—
		Dual/Adaptive	Set-point	Mandatory Minute Volume with Pressure-Limited Ventilation	$VC\text{-}IMV_{DA,S}$	—
		Dual	Adaptive	Automode (Volume Control to Volume Support)	$VC\text{-}IMV_{D,A}$	—
		Adaptive	Set-point	Mandatory Minute Volume Ventilation	$VC\text{-}IMV_{A,S}$	—
Pressure	CMV	Set-point	NA	Pressure Control Assist Control	$PC\text{-}CMV_S$	—
		Adaptive	NA	Pressure Regulated Volume Control	$PC\text{-}CMV_A$	—
	IMV	Set-point	Set-point	Airway Pressure Release Ventilation	$PC\text{-}IMV_{S,S}$	—
		Set-point	NA	High-frequency Oscillatory Ventilation	$PC\text{-}IMV_{S,S}$	Frequency above 150 cycles/min, negative airway pressure possible

	Adaptive	Set-point	Adaptive Pressure Ventilation Synchronized Intermittent Mandatory Ventilation	PC-$IMV_{A,S}$	—
	Adaptive	Adaptive	Automode (Pressure-Regulated Volume Control to Volume Support)	PC-$IMV_{A,A}$	—
	Optimal	Optimal	Adaptive Support Ventilation	PC-$IMV_{O,O}$	—
	Optimal/Intelligent	Optimal/Intelligent	IntelliVent-ASV	PC-$IMV_{CX,OI}$	—
CSV	Set-point	NA	Pressure Support	PC-CSV_S	Set-point constant
	Biovariable	NA	Variable Pressure Support	PC-CSV_B	Set-point automatically adjusted at random
	Servo	NA	Proportional Assist Ventilation	PC-CSV_R	Pressure proportional to volume and flow signals
	Servo	NA	Neurally Adjusted Ventilatory Support	PC-CSV_R	Pressure proportional to diaphragmatic electromyogram
	Adaptive	NA	Volume Support	PC-CSV_A	Pressure adjusted to achieve tidal volume target
	Adaptive	NA	Mandatory Rale Ventilation	PC-CSV_A	Pressure adjusted to achieve rate target
	Intelligent	NA	SmartCare/PS	PC-CSV_I	—

Abbreviations: CMV, continuous mandatory ventilation; CSV, continuous spontaneous ventilation; IMV, intermittent mandatory ventilation; NA, not applicable; PC, pressure control; VC, volume control. Subscripts: A, adaptive; B, biovariable; D, dual; I, intelligent; O, optimal; R, servo; S, set-point.

[a]Included in this table are all the unique modes listed in Table 1.

[b]The Variety level of description may be needed to differentiated between modes that have same order, family, genus, species.

From Mireles-Cabodevila E, Hatipoğlu U, Chatburn RL. A rational framework for selecting modes of ventilation. Respir Care 2013;58(2):351; with permission.

of pressure needed to achieve the target volume. This does not solve our hypoxia, but does ensure the one factor we know saves lives: low tidal volume ventilation. Many clinicians use a pressure-controlled IMV mode with a set-point breath-targeting scheme in airway pressure release ventilation (APRV), also known as Bi-Vent. This mode was described in 1988 [15] and became popular with the rise of open lung ventilation as a treatment for ARDS [16]. This allows an open lung strategy with the lung distended open at a high continuous positive airway pressure (CPAP) most of the time with the occasional release to a low airway pressure for a brief period. The patient can breathe at any point during the high-pressure or low-pressure periods, as they are breathing as they would with CPAP. This continuous high pressure leads to recruitment of alveoli for gas exchange to improve oxygenation as compared with conventional ventilation in randomized controlled trials [17].

To address hypoxia, we still use our standard toolbox of increasing positive end expiratory pressure (which also prevents atelectrauma), and increasing FiO_2. Beyond that, standard advanced modes do not offer new ways to load oxygen onto hemoglobin. We must consider deep sedation, paralysis, prone positioning, nitric oxide, and, possibly extracorporeal membrane oxygenation. High-frequency oscillatory ventilation is a mode of ventilator that is used commonly in the neonatal and pediatric population and had some regional popularity in the adult population. A recent review of studies of high-frequency oscillatory ventilation demonstrated no mortality benefit as a rescue ventilator strategy even though it did show some benefit in observational trials [18]. A recent multicenter, randomized controlled trial of early high-frequency oscillatory ventilation in ARDS was stopped early because of concern for increased mortality in the oscillation group [19].

High pressures

To address high ventilator pressures, one must diagnose the underlying cause of the high-pressure readings on the ventilator. There can be impedance in the ventilator circuit anywhere from the ventilator to the patient's abdomen, and all must be examined. In the tubing, the patient biting the endotracheal tube is the most common cause of the high-pressure alarm, although another kink in the line is unlikely, but possible. A blockage in the inspiratory phase, as in endotracheal tube narrowing with biting or blockage, is visible on the ventilator pressure-volume loop (Fig. 1) with downward widening of the pressure-volume loop.

High intra-abdominal pressures or chest wall rigidity can also cause high-pressure alarms on the ventilator, although true underlying physiology causing this occurs much less often than suspected. Intra-abdominal compartment syndrome is often suspected, and a decompressive laparotomy can be helpful, but should be done only once the patient has proven to have high peak pressures after deep sedation and chemical paralysis. Otherwise, elevated bladder pressures are likely due to patient dyssynchrony and abdominal muscle contraction. Normal intra-abdominal pressures in healthy coughing adults average

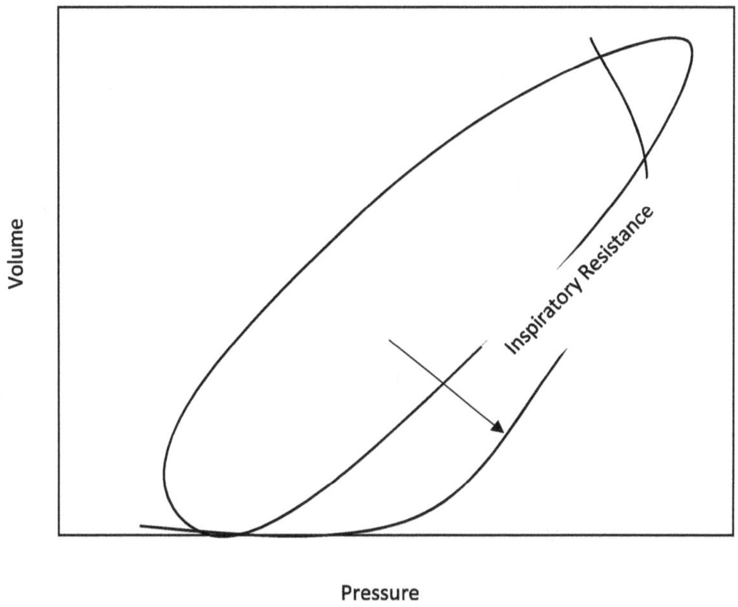

Fig. 1. Change in pressure-volume loop with inspiratory resistance (ie, endotracheal tube obstruction).

81 mm Hg [20]. When laying calmly, intra-abdominal pressures averaged 2 mm Hg, so we should take into account the patient's clinical state when interpreting the reading, as we do with all values [20].

Chest wall rigidity is quite uncommon, but when diagnosed, should be treated rapidly with dantrolene, as it can be a symptom of malignant hyperthermia. It is also a known rare complication of fentanyl administration and is reversible with naloxone.

Finally, we approach poor lung compliance as a possible cause of our high peak pressures and we can look to our new ventilator modes to help manage this. Traditional modes have us use a set-point for volume or pressure and the compliance of the lung determines the resultant dependent variable. In an ill, noncompliant lung, the compliance is constantly changing and the critical care practitioner can use the new ventilator mode to respond to these changes in real time. The adaptive and dual-mode breath-targeting schemes available target the breath volume and pressure goals within set limits according to prior breaths, or current performance within the breath, respectively. Optimal and intelligent breath-targeting schemes can also adjust to changing patient compliance as well as apply broader rules or artificial intelligence programs. Any of these programs can be fooled by a patient not performing as expected despite normal physiology, which is why an experienced clinician at the bedside will always be necessary. A microprocessor will not easily be able to tell the difference between a severely depressed patient unwilling to inspire deeply after a suicide attempt and an incredibly weak patient unable to inspire deeply.

Once we have decided that we have poor lung compliance or expect poor lung compliance, as in the severely contused lung after an motor vehicle collision, we do not have a good way to choose between modes. One must look at the resources in your institution and determine which adaptive or intelligent mode is available. Dräger (Telford, PA) has SmartCare/PS, Maquet has PRVC, and Hamilton (Bonaduz, Switzerland) has Intellivent/Adaptive Support Ventilation. Covidien (Minneapolis, MN) has Proportional Assist Ventilation Plus, but this is not based on compliance as much as it is work of breathing, which is discussed later in this article.

Dyssynchrony and comfort

This is the area in which the newest innovations in mechanical ventilation get interesting. But, we should not forget that the best treatment for dyssynchrony is extubation. The ideal reintubation rate has been debated among the experts, but all agree that it is not zero. In a published prospective observational study of 9 intensive care units, the reintubation rate ranged from 0% to 21% [21]. If the patient cannot be extubated and requires mechanical ventilator assistance, historically we have sedated the patient to tolerance of the set-point ventilation modes. We now have strong and widely accepted data that decreasing sedation improves patient outcomes [22]. Manufacturers have responded with new, more comfortable modes and are marketing them strongly.

No one mode has been proven more comfortable than another in a direct head-to-head trial and the practitioner should look to local resources and equipment for options. The simplest method to ensure patient comfort and synchrony is to set a completely spontaneous mode and every manufacturer has some form of this. Covidien has Pressure Support on the PB 840, Dräger has Continuous Positive Airway Pressure/Pressure Support on the Evita XL, Hamilton has Pressure Support on the G5, and Maquet has Pressure Support on the Servo-i. The difficulty, even in the spontaneous modes, is finding the right triggering mechanism. Most ventilators trigger based on flow within the ventilator itself, but the Neurally Adjusted Ventilatory Assist uses the diaphragm electromyogram via nasogastric tube sensors for triggering and cycling [23]. This has been shown to improve the patient-ventilator interaction [24] and has theoretic cost savings [25], but there has not yet been a study done on patient-centered outcomes.

IMV was initially designed for comfort and to allow spontaneous breathing with underlying mandatory breaths that could be weaned by the physician as the patient improved [26]. There are now modes that have the spontaneous breaths suppress the mandatory breaths, including Mandatory Minute Ventilation (Dräger), Adaptive Support Ventilation (Hamilton), and AutoMode (Maquet). There are no head-to-head trials, or any studies of patient-centered outcomes, including ventilator days, mortality, and morbidity.

Proportional Assist Ventilation (Covidien) is another new mode designed with the intent of increased comfort on the ventilator. It tracks the flow and volume of the patient's breaths to interpret the patient's effort and assists the patient in proportion to the patient's effort [27]. This has been shown to increase exercise tolerance and increase synchrony in the sleeping patient and in patients on the mode for longer than 48 hours [28]. Once again, though, there are no data on improvement in ventilator days or mortality.

Automatic tube compensation is another adjunct to standard modes offered by Covidien that determines the change in flow resistance across the endotracheal tube and compensates for that with additional pressure support. This has been shown to have increased comfort as compared with standard pressure support ventilation settings [29] and have an increased number of passed spontaneous breathing trials with no increase in reintubations [30]. Again, however, there are no data on decreased ventilator days or decreased morbidity and mortality for the patient.

APRV or Bi-Vent allows for spontaneous breaths throughout the ventilator cycle, so no coordination between ventilator and patient is necessary. This mode has a constant positive airway pressure with intermittent release of the high pressure to low pressures to allow release of carbon dioxide. Use of this mode has been shown to decrease sedation requirements as compared with conventional ventilation [17], indicating that it is a more comfortable mode of ventilation.

There are then some advanced rule-based and artificial intelligence–guided systems that are designed for patient comfort by evaluating multiple incoming variables. The SmartCare/PS by Dräger inputs end-tidal CO2, tidal volume, and respiratory rate to adjust pressure support to provide the most comfortable level of support. It is not only a spontaneous breath sequence, but the level of support is adjusted for patient need and comfort and then reduced automatically to challenge the patient toward ventilator liberation [31].

Ventilator liberation

Ventilator liberation is our goal when we apply mechanical ventilation, and ventilator designers have addressed this with new systems and modes. The data have demonstrated success with non–physician driven daily spontaneous breathing-trial protocols [21]. The SmartCare/PS mode by Dräger automatically reduces support, as described previously, and will evaluate the patient's success by its input variables end-tidal CO2, tidal volume, and respiratory rate. Once it gets to a predetermined low level of inspiratory support, the ventilator marks the initiation of a "spontaneous breathing trial" and then reports the results on the screen and recommends ventilator and patient separation if appropriate.

Other modes use the minimum necessary pressure support to reach a target volume, such as PRVC (Maquet) and Volume Control Plus Assist Control (Covidien). These do not go as far as to suggest patient and ventilator separation, but will automatically decrease ventilator support to the patient as the patient improves.

None of these modes can differentiate actual patient ability from patient effort and a good clinician at the bedside can often get a larger tidal volume out of a patient with appropriate encouragement. The incentive spirometer is a prime example of increasing patient tidal volumes in the nonventilated patient by managing expectations and goal setting. Perhaps if the ventilator could provide encouragement to the patient during the recovery process, we would see fewer ventilator days.

Present relevance and future avenues

Current data only demonstrate that low tidal volume ventilation is associated with a mortality benefit in ARDS [3]. All other ventilator interventions are based on physiologic principles of oxygen requirements for cellular mechanics, permissive hypercapnia to a certain degree, and patient comfort as a relative priority in patient care. Based on these priorities, the intensive care provider is given an array of choices to oxygenate and ventilate the patient and liberate the patient from mechanical ventilation as quickly and safely as possible.

Local practices should be examined for adherence to best practices and modified to these, but it is not necessary to align every intensive care unit or every patient to the same mode of ventilation. Practitioners, therapists, and patients will have different levels of comfort with each mode and this flexibility is reasonable until further data are available to alter our behavior. One study estimated that to perform a randomized controlled trial of all current modes would require more than 200 head-to-head comparisons with 4 years per study and $9 billion [1].

Further research would be useful in end-stage hypoxemia rescue. We have recently discovered that high-frequency oscillatory ventilation does not have proven benefit in adults [19] and would benefit from more data on extracorporeal membrane ventilation versus Bi-Vent [18]. It also be useful to know if intelligent design methods are superior to entrained control methods of ventilation. Bundles and guidelines are being prepared in many intensive care units and comparison trials of these for ventilator days, ease of use, and adherence would be an interesting future research avenue.

SUMMARY

The modern intensivist has a huge number of ventilator modes and settings to choose from in managing the patient with respiratory failure, but very few data with which to guide those decisions. In the overall management of the intensive care unit, a non–physician driven guideline has been shown to improve outcomes for the unit as a whole. When the difficult-to-manage patient on a ventilator falls outside of the guideline's abilities, the providers can choose an advanced mode based on the diagnosis of the patient. Patients in ARDS benefit from low tidal volume ventilation in an open lung approach, which can be achieved in a volume-targeted mode or Bi-Vent/APRV. The dyssynchronous patient may benefit from some of the advances in neural adjustments, proportional assist ventilation, or automatic tube compensation. The patient with low lung compliance can take advantage of the modes with optimal and intelligent breath-targeting schemes. Future research can compare guidelines to one another and identify the best therapy for end-stage hypoxemia.

References

[1] Mireles-Cabodevila E, Hatipoğlu U, Chatburn RL. A rational framework for selecting modes of ventilation. Respir Care 2013;58(2):348–66.
[2] Chatburn RL. Classification of ventilator modes: update and proposal for implementation. Respir Care 2007;52(3):301–23.
[3] Ventilation with lower tidal volumes as compared with traditional tidal volumes for acute lung injury and the acute respiratory distress syndrome. The Acute Respiratory Distress Syndrome Network. N Engl J Med 2000;342(18):1301–8.
[4] Dreyfuss D. Acute lung injury and mechanical ventilation: need for quality assurance. Crit Care Med 2004;32(9):1960–1.
[5] Manthous CA, Schmidt GA, Hall JB. Liberation from mechanical ventilation: a decade of progress. Chest 1998;114(3):886–901.
[6] Sinderby C, Beck J. Proportional assist ventilation and neurally adjusted ventilatory assist—better approaches to patient ventilator synchrony? Clin Chest Med 2008;29(2):329–42.
[7] Gruber PC, Gomersall CD, Leung P, et al. Randomized controlled trial comparing adaptive-support ventilation with pressure-regulated volume-controlled ventilation with automode in weaning patients after cardiac surgery. Anesthesiology 2008;109(1):81–7.
[8] Cohen JD, Shapiro M, Grozovski E, et al. Automatic tube compensation-assisted respiratory rate to tidal volume ratio improves the prediction of weaning outcome. Chest 2002;122(3):980–4.
[9] Branson RD, Johannigman JA. What is the evidence base for the newer ventilation modes? Respir Care 2004;49(7):742–60.
[10] Ely EW, Meade MO, Haponik EF, et al. Mechanical ventilator weaning protocols driven by nonphysician health-care professionals: evidence-based clinical practice guidelines. Chest 2001;120(6 Suppl):454S–63S.
[11] Koh Y, Lim CM, Koh SO, et al. A national survey on the practice and outcomes of mechanical ventilation in Korean intensive care units. Anaesth Intensive Care 2009;37(2):272.
[12] Metnitz PGH, Metnitz B, Moreno RP, et al. Epidemiology of mechanical ventilation: analysis of the SAPS 3 database. Intensive Care Med 2009;35(5):816–25.
[13] Farias JA, Frutos F, Esteban A, et al. What is the daily practice of mechanical ventilation in pediatric intensive care units? A multicenter study. Intensive Care Med 2004;30(5):918–25.
[14] Brower RG, Lanken PN, MacIntyre N, et al. Higher versus lower positive end-expiratory pressures in patients with the acute respiratory distress syndrome. N Engl J Med 2004;351(4):327–36.
[15] Garner W, Downs JB, Stock MC. Airway pressure release ventilation (APRV). A human trial. Chest 1988;94(4):779–81.
[16] Daoud EG. Airway pressure release ventilation. Ann Thorac Med 2007;2(4):176.
[17] Habashi NM. Other approaches to open-lung ventilation: airway pressure release ventilation. Crit Care Med 2005;33(3):S228–40.
[18] Shekar K, Davies AR, Mullany DV, et al. To ventilate, oscillate, or cannulate? J Crit Care 2013;28(5):655–62.
[19] Ferguson ND, Cook DJ, Guyatt GH, et al. High-frequency oscillation in early acute respiratory distress syndrome. N Engl J Med 2013;368(9):795–805.

[20] Cobb WS, Burns JM, Kercher KW, et al. Normal intraabdominal pressure in healthy adults. J Surg Res 2005;129(2):231–5.
[21] Robertson TE, Mann HJ, Hyzy R, et al. Multicenter implementation of a consensus-developed, evidence-based, spontaneous breathing trial protocol. Crit Care Med 2008;36(10):2753–62.
[22] Barr J, Fraser GL, Puntillo K, et al. Clinical practice guidelines for the management of pain, agitation, and delirium in adult patients in the intensive care unit. Crit Care Med 2013;41(1):263–306.
[23] Sinderby C, Navalesi P, Beck J, et al. Neural control of mechanical ventilation in respiratory failure. Nat Med 1999;5(12):1433–6.
[24] Piquilloud L, Tassaux D, Bialais E, et al. Neurally adjusted ventilatory assist improves patient–ventilator interaction. Intensive Care Med 2011;37(2):263–71.
[25] Hjelmgren J, Bruce Wirta S, Huetson P, et al. Health economic modeling of the potential cost saving effects of neurally adjusted ventilator assist. Ther Adv Respir Dis 2016;10(1):3–17.
[26] Downs JB, Klein EF Jr, Desautels D, et al. Intermittent mandatory ventilation: a new approach to weaning patients from mechanical ventilators. Chest 1973;64(3):331–5.
[27] Younes M. Proportional assist ventilation, in mechanical ventilation and weaning. New York: Springer; 2002. p. 39–73.
[28] Kacmarek RM. Proportional assist ventilation and neurally adjusted ventilatory assist. Respir Care 2011;56(2):140–52.
[29] Mols G, Rohr E, Benzing A, et al. Breathing pattern associated with respiratory comfort during automatic tube compensation and pressure support ventilation in normal subjects. Acta Anaesthesiol Scand 2000;44(3):223–30.
[30] Cohen JD, Shapiro M, Grozovski E, et al. Extubation outcome following a spontaneous breathing trial with automatic tube compensation versus continuous positive airway pressure. Crit Care Med 2006;34(3):682–6.
[31] Branson RD, Johannigman JA. Innovations in mechanical ventilation. Respir Care 2009;54(7):933–47.

Advances in Surgery 50 (2016) 187–202

ADVANCES IN SURGERY

ELSEVIER
MOSBY

Hernia Management in the Athlete

L. Michael Brunt, MD

Section of Minimally Invasive Surgery, Department of Surgery, Washington University School of Medicine, 660 South Euclid Avenue, Box 8109, St Louis, MO 63110, USA

Keywords

• Sports hernia • Groin pain • Athletic groin pain • Pubalgia

Key points

- Groin injuries are common in sports because of the forces exerted around the pelvis in high-level athletes.
- The approach to athletic groin pain requires a multidisciplinary approach involving sports orthopedists, athletic trainers, and surgeons.
- Surgeons who evaluate athletes with groin pain should be well versed in the differential diagnosis and evaluation strategies.
- Surgery for athletic pubalgia/sport's hernia is appropriate for athletes who fail to respond to conservative management and who have appropriate findings on imaging and physical examination.

Much attention has arisen in recent years regarding the condition in high-performance athletes popularly known as sport's hernia. The term sport's hernia is actually a misnomer in the sense that it does not represent a true herniation of internal contents through the inguinal floor, and this condition is better termed athletic pubalgia or inguinal disruption to more appropriately represent the actual pathophysiology of the condition. Although athletes may have a true inguinal hernia, this is relatively uncommon in comparison with the overall incidence of groin injuries. Therefore, a review of this condition as well as a discussion of the management of inguinal hernia in athletes can better form the basis of a structured approach to this unique population.

There is much confusion around the terminology of sport's hernia, which has been described by various terms listed in Box 1 that include athletic

Disclosure Statement: The author has nothing to disclose.

0065-3411/16/$ – see front matter
http://dx.doi.org/10.1016/j.yasu.2016.03.014

Box 1: Various terminologies for athletic-related groin pain

- Sport's hernia or sportsman's hernia
- Abdominal core injury
- Athletic pubalgia
- Hockey groin syndrome
- Gilmore's groin
- Inguinal disruption
- Posterior abdominal wall deficiency
- Pubic inguinal pain syndrome
- Doha conference terminology [6].
  - Inguinal-related groin pain
  - Adductor-related groin pain
  - Pubic-related groin pain

pubalgia, abdominal core injury, posterior abdominal wall deficiency, Gilmore groin, hockey groin syndrome, and others [1–4]. In 2014, the British Hernia Society convened a consensus conference of experts from across the United Kingdom to address this issue [5]. This group recommended the term "inguinal disruption," which reflects the weakening in the inguinal floor and tension across the pubis and inguinal ligament that results. In November 2014, a world conference on this topic was held in Doha, Qatar, that involved 24 experts and that used a Delphi process and systematic reviews of the literature [6]. This group recommended 3 broad groups of groin pain: (1) defined clinical entities for groin pain with 4 subgroups (adductor-related, iliopsoas-related, inguinal-related, and pubic-related), (2) hip-related groin pain, and (3) other conditions causing groin pain in athletes (eg, neurologic, spine, urologic). For the purposes of this review, the term athletic pubalgia is used to broadly reflect the athletic groin pain conditions that impact the general surgeon with use of inguinal disruption and inguinal and adductor-related pain, as appropriate.

BACKGROUND AND EPIDEMIOLOGY OF GROIN INJURIES

Groin injuries are a common problem in sports because of the forces exerted around the pelvis when athletes move at high speed. Sports such as soccer, football, and ice hockey are the ones most commonly associated with groin injuries because of the frequency that athletes go through sudden cutting, turning, and kicking motions at a high rate of speed. Although these injuries can be related to contact due to a force applied against a muscle when it is eccentrically contracted and a sudden force further stretches that muscle, many of these are actually noncontact in nature. The most common groin injuries are muscular strains, and the adductor muscle group is the most common muscle group injured in this location. In one study of soccer players, groin injuries comprised 5% to 28% of all athletic injuries [7]. Several groups have looked at risk factors for groin injuries. In one study of male soccer players in Norway [8], multivariate analysis showed that an increased risk of groin injury was related to a prior history of an acute groin injury or relative weakness in the adductor muscles on clinical evaluation. Another group demonstrated in a study of National Hockey League (NHL) players that a reduced adductor-to-abductor strength ratio was present on the side of the injury [9]. Moreover, they were able to reduce the incidence of injuries by a factor of 4.5 by instituting a prospective adductor-strengthening program. Finally, in another study of NHL players, a history of previous groin or abdominal strain, veteran player status, and reduced frequency of off-season sports-specific training sessions were all associated with an increased risk of groin injury [10]. These findings suggest strategies with which athletes and athletic trainers can preemptively implement off-season training regimens that may reduce the incidence of these injuries during the rigors of a prolonged regular season.

DIFFERENTIAL DIAGNOSIS

The differential diagnosis of groin pain in athletes is broad and includes disorders of the bony pelvis, muscular strains, hip injuries, and sport's hernia pubalgia and inguinal hernia as reviewed in several recent publications [11–14]. A list of conditions associated with athletic groin pain is given in Box 2. As noted previously, the most common injuries are muscular strains that may consist of adductor, hip flexor, iliopsoas, rectus, and oblique muscular strains. Findings on examination may include palpable areas of tenderness and pain with resisted movements. An effort should be made to isolate different muscle groups to most precisely determine the anatomic basis for the complaints.

A second category of injuries is centered around the pelvis and pubis and includes osteitis pubis and stress-related pubic fractures. Osteitis pubis is a condition in which there is pain localized centrally over the pubic symphysis region. It is thought to be related to overuse and excessive training and can be diagnosed on MRI in which there is evidence of edema throughout the pubic bones on both sides. Treatment is primarily rest and other standard conservative measures, but in some cases this condition can respond to a pubic symphysis injection with local anesthesia plus corticosteroid.

Hip injuries also can overlap with athletic pubalgia, and these include labral tears, femoral acetabular impingement, and osteoarthritis. A careful hip examination should be done in all athletes with groin pain to exclude a hip etiology. Labral tears may appear as an incidental finding on MRI or may be the primary source of groin/hip pain, and so involvement of a sports medicine specialist or hip orthopedist should be undertaken in patients in whom a possible hip etiology is considered.

Athletes may present with a true inguinal hernia, although this is a relatively uncommon occurrence. In our series of more than 250 athletes operated on for

Box 2: Differential diagnosis of athletic groin pain

Abdominal/Inguinal

- Muscular strains (rectus abdominis, oblique)
- Athletic pubalgia injury (rectus aponeurosis tear, inguinal disruption)
- Inguinal hernia
- Nerve entrapment (ilioinguinal)

Pubis

- Osteitis pubis
- Pubic ramus stress fracture

Hip/Thigh Musculature

- Adductor strain, adductor tendinopathy, partial or complete tear
- Hip flexor strain (iliopsoas, rectus femoris)

Hip

- Labral tear
- Femoroacetabular impingement
- Osteoarthritis
- Femoral neck stress fracture
- Avascular necrosis

Urologic

- Urinary tract infection, prostatitis
- Testicular varicocele

Gynecologic

- Endometriosis
- Ovarian cyst
- Round ligament syndrome

chronic groin pain, only 4% had findings of a true inguinal hernia. Symptoms may consist of exertional groin pain or patients may be asymptomatic with the hernia an incidental finding. The diagnosis is usually apparent on physical examination, which should be done with the athlete standing and performing a Valsalva maneuver.

Athletic pubalgia or an inguinal disruption injury (sport's hernia) should be considered in athletes who present with exertional-related pain in the lower abdominal region/distal rectus abdominis or medial inguinal canal that does not respond to initial conservative treatment measures and in whom there is no inguinal hernia. The pain occurs typically at the extremes of exertion, such as sprinting, and can limit quick accelerating movements, such as cutting, turning, and kicking, which are critical to an athlete's success in competition. Other symptoms may include pain with coughing or sneezing and getting in and out of bed or a car. In general, this diagnosis should not be entertained until a period of conservative management of 6 to 8 weeks has been undertaken, unless imaging shows evidence of a rectus aponeurosis tear.

Adductor injuries may be isolated to one muscle group, most commonly the adductor longus, or may involve multiple adductor muscle units, such as the adductor brevis and pectineus. Adductor strains may have a gradual onset or may be associated with a sudden pop or pull if there is a partial or complete tear. Treatment consists of rest, ice, compression, and a graduated stretching and strengthening program and return to sport. The time to recovery can range from a few days to 5 to 6 weeks for complete disruptions. The role of surgical management for adductor-related injuries is gaining increasing interest and is reviewed later in this article (see section on role of adductor tenotomy).

Finally, there are nonathletic causes of groin pain that should be considered, particularly in female athletes. These include various gynecologic etiologies, such as ovarian cyst or endometriosis. Nonathletic causes of groin pain are rare in male athletes.

CLINICAL EVALUATION

The evaluation of the athlete with groin pain should be multidisciplinary, involving the sport medicine physician/orthopedist and/or athletic trainer and should engage the general surgeon only if there is a clinical suspicion of an inguinal hernia or suspected high-grade abdominal injury, or if the athlete fails to improve with conservative management. It is important to obtain a careful history regarding the onset of symptoms, precise anatomic location of the pain, and whether it is inguinal, central abdominal, adductor, hip, or hip flexor related. Any activating or alleviating factors should be identified, such as whether the pain occurs at rest or only with increased physical activity, including running, kicking, skating, cutting/turning movements, and coughing and sneezing. The latter implies a potential abdominal component of the injury. It should be emphasized that pain at rest or with normal light activities is unusual in athletic pubalgia-type injuries. It should be determined if there is a prior history of groin injury, as some athletes have had a lower-level injury the prior season that improved early in the off season, only to have the symptoms reappear with an uptick in activity during training camp or the early part of the next season. In many cases, the onset of symptoms is insidious without a specific precipitating incidence.

Physical examination of the athlete with groin pain should begin with a standard inguinal hernia examination. The athlete should be standing and examined with Valsalva maneuvers both during direct palpation of the inguinal canal and by palpating the external ring by way of invaginating the scrotum. The testicles should be carefully examined as well. The athlete should then be examined supine with palpation over the midline symphysis pubis and pubic bones to identify any areas of tenderness. Palpation of the medial inguinal floor and lateral distal rectus should be done to assess for any inguinal floor weakness or asymmetry between the 2 sides, and this also should be carried out during a sit-up assessing for associated tenderness. Resisted sit-up and trunk rotation should be done to assess for rectus abdominis insertional pain and oblique muscle symptoms. The hip should be examined for range of motion and pain with internal and external rotation and with flexion abduction and external rotation to rule out possible hip pathology. Finally, an examination of the thigh musculature should be carried out by assessment of strength and discomfort with resisted straight leg raising, hip flexion, and resisted adduction and abduction. Palpation should be carried out along the upper adductor muscle tendon junction and tendinous insertion site to assess for any areas of tenderness, thickening, and tightness.

DIAGNOSTIC EVALUATION AND IMAGING

If the presence of an inguinal hernia is demonstrated and corresponds to the area of symptoms, then no further diagnostic evaluation or imaging is indicated. For suspected athletic pubalgia, imaging studies should be carried out to assess for supporting findings of this diagnosis and to exclude other pathology, such as hip abnormalities. The preferred imaging modality for the diagnosis of athletic pubalgia is a pelvic MRI [15]. It is important that this study include high-resolution sagittal sequences, and if adductor pathology is suspected, then oblique transverse T2 images with fat suppression should be included as well. There are several MRI findings that can be associated with athletic pubalgia-type injuries. These include parasymphyseal edema, a secondary cleft at the symphysis pubis, or rectus abdominis or adductor aponeurosis tears or both (Fig. 1) [15,16]. Partial or complete adductor tears can be visualized along with evidence of adductor tendinopathy in the absence of an actual

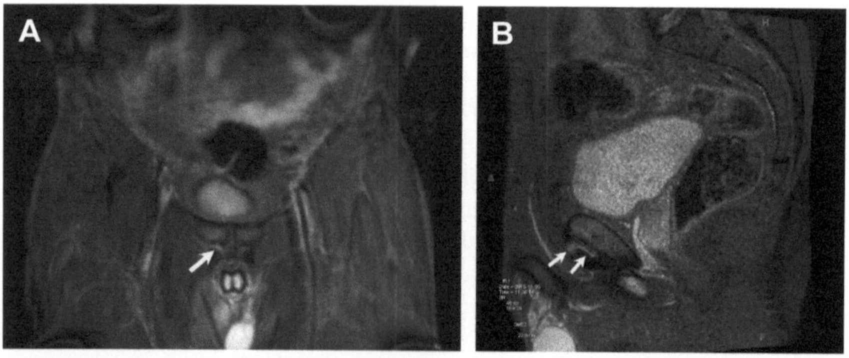

Fig. 1. MRI of rectus aponeurosis tear. (*A*) Coronal view and (*B*) sagittal view, which show a tear (*arrows*) at rectus aponeurosis insertion on pubis.

aponeurotic tear. In addition, the MRI should include images of both hips to exclude obvious hip pathology, such as labral tears or osteoarthritis. The pelvic MRI should also be able to identify stress fractures at the pubis or hip.

There can be overlap between athletic pubalgia and osteitis pubis clinically; on MRI, osteitis pubis is more associated with bone marrow edema that extends across the entire pubic body from anterior to posterior and is symmetric [16]. Some groups have used dynamic ultrasound to detect a bulging or protrusion of the transverse abdominis fascia during a Valsalva maneuver [17]. In one study, a positive correlation was found between ultrasound findings and operative findings of a sport's hernia [14]. A significant limitation of ultrasound is that it is highly operator dependent and it can be difficult for clinicians other than the sonographer to accurately interpret any images obtained, in contrast to MRI, which is readily interpretable by appropriately trained individuals. Plain pelvis radiographs have little role in the evaluation of athletic groin pain except to exclude a possible traumatic pelvic fracture or suspected hip pathology. Abdominal computed tomography (CT) scans similarly have little role because of the limitations of CT in the evaluation of musculotendinous structures and should be reserved for suspected intra-abdominal or pelvic pathology. The presence of an inguinal hernia noted incidentally on MRI should be correlated with clinical findings before recommending surgical intervention, as this may be clinically insignificant.

PATHOPHYSIOLOGY OF ATHLETIC PUBALGIA

The pathophysiology of athletic pubalgia has been postulated to involve principally 1 of 3 different mechanisms or a combination of the 3: (1) rectus tendon injury or injury to the rectus-adductor aponeurosis complex [18,19], (2) posterior abdominal wall/inguinal floor defect [20], and (3) inguinal and/or genital neuropathy [21–23]. Rectus and adductor aponeurosis tendon injuries can be seen on pelvic MRI imaging. Meyers and colleagues [19] proposed the concept of the "pubic joint," in which opposing abdominal and thigh muscular forces act. These primarily involve the rectus on the superior side of the pubis and the adductor muscle group inferiorly. An imbalance in forces across the pubis can lead to weakening of the rectus muscle at the pubic insertion site, which in turn can result in pain at the pubis with exertional movements. Meyers and colleagues [18] described 17 different variants of athletic pubalgia. In the classic variant, the pain is at the lateral rectus abdominis at its insertion on the pubis. The other most common variants involved the adductor longus as a principal site for pain or a combination of rectus and adductor pathology.

The second mechanism associated with inguinal pain in athletes is weakness of the posterior inguinal floor, which has been reported in up to 85% or more of athletes with this condition [5,14,20]. Similar to the previously mentioned concept, this relative weakening of the posterior inguinal floor creates an imbalance of forces across the pubis and may alter the degree of tension on the rectus at its insertion [21]. In addition to defects in the posterior inguinal floor, attenuation or tears in the external oblique aponeurosis are commonly present as well (Fig. 2). Note that these findings are not exclusive of pathology at the rectus insertion site on the pubis and, in fact, they frequently coexist.

A third potential mechanism of pain involves ilioinguinal or genital neuralgia, and some groups have recommended routine resection of the ilioinguinal nerve during inguinal floor repair [22,23]. However, most authorities do not resect the ilioinguinal nerve, including those who do laparoscopic approaches and have good reported outcomes, which argues against this as a primary mechanism. Muschaweck and Berger [21] postulated that pressure on the genital femoral nerve from the bulging posterior inguinal floor can be a source of pain. As a result, selective resection of the genital nerve is performed as a part of their repair. No controlled studies have been carried out to address the impact of ilioinguinal or genital neurectomy on symptomatic response to surgery in athletes with this problem.

It is important to note that athletic pubalgia is not simply one condition, but can represent a spectrum of findings that require an individualized evaluation and assessment of the best therapeutic management approach for these athletes.

SURGICAL INDICATIONS AND OPERATIVE APPROACHES

Inguinal hernia

The presence of a true inguinal hernia in an athlete is an indication for repair regardless of symptoms. However, this generally can be an elective procedure that is undertaken in the off season to avoid missed time from participation in sport. Simply the presence of an inguinal hernia should not be considered a contraindication to playing sports unless the athlete is limited by symptoms or the hernia is locally tender on examination or the hernia is difficult to reduce.

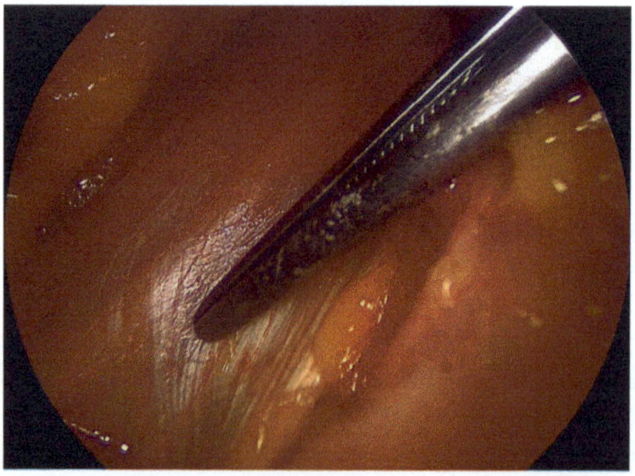

Fig. 2. External oblique aponeurosis weakness and thinning in an athlete undergoing athletic pubalgia surgery.

There are no studies that compare operative approaches for inguinal hernia repair in athletes. A laparoscopic approach may offer some advantages over an open repair in terms of less pain and return to play, but each case should be individualized according to hernia and patient factors and local surgical expertise. Mesh should be avoided in young athletes who are still in their growth phase, and a primary repair should be done instead. Special care should be taken to identify the ilioinguinal nerve if an open repair is done and to avoid mobilizing it from its covering sheath, which may expose the nerve to the subsequent fibrosis around the mesh. If the nerve is going to be compromised in any way, it is better to resect it proximal to the internal ring where the cut end can retract into the muscle to minimize the risk of painful neuroma formation.

Athletic pubalgia

The indications for surgical management of an athletic pubalgia injury include failure of conservative management and symptoms that limit athletic performance. Other potential causes of groin pain, such as hip pathology, that would explain the athlete's pain should be ruled out by examination and imaging (Box 2). It should be noted that other lesions may coexist with an athletic pubalgia, such as osteitis pubis or hip labral tears, and management in those cases should be coordinated with the appropriate other specialists.

Two prospective randomized trials have compared the outcomes of extended physical therapy versus surgical management for this condition [24,25]. In both studies, a higher return to sport and reduction in pain was associated with surgery. Paajanen and colleagues [25] randomized 60 athletes with 3 to 6 months of groin pain who met the criteria for a diagnosis of "sports hernia" to either extended physiotherapy or laparoscopic inguinal floor repair. At 3 months, only 27% of the conservatively managed group had returned to sport compared with 90% of the surgically treated athletes, and at 12 months the return to sport rate was 50% for the conservative group versus 97% for the operative group. Pain scores were also less at each time point for the surgically treated athletes. In addition, 7 of the 30 patients crossed over and underwent surgery after 6 months of failure of conservative treatment. These studies thus favor surgical intervention in appropriately selected athletes.

A variety of operative approaches have been reported for the management of inguinal-related athletic pubalgia, as listed in Box 3. In broad terms, these may be classified as (1) open primary tissue repairs, (2) open tension-free mesh repairs, and (3) laparoscopic posterior mesh repair. Meyers and colleagues [1] advocated a primary tissue repair in which the inferolateral edge of the rectus muscle fascia is sutured to the pubis and adjacent anterior ligaments. This approach is somewhat analogous to a Bassini repair, except the sutures distally are oriented in a near vertical line and the internal ring is not tightened. Muschaweck and Berger [21] used a "minimal repair" technique in which only the weakened section of the posterior inguinal floor is opened. The defect is then is repaired by suturing 2 imbricating running layers of nonabsorbable

Box 3: Surgical approaches to athletic-related groin pain (athletic pubalgia)

- Primary tissue repairs
  - Primary pelvic floor repair (Meyers technique)
  - Minimal repair technique (Muschaweck technique)
- Open tension-free mesh repair
- Laparoscopic posterior mesh repairs
  - Transabdominal preperitoneal (TEP)
  - Total extraperitoneal preperitoneal (TAPP)
  - Inguinal ligament release with TAPP repair (Lloyd technique)
- Adductor tenotomy (partial or complete)[a]

[a]Note: an adductor release may be performed in isolation or in conjunction with any of the inguinal floor repair techniques.

monofilament suture between the transversalis/internal layers and the iliopubic tract/inguinal ligament with lateralization of the rectus somewhat analogous to a Shouldice repair. The open tissue free mesh repair is analogous to the Lichtenstein tension-free mesh hernioplasty and accomplishes the similar purpose of providing strength and support across a weakened posterior inguinal floor and stabilizing the distal lateral rectus (Fig. 3) [26]. Laparoscopically, both transabdominal preperitoneal (TAPP) and total extraperitoneal (TEP) approaches have been used. Lloyd and colleagues [27] advocated a ligament release in addition to laparoscopic repair of the inguinal floor based on the concept that tension in the ligament as the principal source of pain in these athletes. The inguinal ligament is "released" close to its attachment to the pubis and the entire inguinal floor is reinforced with a lightweight polypropylene mesh

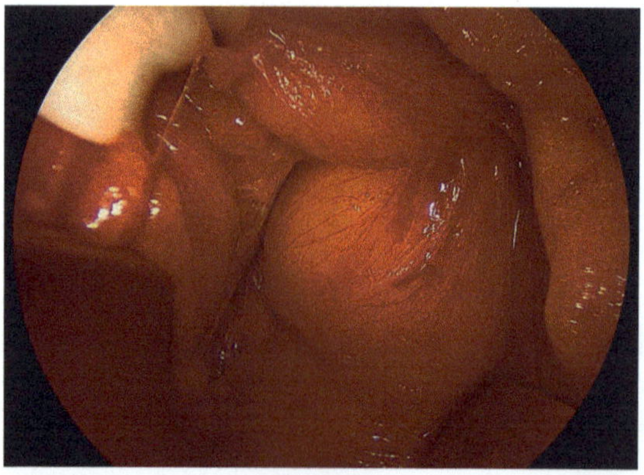

Fig. 3. Posterior inguinal floor weakness in an athlete undergoing athletic pubalgia surgery.

(Figs. 4 and 5). A successful return to sport was reported in 92% of athletes who underwent this procedure but follow-up was short, at an average of 28 days.

The largest experience with surgical repair in patients with athletic pubalgia was reported by Meyers and colleagues (Philadelphia) in 2008 [28]. More than 5200 athletes were operated on between 1986 and 2008. Return to sport within 3 months was accomplished in 95.3% of athletes. Reoperation for significant postoperative hematoma was necessary in 14 patients (0.3%) and the wound infection rate was 0.4%. Reoperation was undertaken for development of symptoms on the contralateral side in 182 athletes and 28 athletes required additional adductor surgery. The precise incidence of adductor release in this series was not stated, but overall approximately 60% of patents had an adductor component of their athletic pubalgia syndrome. Of note is that 241 patients (4.6%) had failed prior traditional hernia surgery.

Muschaweck and Berger [21] (Munich, Germany) reported 129 athletes operated on from 2008 to 2009 with the minimal repair technique. Patients were allowed to lift up to 20 kg immediately after surgery, resume running/cycling at 2 days, and begin specific training on the third to fourth postoperative days. The results at the 4-week follow-up after surgery were a resumption of training resumed at 7 days in 96.1% of athletes and an overall median time to return to sport of 18.5 days. These results highlight the value of allowing early rehabilitation and return to sport after surgical repair, although longer-term results and the durability of this approach have not yet been reported.

Open tension-free mesh repairs, as described by several groups, also have achieved successful return to sport in more than 90% of cases [23,29]. Theoretically, this approach should allow early resumption of sport as well, without concerns for reinjury because of the tension-free method of repairing the inguinal floor. Brown and colleagues [23] in Montreal operated on 98 elite/professional hockey players over an 18-year time frame. They used a polytetrafluoroethylene (PTFE) patch technique placed underneath the external oblique aponeurosis in conjunction with ilioinguinal neurectomy. Overall, 97

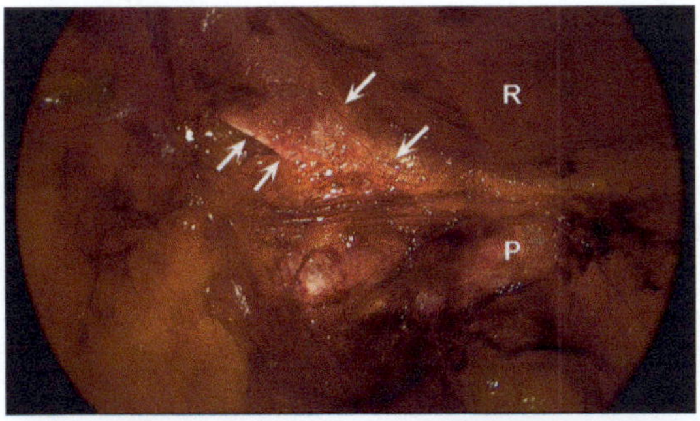

Fig. 4. Laparoscopic view of weakened left posterior inguinal floor. R, rectus; P, pubis. Arrows point to area of floor weakness.

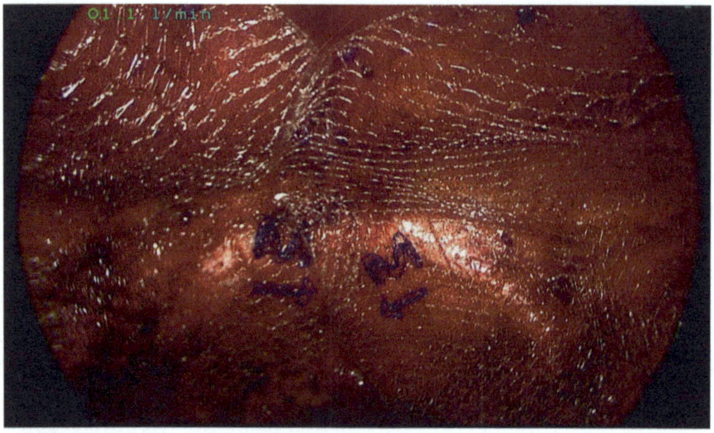

Fig. 5. Laparoscopic view of bilateral posterior mesh repair for athletic pubalgia, total extraperitoneal approach.

of 98 players returned to playing hockey with recurrent symptoms being seen in 3 athletes.

Success with laparoscopic repair has been reported by several groups [30–32]. The largest series reported is from Evans [31], who carried out a laparoscopic TAPP repair with mesh in 287 athletes. The repairs were bilateral in a high percentage of cases (56%), although nearly one-third of those patients were asymptomatic on the side contralateral to the primary injury. Return to sport data were available in 192 patients, of whom 90% were playing sport by 4 weeks. Eight patients required reoperation for recurrences on longer-term follow-up. Genitsaris and associates [32] carried out a bilateral laparoscopic TAPP repair in 131 patients who had failed conservative management of athletic groin pain. The reason for the bilateral repair was a finding of a posterior wall weakness on the contralateral side, although 33 of these patients had unilateral symptoms only. Return to sport was accomplished at 3 weeks after surgery, with 1 failure (0.76%) noted during follow-up.

At the present time, there is no consensus on 1 single surgical approach to the management of athletic groin pain. In the 2014 British Hernia Society consensus conference, it was noted that although the laparoscopic repair was associated with a somewhat earlier return to activity, this has not been analyzed in any controlled or case-matched comparison study [5]. It was stated that the type of repair undertaken is primarily related to the individual surgeon's expertise.

Given the data supporting good outcomes for both open and laparoscopic repairs, the author has undertaken an individualized approach to the management of these athletes that takes into consideration the examination findings, imaging results, presence of a rectus aponeurosis tear, and the extent of any associated adductor-related groin symptoms and findings, and history of prior inguinal surgery. In the author's series of 257 cases operated on over the past 12 years, open tension-free mesh repair has been carried out in 82.8%, laparoscopic TEP mesh repairs in 12.5%, and primary tissue repairs in 4.7%. A partial adductor tenotomy selectively in athletes with predominately chronic adductor symptoms and associated MRI findings was performed in 94 athletes. One-year follow-up was available for 97 athletes, of whom 94.5% had returned to sport. Time to return to play data are not consistently available in this analysis, but in general has ranged from 5 to 8 weeks in most cases.

ROLE OF ADDUCTOR TENOTOMY

In athletes with predominately adductor-related symptoms, and examination and imaging findings that do not respond to maximal conservative treatment measures, adductor tenotomy has been advocated to reduce the tension in the adductor compartment and facilitate resolution of symptoms. Several groups have reported results with either partial or complete adductor tenotomy with or without concomitant repair of the ipsilateral inguinal floor. Meyers and colleagues [1] described division of the anterior epimysial fibers of the adductor longus in selected athletes in conjunction with a primary pelvic floor repair. Schilders and colleagues [33] reported outcomes of a selective partial adductor release in professional soccer and rugby players with chronic adductor tendinopathy. All athletes had undergone 3 months of active adductor therapy and a pubic cleft injection. The procedure consisted of division of the superficial fibers of the adductor tendon 2 to 3 cm from its origin. Return to preinjury level of sport was achieved in 42 of 43 athletes at a mean of 9.2 weeks postoperatively. Ten of their athletes had undergone prior inguinal floor repairs and an additional 3 had a groin repair between 1.0 and 3.5 years postoperatively.

"Percutaneous" adductor tenotomy via a 1-cm stab incision just distal to the adductor longus insertion was carried out by Atkinson and colleagues [34] in a study of 48 patients. The mean time to return to sport was 18.5 weeks with 54% returning to preinjury levels. Improvement in function was rated at 78.1% and improvement in pain at 86.5%. Concomitant laparoscopic inguinal floor repair with mesh and ipsilateral adductor tenotomy was carried out in 54 patients in another study [35]. A rectus injury on MRI was seen in 26% of those undergoing MRI. The tenotomy was performed 1 cm distal to the insertion on the pubis. On average, sports-related activity was resumed at 24 days in all athletes. Over a mean follow-up of 18 months, one athlete required contralateral tenotomy and another developed an adductor brevis hematoma. Vezeridis and Gill [36] performed a complete adductor release in 15 athletes with a follow-up of 7.2 years. More than 90% had significant improvement in symptoms and 80% were asymptomatic. The average time to return to sport was 14.3 weeks.

Whether acute adductor avulsions should be managed conservatively or be repaired is controversial. Schlegel and colleagues [37] analyzed conservative management ($n = 14$) versus surgical repair ($n = 5$) in a study of National Football League players. Mean time to return to play was 6.1 ± 3.1 weeks in the conservatively treated group compared with 12.0 ± 2.5 weeks in the surgically managed patients. In another study of 15 high-level athletes, adductor repair was performed between 5 and 34 days of their injury [38]. The repair was done by using bone anchors to reattach the torn tendon to the pubis. Return to sport occurred at a mean of 13 weeks (range 10–21 weeks). An accompanying mesh reinforcement of the abdominal wall was done in 7 of these cases. No recurrences were observed over 1 year of follow-up.

POSTOPERATIVE MANAGEMENT AND RETURN TO SPORT

Just like with any orthopedic surgical procedure in a high-performance athlete, it is important to have a structured approach to physical therapy and rehabilitation after surgery for athletic pubalgia and also for conventional inguinal hernia repair. The guiding principles should include a stepwise return to activity based on symptomatic progression with an emphasis on strength, flexibility, and balance in the lower extremity muscle units and a strong stable abdominal core. Our protocol [29] consists of normal light activities, including walking the first 3 to 5 days, with resumption of brisk walking progressing to light running and stationary biking as soon as comfort allows. Resistance exercises, including pool therapy, can be introduced within 10 to 12 days of surgery. Sports-specific activity, such as running easy pass routes, skating, dribbling a soccer ball, throwing, and catching should be initiated by 2 to 2.5 weeks. Scar mobilization and massage can be implemented as soon as is comfortable, but usually by 3 weeks. Progression from that point should be based on functional performance and symptoms with progressive increase in speed, intensity, and quickness toward scrimmaging and then game play. Recently, an accelerated recovery protocol was advocated by Muschaweck and coworkers [14,21] that allows a resumption of full sports training within less than 2 weeks and return to competitive play by 3 to 4 weeks. For many athletes, surgery is undertaken in the off season and a more gradual return to intense sports activity is appropriate. It should be emphasized that the degree of underlying pathology and level of injury are also important determinants of the timetable for return to play and may result in a more extended recovery time in any given athlete.

SUMMARY

In summary, the evaluation of the athlete with groin pain and suspected athletic pubalgia requires a multidisciplinary approach that should involve the athletic trainer, sports orthopedist, and surgeon. The presence of a true inguinal hernia is an indication for repair, preferably in the off season to minimize time away from sport. For athletes with a diagnosis of athletic pubalgia who have failed conservative management, several surgical options may be considered and the repair should be tailored to the particular pathology and symptomatic findings. Surgeons who undertake management of these athletes should be well versed in the varied pathology of this condition and related musculoskeletal causes of groin pain.

References

[1] Meyers W, Foley D, Garrett W, et al. Management of severe lower abdominal or inguinal pain in high-performance athletes. PAIN (Performing Athletes with Abdominal or Inguinal Neuromuscular Pain Study Group). Am J Sports Med 2000;28:2–8.
[2] Steele P, Annear P, Grove JR. Surgery for posterior inguinal wall deficiency in athletes. J Sci Med Sport 2004;7(4):415–21.
[3] Gilmore OJA. Gilmore's groin: ten years experience of groin disruption-a previously unsolved problem in sportsmen. Sports Med Soft Tissue Trauma 1991;3:12–4.
[4] Irshad K, Feldman L, Lavoie C, et al. Operative management of "hockey groin syndrome": 12 years of experience in National Hockey League players. Surgery 2001;130:759–64.
[5] Sheen AJ, Stephenson BM, Lloyd DM, et al. Treatment of the sportsman's groin: British Hernia Society's 2014 position statement based on the Manchester Consensus Conference. Br J Sports Med 2014;48:1079–87.
[6] Weir A, Brikner P, Delahunt E, et al. Doha agreement meeting on terminology and definitions in groin pain in athletes. Br J Sports Med 2015;49:768–74.
[7] Ekstrand J, Hilding J. The incidence and differential diagnosis of acute groin injuries in male soccer players. Scand J Med Sci Sports 1999;9:98–103.
[8] Engebretson AH, Myklebust G, Holme I, et al. Intrinsic risk factors for groin injuries among male soccer players: a prospective cohort study. Am J Sports Med 2010;38(10):2051–7.
[9] Tyler TF, Nicholas SJ, Campbell RJ, et al. The association of hip strength and flexibility with the incidence of adductor muscle strains in professional ice hockey players. Am J Sports Med 2001;29:124–8.
[10] Emery CA, Meeuwisse W. Risk factors for groin injuries in hockey. Med Sci Sports Exerc 2001;33(9):1423–33.
[11] Swan KG, Wolcott M. The athletic hernia: a systematic review. Clin Orthop Relat Res 2007;455:78–87.
[12] Caudill P, Nyland J, Smith C, et al. Sports hernias: a systematic literature review. Br J Sports Med 2008;42:954–64.
[13] Nam A, Brody F. Management and therapy for sports hernia. J Am Coll Surg 2008;206: 154–64.
[14] Minnich JM, Hanks JB, Muschaweck U, et al. Sports hernia: diagnosis and treatment highlighting a minimal repair surgical technique. Am J Sports Med 2011;39:1341–9.
[15] Zoga AC, Kavanagh EC, Morrison WB, et al. Athletic pubalgia and the "sports hernia": MR imaging findings. Radiology 2008;247:797–807.
[16] Rubin DA. Imaging of athletic groin pain. In: Diduch DR, Brunt LM, editors. Sports hernia and athletic pubalgia. New York: Springer; 2014. p. 87–105.
[17] Muschaweck U, Berger LM. Sportsmen's groin–diagnostic approach and treatment: with the minimal repair technique: a single center uncontrolled review. Sports Health 2010;2:216–21.
[18] Meyers WC, Greenleaf R, Saad A. Anatomic basis for evaluation of abdominal and groin pain in athletes. Oper Tech Sports Med 2005;13:55–61.
[19] Meyers WC, Yoo E, Devon ON, et al. Understanding "sports hernia" (athletic pubalgia): the anatomic and pathophysiologic basis for abdominal and groin pain in athletes. Oper Tech Sports Med 2007;15:165–77.
[20] Steele P, Annear P, Grove JR. Surgery for posterior inguinal wall deficiency in athletes. J Sci Med Sport 2004;7(4):415–21.
[21] Muschaweck U, Berger L. Minimal repair technique of sportsmen's groin: an innovative open-suture repair to treat chronic inguinal pain. Hernia 2010;14:27–33.
[22] Ziprin P, Williams P, Foster ME. External oblique aponeurosis nerve entrapment as a cause of groin pain in the athlete. Br J Surg 1999;86:566–8.
[23] Brown R, Mascia A, Kinnear DG, et al. An 18 year review of sports groin injuries in the elite hockey player: clinical presentation, new diagnostic imaging, treatment, and results. Clin J Sport Med 2008;18:221–6.

[24] Ekstrand J, Ringbog S. Surgery versus conservative treatment in soccer players with chronic groin pain: a prospective, randomized study in soccer players. Eur J Sports Traumatol Rel Res 2001;23:141–5.
[25] Paajanen H, Brinck T, Hermunen H, et al. Laparoscopic surgery for chronic groin pain in athletes is more effective than nonoperative treatment: a randomized clinical trial with magnetic resonance imaging of 60 patients with sportsman's hernia (athletic pubalgia). Surgery 2011;150:99–107.
[26] Brunt LM. Surgical treatment of sports hernia: open mesh approach. In: Diduch D, Brunt LM, editors. Sports hernia and athletic pubalgia: diagnosis and treatment. New York: Springer; 2014. p. 133–42.
[27] Lloyd DM, Sutton CD, Altafa A, et al. Laparoscopic inguinal ligament tenotomy and mesh reinforcement of the anterior abdominal wall: a new approach for the management of chronic groin pain. Surg Laparosc Endosc Percutan Tech 2008;18(4):363–8.
[28] Meyers WC, McKechnie A, Philippon MJ, et al. Experience with "sports hernia" spanning two decades. Ann Surg 2008;248:656–65.
[29] Brunt LM, Barile R. My approach to athletic pubalgia. In: Byrd TW, editor. Operative hip arthroscopy. 3rd edition. New York: Springer; 2013. p. 55–65.
[30] Azurin DJ, Go LS, Schuricht A, et al. Endoscopic preperitoneal herniorrhaphy in professional athletes with groin pain. J Laparoendosc Adv Surg Tech A 1997;7:7–12.
[31] Evans DS. Hunterian lecture. Laparoscopic transabdominal pre-peritoneal (TAPP) repair of groin hernia: one surgeon's experience of a developing technique. Ann R Coll Surg Engl 2002;84:393–8.
[32] Genitsaris M, Goulimaris I, Sikas N. Laparoscopic repair of groin pain in athletes. Am J Sports Med 2004;32:1238–42.
[33] Schilders E, Dmitrakopoulou A, Cooke M, et al. Effectiveness of a selective partial adductor release for chronic adductor-related groin pain in professional athletes. Am J Sports Med 2013;41:603–7.
[34] Atkinson HD, Johal P, Falworth MS, et al. Adductor tenotomy: Its role in the management of sports-related groin pain. Arch Orthop Trauma Surg 2010;130:965–70.
[35] Rossidis G, Perry A, Abbas H, et al. Laparoscopic hernia repair with adductor tenotomy for athletic pubalgia: an established procedure for an obscure entity. Surg Endosc 2015;29:381–6.
[36] Vezeridis P, Gill TJ. Adductor injuries and the role of adductor tenotomy for groin pain in athletes. In: Diduch D, Brunt LM, editors. Sports hernia and athletic pubalgia: diagnosis and treatment. New York: Springer; 2014. p. 173–81.
[37] Schlegel TF, Bushnell BD, Godfery J, et al. Success of nonoperative management of adductor longus tendon ruptures in National Football League athletes. Am J Sports Med 2009;37:1394–9.
[38] Tansey RJ, Benjamin-Lang H, Jassim S, et al. Successful return to high-level sports following early surgical repair of combined adductor complex and rectus abdominis avulsion. Bone Joint J 2015;97-B:1488–92.

Advances in Surgery 50 (2016) 203–220

ADVANCES IN SURGERY

Groin Pain After Inguinal Hernia Repair

David K. Nguyen, MD[a], Parviz K. Amid, MD[a,b], David C. Chen, MD[a,b,*]

[a]Department of Surgery, David Geffen School of Medicine at UCLA, 10833 Le Conte Avenue, Los Angeles, CA 90095, USA; [b]Lichtenstein Amid Hernia Clinic at UCLA, 1304 15th Street, Suite 102, Santa Monica, CA 90404, USA

Keywords

• Chronic pain • Inguinal hernia • Lichtenstein • Neurectomy • CPIP
• Chronic postoperative inguinal pain • Inguinodynia

Key points

- Quality of life and avoidance of chronic postoperative inguinal pain (CPIP) are now primary outcomes of elective inguinal herniorrhaphy because of the success of tension-free mesh-based repairs.
- Multidisciplinary approach with a pain management team is indicated if several months of expectant management of CPIP do not result in amelioration of symptoms.
- Conservative treatment with topical, pharmacologic, behavioral, and expectant measures is advocated in all patients.
- Triple neurectomy is the recommended surgical treatment of neuropathic inguinal pain refractory to conservative measures.
- Reoperation for CPIP is best performed by experienced herniologists; less experienced clinicians should refer patients with CPIP who fail conservative management to a multidisciplinary team.

INTRODUCTION

Inguinal hernia repair is one of the most common surgical procedures performed in the world, with 20 million performed worldwide and 800,000 in the United States annually [1–4]. Refinement of techniques and mesh-based

Disclosure Statement: The authors have nothing to disclose.

*Corresponding author. Lichtenstein Amid Hernia Clinic at UCLA, 1304 15th Street, Suite 102, Santa Monica, CA 90404. *E-mail address*: dcchen@mednet.ucla.edu

0065-3411/16/$ – see front matter
http://dx.doi.org/10.1016/j.yasu.2016.04.003

tension-free repairs has resulted in a decrease of hernia recurrence rates to between 1% and 5% [5]. Chronic postoperative inguinal pain (CPIP) is now the most significant complication and quality of life is the most relevant outcome of inguinal hernia repair [6,7]. CPIP affects the daily life of 5% to 10% of patients, with downstream effects on patient satisfaction, health care utilization, societal cost, and quality of life [8–10].

The high prevalence of CPIP requires a systematic approach for optimal management of these patients. This article reviews the current literature regarding causes of CPIP along with up-to-date Delphi consensus statements on management of CPIP proposed by expert herniologists and pain management physicians.

SIGNIFICANCE

Definition

CPIP was formally defined in 2008 as new or different quality of pain (if pain existed before hernia repair) arising as a direct consequence of a nerve lesion or disease affecting the somatosensory system after inguinal hernia repair [11]. The estimated risk of moderate to severe CPIP is 10% to 12% with CPIP affecting daily life in 0.5% to 6% of patients [4,12,13]. This translates to 4000 to 48,000 new cases in the United States annually [7]. Downstream effects of CPIP include the following:

- Depression and anxiety [10,14–17]
- Cognitive impairment
- Somatic comorbidities
- Sleep deprivation leading to worsening of pain
- Reduced quality of life
- Total annual indirect and direct health care cost of CPIP: $9000 to $40,000 per patient

Etiology

The cause of CPIP is complex and variable. Patients often exhibit overlapping signs and symptoms of pain types. Diagnosis and management is challenging because of the significant overlap and combinations. Distinguishing between neuropathic and nonneuropathic or visceral pain is complicated by excitatory coupling between sympathetic and afferent nociceptive nerve fibers; neuroplasticity; deafferentation hyperalgesia; pain centralization; and socioeconomic, genetic, and patient-related factors. CPIP types include neuropathic, nonneuropathic, somatic, and visceral [7].

Neuropathic pain

Neuropathic pain in CPIP is postulated to arise from damage or trauma to the inguinal nerves. The pain is typically experienced in the sensory distribution of the affected nerves. Classic symptoms include hypoesthesia or hyperesthesia, allodynia, and parasthesias.

The relevant nerves in CPIP are the iliohypogastric nerve (IHN), ilioinguinal nerve (IIN), and the genital branch of the genitofemoral nerve (GFN) with anterior-based repair and the addition of the femoral branch of the GFN or the lateral femoral cutaneous nerve with posterior-based preperitoneal repair.

Relevant anatomy

The IIN is located over the spermatic cord and covered and protected from mesh by the investing fascia of the internal oblique muscle (Fig. 1). Removal of the nerve from its natural bed through neurolysis risks perineural scarring and direct contact of the nerve to the mesh. The genital branch of the GFN is located under the cord and covered and protected from direct contact with mesh by the deep cremasteric fascia and is easily identified by the blue line of the external spermatic vein adjacent to the nerve. The IHN is located between the external and internal oblique layers covered by the investing fascia of the internal oblique muscle. One can expose the IHN by opening the anatomic cleavage between the internal and external oblique layers high enough to expose the internal oblique aponeurosis. The IHN has a segment that runs intramuscularly inferiorly and laterally that is vulnerable to injury when passing suture through the internal oblique muscle or conjoined tendon to fix it to the inguinal ligament, flat mesh, or plug.

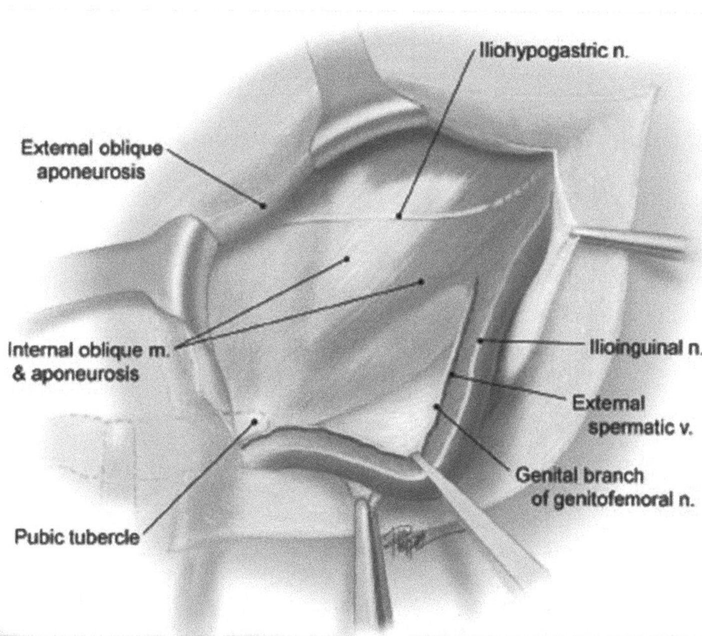

Fig. 1. Inguinal nerve anatomy (anterior approach via inguinal canal). (*Courtesy of* Parviz K. Amid, MD, Los Angeles, CA.)

In the preperitoneal space used for open and laparoscopic posterior repairs, the genital and femoral branches of the GFN and the lateral femoral cutaneous nerve may be injured from direct dissection, direct apposition of the mesh causing perineural scarring, or fixation with tacks or suture. The IIN and IHN have exited proximal to this operative field and are injured only through traumatic fixation with tacks or suture penetrating through the muscular floor of the inguinal canal.

Box 1 describes the intraoperative and postoperative events that contribute to nerve trauma and damage.

Nonneuropathic pain

Structural issues, such as hernia recurrence, muscle strain, excessive scar tissue formation, meshoma formation, or mesh-related excess fibrosis, can lead to nonneuropathic pain [18,19].

Visceral pain

Hernia recurrence with intestinal involvement, incarceration, or mesh adherence to the intestine can contribute to visceral pain. Additionally, involvement of the spermatic cord (funiculodynia), periurethral structures, venous congestion of the spermatic cord, dyssynergia of the ejaculatory effector muscles, stricture of the vas deferens, or twisting of the spermatic cord can cause visceral pain [12,18–20].

Somatic pain

The most commonly and well-described pain syndrome to fall under somatic pain is periostitis pubis. This is commonly caused by deeply placed anchoring

Box 1: Events leading to inguinal nerve trauma and damage

Intraoperative events

Surgical manipulation

Stretching/crushing

Electrical/thermal damage

Partial/complete transection

Suture entrapment in open repair

Tack, suture, or fixation entrapment in laparoscopic repair

Postoperative events

Envelopment in meshoma

Irritation secondary to excessive fibrotic reaction

Granuloma or neuroma formation

Data from Poobalan AS, Bruce J, Smith WC, et al. A review of chronic pain after inguinal herniorrhaphy. Clin J Pain 2003;19:48–54 and Hakeem A, Shanmugam V. Current trends in the diagnosis and management of post-herniorraphy chronic groin pain. World J Gastrointest Surg 2011;3:73–81.

sutures or actual periosteal anchoring of the mesh to the pubic tubercle [12,20–22].

Risk factors

Preoperative, perioperative, and postoperative risk factors have been identified for chronic postsurgical pain. Two reviews from nationwide hernia databases of Scandinavian countries and Scotland, and several meta-analyses and a prospective study have identified chronic postsurgical pain risk factors in patients with inguinal hernia and identified risk factors for CPIP. These are listed in Box 2.

From a surgeon's standpoint, development of CPIP is independent of repair technique. However, identification and protection of the inguinal nerves is of utmost importance [4]. Although CPIP predates the use of mesh, the presence

Box 2: Risk factors for CPIP

Preoperative factors

Young age
Female gender
High pain intensity level (inguinal or elsewhere)
Lower preoperative optimism
Impairment of everyday activities
Operation for a recurrent hernia
Genetic predisposition (DQB I*03:02 HLA haplotype)

Experimentally induced pain

High pain intensity to tonic heat stimulation

Perioperative factors

Less experienced surgeon/not dedicated hernia center
Open repair technique
Mesh type: heavyweight (open, laparoscopic)
Mesh fixation: suture (open), staple (laparoscopic)
IIN neurolysis in Lichtenstein repair

Postoperative factors

Postoperative complications (hematoma, infection)
High early postoperative pain intensity
Lower perceived control over pain
Sensory dysfunction in the groin

Adapted from Bjurstrom MF, Nicol AL, Amid PK, et al. Pain control following inguinal herniorrhaphy: current perspectives. J Pain Res 2014;7:277–90; with permission.

and type of mesh certainly can contribute to the development of chronic pain. Studies have demonstrated significant reduction of CPIP in laparoscopic and open repairs with lightweight compared with heavyweight mesh [23,24]. The mechanism is thought to be greater biocompatibility resulting in less inflammation, increased elasticity, decreased stiffness, and reduction in foreign body sensation [7]. Mesh fixation techniques in open and laparoscopic repairs have been studied extensively. Avoidance of sutures and tacks can ostensibly reduce the incidence of CPIP [25,26]. Proposed alternatives include glue fixation but this has not been adequately studied [27,28]. Use of regional (epidural or spinal) anesthesia is not recommended, especially in older patients, because of an increased risk of urinary retention and other rare, but severe complications [29–32]. Local infiltration of anesthetic is the preferred method for open repair [29–32]. Atraumatic mesh fixation in laparoscopic inguinal hernia repair may reduce the frequency of entrapment neuropathy.

SYMPTOMATOLOGY AND DIAGNOSIS

The signs and symptoms of CPIP reflect the variable and overlapping nature of its causes and depend on the types of pain experienced by the patient. Box 3 lists various signs and symptoms based on the different types of CPIP. One must consider hernia recurrence as a source of CPIP. It is easily diagnosed and should be ruled out early in the evaluation. Differential diagnoses should also include other surgical, orthopedic, neurologic, infectious, urologic, or gynecologic causes.

The evaluation and diagnosis of CPIP should characterize the causes and types of pain and exclude other potential diagnoses. A detailed history and physical examination is essential.

History

In addition to obtaining a thorough past medical and surgical history, administration of validated pain, function, and quality of life instruments may help to delineate the type and severity of pain. These include the Short Form McGill Pain Questionnaire, Neuropathic Pain Questionnaire, Douleur Neuropathique 4 Questions, 36-Item Short Form Health Survey, and Activity Assessment Scale. Neuropathic Pain Questionnaire and Douleur Neuropathique 4 Questions tools have high specificity for neuropathic pain and if a neuropathic component is identified, then it can be further characterized using the Neuropathic Pain Scale or Short Form McGill Pain Questionnaire [34].

Knowledge of the original operative technique and detailed evaluation of the original operative report helps determine the likely causes and which nerves are at risk (Fig. 2).

Physical examination

A thorough physical examination is predicated on in-depth knowledge of the groin neuroanatomy. An understanding of the anatomic course of the three inguinal nerves, their dermatomes, and the presence of hernia recurrence or mesh is crucial to successfully evaluating the patient with CPIP [1,4]. Tinel

Box 3: Symptoms and descriptors of CPIP

Neuropathic pain
Pain (neuralgia)
Reduced sensation (hypoesthesia)
Increased sensation (hyperesthesia)
Burning sensation (parasthesia)
Pain in response to nonpainful stimulus (allodynia)
Increased pain response to painful stimuli (hyperalgesia)
Stabbing/burning/pulling/throbbing/shooting/prickling/sharp
Localized
Radiating to scrotum, labium, upper thigh
Trigger point with positive Tinel sign
Worse with ambulation, twisting/stretching of upper body
Worse with stooping/sitting and hyperextension of hip
Worse with sexual intercourse
Improves with lying down or flexion of hip and thigh

Nonneuropathic pain
Dull, constant ache
Entirety of groin area
No specific trigger point or radiating component
Gnawing/tender/pounding/pulling

Somatic pain
Maximal pain at the pubic tubercle

Visceral pain
Related to sexual dysfunction/ejaculatory pain
Located at superficial ring or testicular/labial regions
Aching without specific trigger point
Diffusely tender spermatic cord (anterior operative approach)

Adapted from Refs. [12, 20–22, 33]

test (tapping skin medial to anterior superior iliac spine or over the area of maximal tenderness) can reproduce neuropathic pain along the sensory distribution of the affected nerves. These findings help to distinguish between neuropathic, nonneuropathic, or mixed pain. Distinguishing between individual inguinal nerves is often more difficult because of overlapping sensory innervations, peripheral communication, and common routes of origin [34–36].

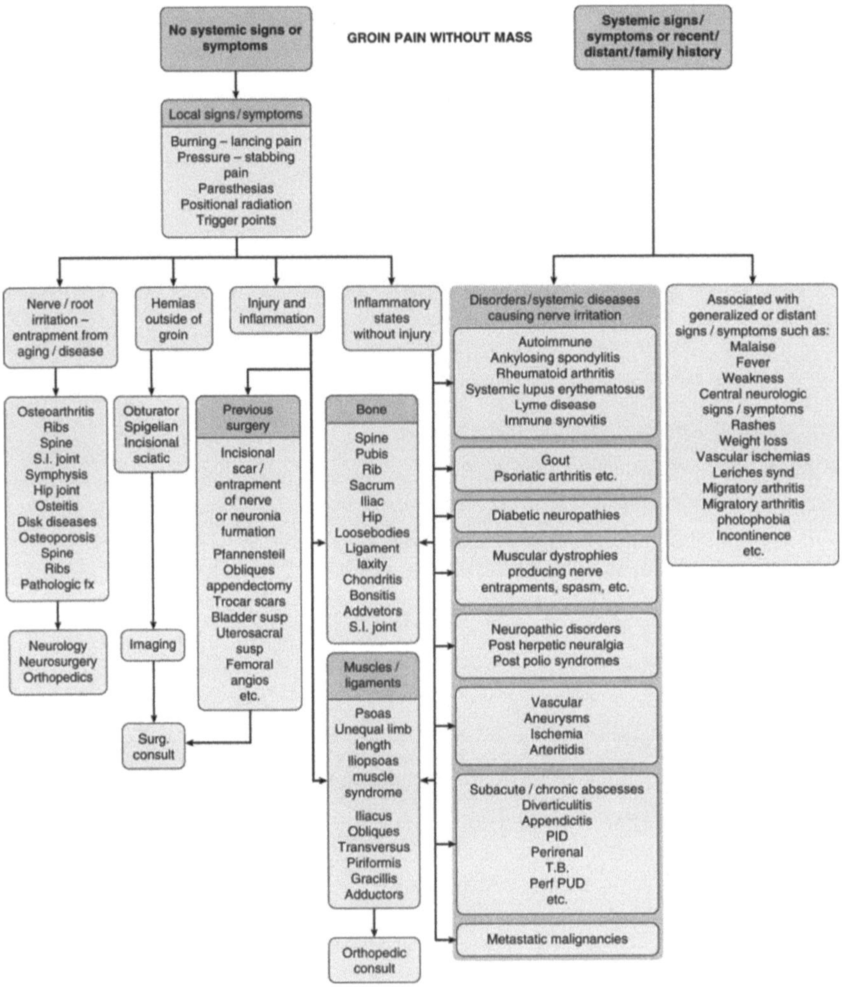

Fig. 2. Differential diagnosis of groin pain. PID, pelvic inflammatory disease; PUD, peptic ulcer disease; T.B., tuberculosis. (*From* Ramshaw B, Mirmedhi I. Athletic pubalgia: the sports hernia. In: Cameron JL, Cameron AM, editors. Current surgical therapy. 11th edition. St. Louis, MO: Elsevier; 2014. p. 553–7.)

Diagnostic imaging and tests

Ultrasonography is a common initial modality to detect recurrence or meshoma [37]. Cross-sectional computed tomography or MRI of the abdominal wall can be used to exclude recurrence or meshoma and investigate other differential diagnoses of CPIP. MRI is considered the best valid diagnostic imaging tool for differentiating causes of uncertain inguinal pain; however, this modality is radiologist dependent [37–40].

Local anesthetic block can help identify IIN, IHN, or GFN neuralgia. In the setting of equivocal diagnostic nerve blocks, needle electromyogram can provide additional information through revealing denervation and abnormalities of the abdominal wall muscles specific to IHN/IIN injury [41,42].

Magnetic resonance neurography can identify peripheral nerve compression that improves with surgical decompression. This is also technique and radiologist dependent [43].

TREATMENT

CPIP is a product of neuropathic and nociceptive pain and is also influenced by socioeconomic, emotional, cognitive, and genetic factors. A multimodal, multidisciplinary approach to CPIP is therefore necessary. Early involvement and cooperation with pain management specialists is important for the optimal management of these patients.

Nonsurgical management

Nonsurgical management includes expectant, behavioral, topical, pharmacologic, and interventional measures. Physiotherapy, acupuncture, and mind-body therapies can ameliorate pain conditions without medications or more invasive interventions. Adopting recumbent position or flexion of the hip and thigh can provide temporary relief; however, it is important to emphasize the harm associated with inactivity [44].

There are numerous pharmacologic therapies available for neuropathic and nonneuropathic pain, but the data behind these therapies are not specific for CPIP (Box 4). Rather, they are extrapolated from studies in the context of post-herpetic neuralgia or painful diabetic peripheral neuropathy [45–49]. Treatment should be individualized and based on potential side effects, concomitant treatment of other comorbidities (anxiety, depression, insomnia), drug interactions, risk of abuse, and cost. Furthermore, these drugs should only be prescribed with input from pain management physicians.

Topical medications, such as lidocaine patches or capsaicin, can be considered as second-line treatment or when comorbidities limit the use of first-line pharmacologic therapies.

Interventional pain management

Interventional pain management techniques are also included in the armamentarium of nonsurgical approaches. The existing data are limited to case reports and case series because few prospective, randomized controlled trials have been performed.

Nerve blocks

Historically, nerve blocks to the IIN and IHN have been performed using anatomic landmarks. Recent technologic advances in imaging have led to ultrasound-guided IIN/IHN blocks. These are often done for diagnostic purposes. The data regarding these techniques for amelioration of symptoms are mixed [57,58]. Thomassen and colleagues [59] found ultrasound-guided IIN/IHN nerve blocks to be effective in treating CPIP with prolonged pain relief after median follow-up time of 20 months. Conversely, a randomized,

Box 4: Pharmacologic therapy for CPIP

Nonneuropathic pain
Nonsteroidal anti-inflammatory drugs
Steroids

Neuropathic pain
Gabapentin/pregabalin
Selective serotonin-norepinephrine reuptake inhibitor (duloxetine/venlafaxine)
Tricyclic antidepressant
Opioids
Tramadol
Selective serotonin reuptake inhibitor (citalopram/paroxetine)
Buproprion
Cannabinoids
Anticonvulsants
Clonidine
Mexiletine
Memantine

Adapted from Refs. [45–56]

double-blinded, placebo-controlled study of IIN/IHN blocks using a CPIP and healthy patient cohort with crossover design failed to provide substantial evidence to support the use of nerve blocks in the treatment of CPIP [57].

Neuroablative techniques
If nerve blocks do provide short-term relief, the patient may subsequently benefit from neurolytic or neuroablative techniques. These include chemical neurolysis with alcohol or phenol, cryoablation, or pulsed radiofrequency ablation. Cryoablation and radiofrequency ablation in small series have demonstrated at least 75% reduction in symptoms [60–62]. More prospective, randomized studies are needed to validate these techniques but they are certainly useful adjuncts in patients who are poor surgical candidates.

Neuromodulation
There is a subset of patients for which all interventions, surgical and nonsurgical, are ineffective at ameliorating their symptoms of CPIP. Neuromodulation with peripheral nerve field stimulation or spinal cord stimulation may be appropriate for this select group of patients. Neuromodulation works by producing gentle parasthesias in the concordant areas of pain. Again, patient selection is crucial to the success of these modalities. Patients who are well-motivated, young, not involved in litigation, have success with a preimplantation trial

period, favorable spinal anatomy, and pass a preimplantation psychiatric evaluation are deemed good candidates [63].

Surgical management

Patients with CPIP who are refractory to a systematic regimen of diagnostic and interventional measures can be considered for operative intervention. However, successful surgical management is entirely dependent on selecting patients with discrete, neuroanatomic problems that can be corrected with surgery [1,4,9,64]. Failure of conservative management, in and of itself, is not an indication to proceed with surgery.

In-depth knowledge of groin neuroanatomy, technical details of the original operation, and an understanding of the causes of the patient's current symptoms are necessary to determine the optimal surgical approach [1,4,18,64–67].

The recommended timing of surgical treatment of CPIP not responding to nonsurgical treatment is 6 months to 1 year after the original inguinal hernia repair [1,4]. A systematic evaluation as described in previous sections is imperative to accurately identify the specific causes of pain. Type of repair, type of mesh, position of mesh, method of fixation, nerve handling, and neurolysis or neurectomy are all important details to note in the original operative report or when speaking with the referring surgeon [4,21,68]. Imaging studies to evaluate for recurrence or meshoma are also important [68]. Neuropathic pain not present before the operation, isolated to the inguinal distribution, with demonstrated improvement from diagnostic and therapeutic nerve blocks is most likely to benefit from operative neurectomy (Box 5).

Selective versus triple neurectomy

Common options for the treatment of CPIP include selective IIN, IHN, and GFN neurolysis or neurectomy along with removal of mesh and fixation material with revision of prior hernia repair [69–74]. Removal of mesh and fixation material eliminates the immediate cause of CPIP, but fails to address the injured nerves that are left behind. Selective neurolysis or neurectomy may improve a small subset of patients with CPIP [69–73]. However, electron microscopy of grossly normal nerves resected during triple neurectomy for CPIP demonstrate ultrastructural damage contributing to CPIP but unseen to the naked eye [69–73]. There is also significant variation and cross-innervation of the inguinal nerves in the retroperitoneum and inguinal canal that make selective neurectomy less reliable [4,35,75]. Lastly, reoperation in a scarred field only makes nerve identification more unreliable, and increases the risk of recurrence, vascular injury, testicular compromise, and visceral injury. Experienced clinicians with CPIP can sometimes isolate single affected nerves based on clinical presentation, dermatomal somatosensory mapping, and operative mechanism achieving successful remediation with selective neurectomy. However, pain presenting in overlapping dermatomal distributions found within the inguinal canal is best addressed with triple neurectomy based on technical and neuroanatomic considerations.

Box 5: Locations of potential nerve injury and associated operations

Anterior to transversalis fascia

IIN/visible and intramuscular segment IHN/inguinal segment of genital branch of GFN

Open anterior repair (tissue, Lichtenstein, PHS [Prolene hernia system], plug and patch)

Laparoscopic repair (mesh fixation)

Posterior to transversalis fascia (preperitoneal space)

Main trunk of GFN

Preperitoneal segment of genital branch of GFN

Open preperitoneal repair (plug, PHS, Kugel)

Laparoscopic repair

Retroperitoneal space

Main trunk of GFN over psoas muscle

Lateral femoral cutaneous nerve

Data from Starling JR, Harms BA. Diagnosis and treatment of genitofemoral and ilioinguinal neuralgia. World J Surg 1989;13:586–91 and Klaassen Z, Marshall E, Tubbs RS, et al. Anatomy of the ilioinguinal and iliohypogastric nerves with observations of their spinal nerve contributions. Clin Anat 2011;24(4):454–61.

Approach to open triple neurectomy

This approach involves re-exploration through the prior operative field. It is indicated for neuropathic CPIP when a recurrence or meshoma is present or for patients that underwent anterior repair without placement of preperitoneal mesh [66]. It is more complex and technically challenging to proceed in a reoperative field, and morbidity is increased. Steps of open triple neurectomy are as follows:

- Identify IIN lateral to internal ring between the ring and anterior superior iliac spine [4,65–67]
- Identify IHN with anatomic cleavage between external and internal oblique
- Trace nerve proximally within fibers of internal oblique lateral to prior operative field
- Subaponeurotic IHN is found by splitting internal oblique aponeurosis
- Identify inguinal segment genital branch of the GFN between cord and inguinal ligament and trace laterally to the internal ring
- Nerves should be resected proximal to prior operative field
- Ligate cut ends to avoid neuroma formation
- Insert cut ends into muscle to keep nerve stumps away from future scarring
- If plug or meshoma is present, remove during operation
- Resect main trunk of GFN over psoas muscle by dividing floor of inguinal canal and accessing retroperitoneum (extended triple neurectomy)
- Resection of paravasal nerves if orchialgia is present

Approach to endoscopic retroperitoneal triple neurectomy

This approach allows for proximal access to potential sites of peripheral neuropathy and overcomes the limitations that exist with open triple neurectomy after laparoscopic or open preperitoneal repair. Endoscopic access in the retroperitoneum allows for identification of the IIN and IHN at the L1 nerve root overlying the quadratus lumborum and the genital and femoral branches of the GFN exiting from the psoas muscle [76–78]. The advantage of this operation is safety and separation from the scar tissue of any prior inguinal hernia repair. In addition, the anatomy is consistent and the operation itself is simple. Disadvantages can include deafferentation hypersensitivity, numbness in groin region and flank, and bulging of the lateral abdominal wall secondary to loss of motor function of the IIN and IHN to the transversus abdominus muscle [76–78]. Furthermore, mesh or plug removal may not be feasible with a retroperitoneal endoscopic approach [76–78].

Surgical management of chronic postoperative inguinal pain with recurrence or meshoma

The approach to this problem depends on the type of hernia repair the patient has had in the past and whether a meshoma is present. If recurrence is identified, surgical revision using an alternative approach is recommended. If accompanied by neuropathic pain, an open anterior approach allows correction of the hernia and access to the nerves. [67]. If a meshoma is present, removal is indicated if there is pain refractory to conservative management [4]. If one proceeds with meshoma removal, then systematic triple neurectomy is recommended. Figs. 3 and 4 reflect the most current, comprehensive consensus algorithm using the Delphi method and involving 26 world authorities on CPIP [6].

One must explicitly communicate with the patient the potential benefits and complications for operative intervention of CPIP. The ability to do so helps with managing patient expectations. Patients should be advised of permanent numbness, inability to identify or access the nerves, abdominal wall laxity, testicular atrophy, labial numbness, potential for ongoing pain, continued disability, and testicular pain caused by nociceptive component.

FUTURE DIRECTIONS

CPIP is now recognized as the most significant complication after open or laparoscopic inguinal hernia repair. Until recently, there was no universally accepted definition, cause, classification, or standard surgical treatment of this problem. Recently, a consensus statement by expert herniologists was created using the Delphi method.

Surgeons who treat inguinal hernias should possess an in-depth knowledge of the groin neuroanatomy to refine their technique and prevent this disabling complication from befalling a patient. Adhering to surgical principles that include three-nerve identification, preservation, or pragmatic neurectomy during open repair decreases the incidence of CPIP. Avoiding the preperitoneal

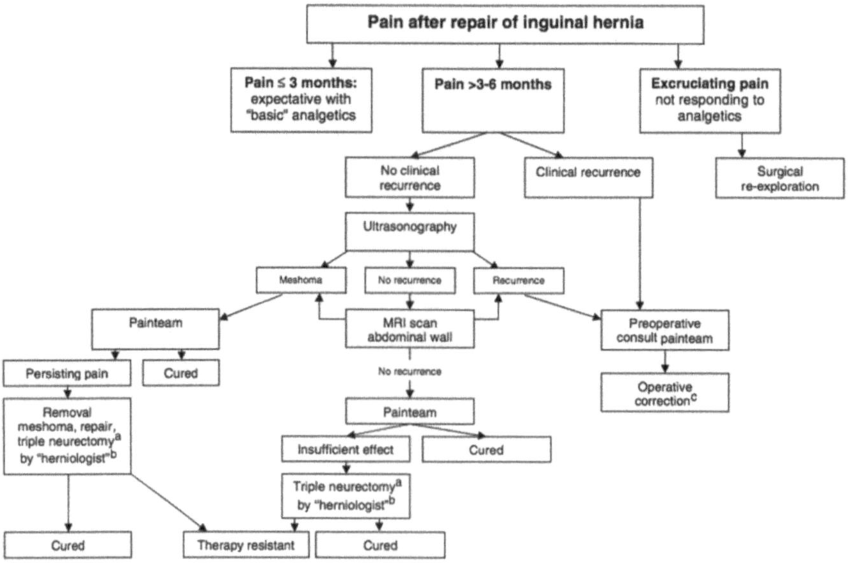

Fig. 3. International consensus algorithm for management of chronic postoperative inguinal pain. [a] Including proximal genitofemoral nerve-neurectomy in case of chronic pain after open or laparoscopic preperitoneal mesh technique. [b] Open or endoscopic procedure. [c] In case of neuropathic pain anterior correction in combination with triple neurectomy is optional. (*Adapted from* Lange JF, Kaufmann R, Wijsmuller AR, et al. An international consensus algorithm for management of chronic postoperative inguinal pain. Hernia 2015;19(1):33–43.)

nerves below the iliopubic tract with minimal to no mesh fixation decreases the risk of CPIP after laparoscopic repair.

All patients with CPIP should undergo a multidisciplinary evaluation with a pain management team and a surgeon. Pharmacologic therapies and diagnostic

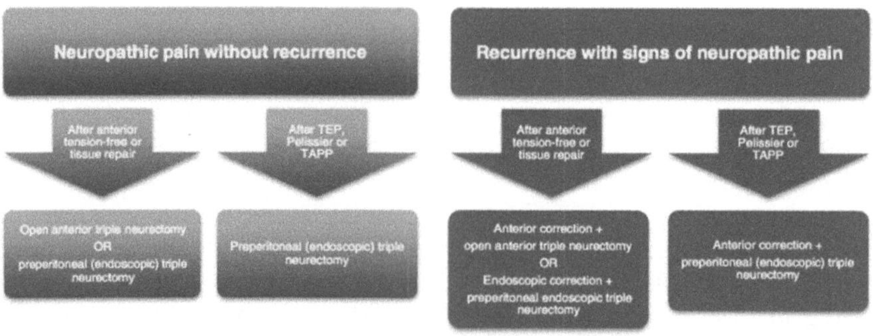

Fig. 4. Management of chronic postoperative inguinal pain with and without recurrence. TAPP, transabdominal preperitoneal; TEP, totally extraperitoneal. (*Adapted from* Lange JF, Kaufmann R, Wijsmuller AR, et al. An international consensus algorithm for management of chronic postoperative inguinal pain. Hernia 2015;19(1):33–43.)

and therapeutic nerve blocks should be used in all patients as part of an appropriate multimodal approach. Patients who are refractory conservative management should undergo operative intervention 6 months to 1 year after the original inguinal hernia repair. Reoperative candidates should be seen and operated on by experienced herniologists.

Moving forward, methods should be developed to identify patients who are at high risk of developing CPIP before any operation. Patient expectations should be appropriately developed and preventive multimodal analgesia and anesthesia given high priority. Preventive measures and administration of perioperative and postoperative gabapentinoids, ketamine, or local anesthetic may serve to minimize the inflammatory cascade, and decrease central sensitization, ultimately preventing the development of CPIP. Patients with CPIP who are optimally managed with a multidisciplinary, logical, and stepwise approach have the best opportunity to minimize their symptoms, manage their pain, decrease additional morbidity, and improve their quality of life.

References

[1] Aasvang E, Kehlet H. Surgical management of chronic pain after inguinal hernia repair. Br J Surg 2005;92:795–801.

[2] Aasvang EK, Bay-Nielsen M, Kehlet H. Pain and functional impairment 6 years after inguinal herniorrhaphy. Hernia 2006;10:316–21.

[3] Bay-Nielsen M, Perkins FM, Kehlet H. Pain and functional impairment 1 year after inguinal herniorrhaphy: a nationwide questionnaire study. Ann Surg 2001;233:1–7.

[4] Alfieri S, Amid PK, Campanelli G, et al. International guidelines for prevention and management of post-operative chronic pain following inguinal hernia surgery. Hernia 2011;15: 239–49.

[5] Bittner R, Schwarz J. Inguinal hernia repair: current surgical techniques. Langenbecks Arch Surg 2012;397:271–82.

[6] Lange JF, Kaufmann R, Wijsmuller AR, et al. An international consensus algorithm for management of chronic postoperative inguinal pain. Hernia 2015;19(1):33–43.

[7] Bjurstrom MF, Nicol AL, Amid PK, et al. Pain control following inguinal herniorrhaphy: current perspectives. J Pain Res 2014;7:277–90.

[8] Kehlet H, Jensen TS, Woolf CJ. Persistent postsurgical pain: risk factors and prevention. Lancet 2006;367(9522):1618–25.

[9] Kehlet H. Chronic pain after groin hernia repair. Br J Surg 2008;95(2):135–6.

[10] Parsons B, Schaefer C, Mann R, et al. Economic and humanistic burden of post-trauma and post-surgical neuropathic pain among adults in the United States. J Pain Res 2013;6: 459–69.

[11] Aasvang E, Kehlet H. Chronic postoperative pain: the case of inguinal herniorrhaphy. Br J Anaesth 2005;95:69–76.

[12] Poobalan AS, Bruce J, Smith WC, et al. A review of chronic pain after inguinal herniorrhaphy. Clin J Pain 2003;19:48–54.

[13] Nienhuijs S, Staal E, Strobbe L, et al. Chronic pain after mesh repair of inguinal hernia: a systematic review. Am J Surg 2007;194:394–400.

[14] Fine PG. Long-term consequences of chronic pain: mounting evidence for pain as a neurological disease and parallels with other chronic disease states. Pain Med 2011;12: 996–1004.

[15] Tsang A, Von Korff M, Lee S, et al. Common chronic pain conditions in developed and developing countries: gender and age differences and comorbidity with depression-anxiety disorders. J Pain 2008;9:883–91.

[16] Courtney CA, Duffy K, Serpell MG, et al. Outcome of patients with severe chronic pain following repair of groin hernia. Br J Surg 2002;89:1310–4.
[17] Kalliomaki ML, Sandblom G, Gunnarsson U, et al. Persistent pain after groin hernia surgery: a qualitative analysis of pain and its consequences for quality of life. Acta Anaesthesiol Scand 2009;53:236–46.
[18] Amid PK, Hiatt JR. New understanding of the causes and surgical treatment of postherniorrhaphy inguinodynia and orchalgia. J Am Coll Surg 2007;205:381–5.
[19] Heise CP, Starling JR. Mesh inguinodynia: a new clinical syndrome after inguinal herniorrhaphy? J Am Coll Surg 1998;187:514–8.
[20] Hakeem A, Shanmugam V. Current trends in the diagnosis and management of post-herniorraphy chronic groin pain. World J Gastrointest Surg 2011;3:73–81.
[21] Cunningham J, Temple WJ, Mitchell P, et al. Cooperative hernia study. Pain in the postrepair patient. Ann Surg 1996;224:598–602.
[22] Loos MJ, Roumen RM, Scheltinga MR. Classifying post-herniorrhaphy pain syndromes following elective inguinal hernia repair. World J Surg 2007;31:1760–5 [discussion: 1766–7].
[23] Sajid MS, Leaver C, Baig MK, et al. Systematic review and metaanalysis of the use of lightweight versus heavyweight mesh in open inguinal hernia repair. Br J Surg 2012;99:29–37.
[24] Sajid MS, Kalra L, Parampalli U, et al. A systematic review and meta-analysis evaluating the effectiveness of lightweight mesh against heavyweight mesh in influencing the incidence of chronic groin pain following laparoscopic inguinal hernia repair. Am J Surg 2013;205: 726–36.
[25] Colvin HS, Rao A, Cavali M, et al. Glue versus suture fixation of mesh during open repair of inguinal hernias: a systematic review and meta-analysis. World J Surg 2013;37:2282–92.
[26] de Goede B, Klitsie PJ, van Kempen BJ, et al. Meta-analysis of glue versus sutured mesh fixation for Lichtenstein inguinal hernia repair. Br J Surg 2013;100:735–42.
[27] Ladwa N, Sajid MS, Sains P, et al. Suture mesh fixation versus glue mesh fixation in open inguinal hernia repair: a systematic review and meta-analysis. Int J Surg 2013;11:128–35.
[28] Sanders DL, Waydia S. A systematic review of randomised control trials assessing mesh fixation in open inguinal hernia repair. Hernia 2014;18(2):165–76.
[29] Bay-Nielsen M, Kehlet H. Anaesthesia and post-operative morbidity after elective groin hernia repair: a nation-wide study. Acta Anaesthesiol Scand 2008;52:169–74.
[30] Kehlet H, Aasvang E. Groin hernia repair: anesthesia. World J Surg 2005;29:1058–61.
[31] Nordin P, Zetterstrom H, Carlsson P, et al. Cost-effectiveness analysis of local, regional and general anaesthesia for inguinal hernia repair using data from a randomized clinical trial. Br J Surg 2007;94:500–5.
[32] Nordin P, Zetterstrom H, Gunnarsson U, et al. Local, regional, or general anaesthesia in groin hernia repair: multicentre randomised trial. Lancet 2003;362:853–8.
[33] Choi PD, Nath R, Mackinnon SE. Iatrogenic injury to the ilioinguinal and iliohypogastric nerves in the groin: a case report, diagnosis, and management. Ann Plast Surg 1996;37:60–5.
[34] Jones RC 3rd, Backonja MM. Review of neuropathic pain screening and assessment tools. Curr Pain Headache Rep 2013;17(9):363.
[35] Starling JR, Harms BA. Diagnosis and treatment of genitofemoral and ilioinguinal neuralgia. World J Surg 1989;13:586–91.
[36] Harms BA, DeHaas DR Jr, Starling JR. Diagnosis and management of genitofemoral neuralgia. Arch Surg 1984;119:339–41.
[37] Bradley M, Morgan D, Pentlow B, et al. The groin hernia: an ultrasound diagnosis? Ann R Coll Surg Engl 2003;85:178–80.
[38] Ferzli GS, Edwards ED, Khoury GE. Chronic pain after inguinal herniorrhaphy. J Am Coll Surg 2007;205:333–41.

[39] van den Berg JC, de Valois JC, Go PM, et al. Detection of groin hernia with physical examination, ultrasound, and MRI compared with laparoscopic findings. Invest Radiol 1999;34: 739–43.
[40] Aasvang EK, Jensen KE, Fiirgaard B, et al. MRI and pathology in persistent postherniotomy pain. J Am Coll Surg 2009;208:1023–8 [discussion: 1028–9].
[41] Ellis RJ, Ceisse H, Holub BA. Ilioinguinal nerve conduction. Muscle Nerve 1992;15:1195.
[42] Knockaert DC, Boonen AL, Bruyninckx FL, et al. Electromyographic findings in ilioinguinal-iliohypogastric nerve entrapment syndrome. Acta Clin Belg 1996;51:156–60.
[43] Filler A. Magnetic resonance neurography and diffusion tensor imaging: origins, history, and clinical impact of the first 50,000 cases with an assessment of efficacy and utility in a prospective 5000-patient study group. Neurosurgery 2009;65:A29–43.
[44] Astin JA. Mind-body therapies for the management of pain. Clin J Pain 2004;20:27–32.
[45] Dworkin RH, O'Connor AB, Backonja M, et al. Pharmacologic management of neuropathic pain: evidence-based recommendations. Pain 2007;132:237–51.
[46] Attal N, Cruccu G, Baron R, et al. EFNS guidelines on the pharmacological treatment of neuropathic pain: 2010 revision. Eur J Neurol 2010;17(1113):e88.
[47] Attal N, Cruccu G, Haanpää M, et al. EFNS guidelines on pharmacological treatment of neuropathic pain. Eur J Neurol 2006;13:1153–69.
[48] Moulin DE, Clark AJ, Gilron I, et al. Pharmacological management of chronic neuropathic pain: consensus statement and guidelines from the Canadian Pain Society. Pain Res Manag 2007;12:13–21.
[49] O'Connor AB, Dworkin RH. Treatment of neuropathic pain: an overview of recent guidelines. Am J Med 2009;122:S22–32.
[50] Clarke H, Bonin RP, Orser BA, et al. The prevention of chronic postsurgical pain using gabapentin and pregabalin: a combined systematic review and meta-analysis. Anesth Analg 2012;115:428–42.
[51] Benito-Leon J, Picardo A, Garrido A, et al. Gabapentin therapy for genitofemoral and ilioinguinal neuralgia. J Neurol 2001;248:907–8.
[52] Sen H, Sizlan A, Yanarateş O, et al. The effects of gabapentin on acute and chronic pain after inguinal herniorrhaphy. Eur J Anaesthesiol 2009;26:772–6.
[53] Cohen SP, Galvagno SM, Plunkett A, et al. A multicenter, randomized, controlled study evaluating preventive etanercept on postoperative pain after inguinal hernia repair. Anesth Analg 2013;116:455–62.
[54] Finnerup NB, Otto M, McQuay HJ, et al. Algorithm for neuropathic pain treatment: an evidence based proposal. Pain 2005;118:289–305.
[55] Bischoff JM, Petersen M, Uçeyler N, et al. Lidocaine patch (5%) in treatment of persistent inguinal postherniorrhaphy pain: a randomized, double-blind, placebo-controlled, crossover trial. Anesthesiology 2013;119(6):1444–52.
[56] Derry S, Sven-Rice A, Cole P, et al. Topical capsaicin (high concentration) for chronic neuropathic pain in adults. Cochrane Database Syst Rev 2013;(2):CD007393.
[57] Bischoff JM, Koscielniak-Nielsen ZJ, Kehlet H, et al. Ultrasound-guided ilioinguinal/iliohypogastric nerve blocks for persistent inguinal postherniorrhaphy pain: a randomized, double-blind, placebo-controlled, crossover trial. Anesth Analg 2012;114:1323–9.
[58] Peng PW, Tumber PS. Ultrasound-guided interventional procedures for patients with chronic pelvic pain: a description of techniques and review of literature. Pain Physician 2008;11: 215–24.
[59] Thomassen I, van Suijlekom JA, van de Gaag A, et al. Ultrasound-guided ilioinguinal/iliohypogastric nerve blocks for chronic pain after inguinal hernia repair. Hernia 2013;17: 329–32.
[60] Rozen D, Ahn J. Pulsed radiofrequency for the treatment of ilioinguinal neuralgia after inguinal herniorrhaphy. Mt Sinai J Med 2006;73:716–8.
[61] Rozen D, Parvez U. Pulsed radiofrequency of lumbar nerve roots for treatment of chronic inguinal herniorraphy pain. Pain Physician 2006;9:153–6.

[62] Werner MU, Bischoff JM, Rathmell JP, et al. Pulsed radiofrequency in the treatment of persistent pain after inguinal herniotomy: a systematic review. Reg Anesth Pain Med 2012;37:340–3.
[63] Rosendal F, Moir L, de Pennington N, et al. Successful treatment of testicular pain with peripheral nerve stimulation of the cutaneous branch of the ilioinguinal and genital branch of the genitofemoral nerves. Neuromodulation 2013;16:121–4.
[64] Lichtenstein IL, Shulman AG, Amid PK, et al. Cause and prevention of postherniorrhaphy neuralgia: a proposed protocol for treatment. Am J Surg 1988;155(6):786–90.
[65] Amid PK. A 1-stage surgical treatment for postherniorrhaphy neuropathic pain: triple neurectomy and proximal end implantation without mobilization of the cord. Arch Surg 2002;137(1):100–4.
[66] Amid PK. Causes, prevention, and surgical treatment of postherniorrhaphy neuropathic inguinodynia: triple neurectomy with proximal end implantation. Hernia 2004;8(4):343–9.
[67] Amid PK, Chen DC. Surgical treatment of chronic groin and testicular pain after laparoscopic and open preperitoneal inguinal hernia repair. J Am Coll Surg 2011;213(4):531–6.
[68] Amid PK. Radiologic images of meshoma: a new phenomenon causing chronic pain after prosthetic repair of abdominal wall hernias. Arch Surg 2004;139:1297–8.
[69] Aasvang EK, Kehlet H. The effect of mesh removal and selective neurectomy on persistent postherniotomy pain. Ann Surg 2009;249(2):327–34.
[70] Starling JR, Harms BA. Ilioinguinal, iliohypogastric, and genitofemoral neuralgia. In: Bendavid R, editor. Prostheses and abdominal wall hernia. Austin (TX): RG Landes Co; 1994. p. 351–6.
[71] Zacest AC, Magill ST, Anderson VC, et al. Long-term outcome following ilioinguinal neurectomy for chronic pain. J Neurosurg 2010;112(4):784–9.
[72] Loos MJ, Scheltinga MR, Roumen RM. Tailored neurectomy for treatment of postherniorrhaphy inguinal neuralgia. Surgery 2010;147(2):275–81.
[73] Madura JA, Madura JA 2nd, Copper CM, et al. Inguinal neurectomy for inguinal nerve entrapment: an experience with 100 patients. Am J Surg 2005;189(3):283–7.
[74] Keller JE, Stefanidis D, Dolce CJ, et al. Combined open and laparoscopic approach to chronic pain after inguinal hernia repair. Am Surg 2008;74:695–700.
[75] Klaassen Z, Marshall E, Tubbs RS, et al. Anatomy of the ilioinguinal and iliohypogastric nerves with observations of their spinal nerve contributions. Clin Anat 2011;24(4):454–61.
[76] Chen DC, Hiatt JR, Amid PK. Operative management of refractory neuropathic inguinodynia by a laparoscopic retroperitoneal approach. JAMA Surg 2013;148(10):962–7.
[77] Song JW, Wolf JS Jr, McGillicuddy JE, et al. Laparoscopic triple neurectomy for intractable groin pain: technical report of 3 cases. Neurosurgery 2011;68(2):339–46 [discussion: 346].
[78] Giger U, Wente MN, Büchler MW, et al. Endoscopic retroperitoneal neurectomy for chronic pain after groin surgery. Br J Surg 2009;96(9):1076–81.

Advances in Surgery 50 (2016) 221–234

ADVANCES IN SURGERY

Evolution of Sepsis Management

From Early Goal-Directed Therapy to Personalized Care

Lyndsay W. Head, MD[a], Craig M. Coopersmith, MD[b,*]

[a]Emory University School of Medicine, 3B South, Emory University Hospital, 1364 Clifton Road, NE, Atlanta, GA 30322, USA; [b]Department of Surgery, Emory Critical Care Center, Emory University School of Medicine, 101 Woodruff Circle, Suite WMB 5105, Atlanta, GA 30322, USA

Keywords

• Sepsis • Sepsis management • Early goal-directed therapy • Antibiotics • Resuscitation • Fluids • Surviving sepsis campaign • Sepsis bundles

Key points

- Sepsis is defined as life-threatening organ dysfunction caused by a dysregulated host response to infection.
- A specific protocol termed, "early goal-directed therapy," has not been shown to improve survival in sepsis compared with "usual care."
- Although this specific protocol is not beneficial if applied to all patients with sepsis, key tenets of sepsis management, including early fluid resuscitation, cultures, antibiotic therapy, lactate measurement, and vasopressors (if indicated), are indicated in all septic patients.
- Compliance with 3- and 6-hour bundles of sepsis management is associated with improved outcomes in septic patients.

In 1843, pathologist Dr Johann Scherer first noted the presence of lactic acidosis in septic shock. His patient, a 23-year-old woman, became septic following childbirth. She was prescribed a regimen of bloodletting and clystering and died 36 hours later. Her autopsy findings were consistent with severe purulent endometritis, and blood samples revealed an elevated lactic

Disclosure: Dr. Craig M. Coopersmith is a member of the Steering Committee of the Surviving Sepsis Campaign.

*Corresponding author. *E-mail address:* cmcoop3@emory.edu

0065-3411/16/$ – see front matter
http://dx.doi.org/10.1016/j.yasu.2016.04.002

acid level [1]. This case was perhaps one of the initial cases to show an association between tissue hypoperfusion and septic shock. Despite many advances in medical technology since this time, the question of how best to manage and prevent the destructive host response of sepsis is still being evaluated today.

DEFINITION OF SEPSIS

In modern critical care, sepsis was first defined by the Society of Critical Care Medicine/American College of Chest Physician consensus conference in 1991 [2]. Sepsis was defined as having at least 2 of 4 components of the systemic inflammatory response syndrome (SIRS) in the setting of a suspected infection. SIRS was defined as (a) temperature greater than 38°C or less than 36°C, (b) heart rate greater than 90 beats per minute, (c) respiratory rate greater than 20 per minute or $PaCO_2$ less than 32 mm Hg, and (d) white blood cell count greater than 12,000/mm^3 or less than 4000/mm^3 or greater than 10% of immature bands. Sepsis in the setting of organ dysfunction was further defined as severe sepsis, and sepsis-induced hypotension persisting despite adequate fluid resuscitation was defined as septic shock. Despite numerous limitations with this definition, a subsequent consensus conference in 2001 expanded the list of diagnostic criteria, but the definition remained unchanged [3].

In 2016, a consensus conference between the Society of Critical Care Medicine and the European Society of Intensive Care Medicine (endorsed by 30 international organizations) proposed a new definition of sepsis. The new definition is that sepsis is life-threatening organ dysfunction caused by a dysregulated host response to infection [4]. The clinical criterion used to operationalize organ failure is an increase in the Sequential Organ Failure Assessment (SOFA) score of 2 points or more. Notably, septic shock was defined as a subset of patients with particularly severe circulatory, cellular, and metabolic abnormalities associated with a higher risk of death than sepsis alone. Patients with septic shock at the bedside can be identified as requiring vasopressors to maintain a mean arterial pressure of 65 mm Hg or greater and a serum lactate level of greater than 2 mmol/L. This combination was associated with a mortality of greater than 40% [5].

Notably, the term severe sepsis was eliminated from the new definition. The rationale is that sepsis carries a mortality of approximately 10%–greater than that of myocardial infarction, stroke, or trauma–and the term "severe" is therefore redundant in a syndrome that is potentially life-threatening by definition. In the new paradigm, what was called "sepsis" in earlier definitions is now referred to as "infection" (where the host response may be adaptive) and what was called "severe sepsis" in earlier definitions is now referred to as "sepsis." SIRS continues to be an appropriate method of screening for infection. However, a new screen called quick SOFA (qSOFA) has recently been identified that involves evaluating infected patients for (a) altered mental status, (b) respiratory rate $>$ 22 per minute, and (c) systolic hypotension $<$ 100 mm Hg

[6]. Patients with at least 2 of 3 qSOFA points have a markedly elevated risk of either mortality or intensive care unit (ICU) stay of greater than 3 days, and therefore, patients with suspected infection with at least 2 qSOFA points should be screened for organ failure and the presence of sepsis (Fig. 1).

Notably, unlike the 2 previous iterations of sepsis definitions, which were entirely based on expert opinion, the clinical criteria used in the new sepsis definitions as well as for qSOFA (as a prompt to screen for sepsis) reflect a combination of expert consensus as well as large database analysis of well over 1 million patients from the United States and Europe, academic and community hospitals, and different types of health care systems.

This era is currently a complex time in sepsis evaluation because billing codes in International Classification of Diseases, 10th edition, and public reporting to the federal government in the United States use the older term "severe sepsis," which is not present in the new definition. However, it is important to note that different definitions serve different purposes (ie, bedside evaluation and management, surveillance, clinical or basic research), and each currently used and proposed definition of sepsis has utility depending on the context in which is used [7,8].

Regardless, it is an unfortunate reality that sepsis is one of the leading causes of death worldwide. Recent estimates suggest that between 230,000 and 370,000 people die of sepsis per year in the United States [9]. In addition, despite a decrease in mortalities over the past decade, the incidence of sepsis in developed countries is increasing [10,11].

PATHOBIOLOGY OF SEPSIS

The sepsis syndrome is determined by the complex interaction between an invading micro-organism and how the host responds to that organism. A host response to an infection does not need to be maladaptive. In fact, many components of the host response (including some components of SIRS such as fever and elevated white blood cell count) are, in fact, both appropriate and adaptive and serve to assist the host in eradicating the infection while preserving overall host integrity. However, when the body's response to infection is maladaptive, organ failure can ensue, which greatly increases the risk of either mortality or prolonged stay in the ICU.

Any microbiological stimulus (bacterial, fungal, or viral) can incite the sepsis syndrome. Although proinflammatory and anti-inflammatory mediators are both simultaneously elevated in sepsis, the early phases of sepsis are stereotypically proinflammatory in nature. For patients who do not rapidly improve, this is typically followed by progression to a more immunosuppressed state characterized by increased lymphocyte apoptosis and immunoparalysis, wherein patients are at increased risk of secondary infection as well as reactivation of latent viruses (Fig. 2) [12,13]. Simultaneously, sepsis induces microcirculatory dysfunction on a cellular level as well as mitochondrial dysfunction on a subcellular level. Of note, an individual host's response to sepsis can be highly

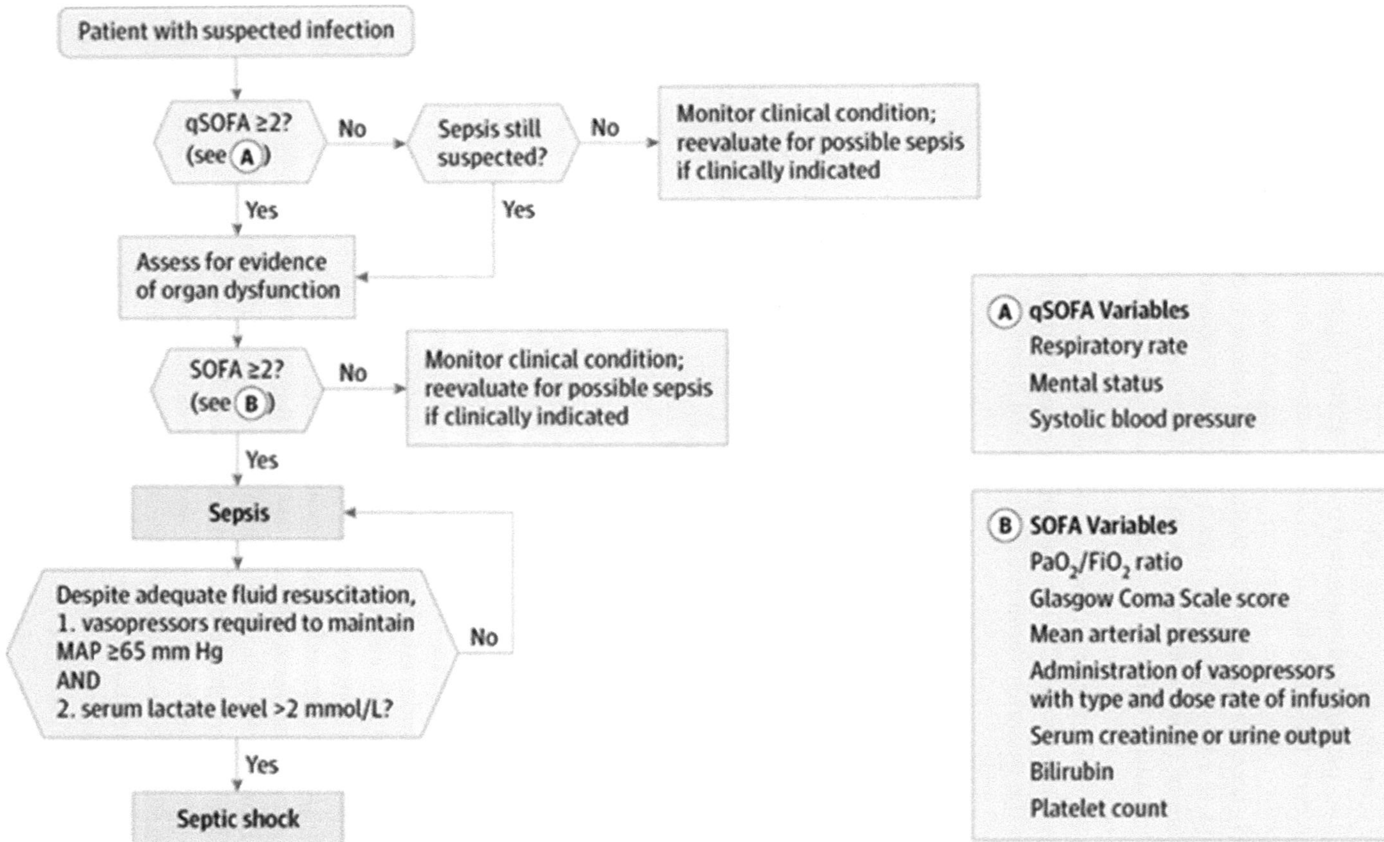

Fig. 1. Operationalization of clinical criteria identifying patients with sepsis and septic shock. The baseline SOFA score should be assumed to be zero unless the patient is known to have pre-existing (acute or chronic) organ dysfunction before the onset of infection. MAP, mean arterial pressure. (*From* Singer M, Deutschman CS, Seymour CW, et al. The third international consensus definitions for sepsis and septic shock (sepsis-3). JAMA 2016;315(8):801–10; with permission.)

variable and depends on both host (age, comorbidities, genetics) and pathogen factors [14–16].

THERAPY FOR SEPSIS

The success of sepsis therapy, resulting in survival being higher than ever before, is a paradox on the surface. On the one hand, despite decades of intensive basic research and well over 100 clinical trials, there are no adjunctive treatments for sepsis that have been demonstrated to be beneficial at the bedside. However, administration of broad spectrum antibiotics and rapid resuscitation has been remarkably successful in decreasing mortality.

The gold-standard initial therapy for sepsis is the Surviving Sepsis Campaign bundles [17]. Within 3 hours of the diagnosis of sepsis, health care providers should (a) measure a serum lactate level, (b) obtain blood cultures (before starting antibiotics), (c) start broad spectrum antibiotics, and (d) bolus a patient with 30 mL/kg of crystalloid for patients who are hypotensive or have an elevated serum lactate. Within 6 hours, the following interventions should be initiated: (a) start vasopressors for hypotension that is refractory to volume resuscitation to maintain a mean arterial pressure greater than 65 mm Hg, (b) reassess intravascular volume status, and (c) remeasure lactate if initial lactate was elevated. These simple interventions have been demonstrated to markedly decrease mortality in a database of nearly 30,000 patients [18] and form the basis for the first-quality metric for sepsis from the National Quality Forum and from the Centers for Medicare and Medicaid Services.

EARLY GOAL-DIRECTED THERAPY

The combination of intravascular volume depletion, vasodilation, myocardial depression, and increased metabolism in sepsis can lead to a state of imbalance between systemic oxygen delivery and oxygen demand; this led to the concept that optimizing this balance early in the course of sepsis treatment could improve outcomes. In 2001, Rivers and colleagues [19] published a groundbreaking single-center study showing that early goal-directed therapy (EGDT) decreased mortality from 46.5% to 30.5% in a cohort of 263 patients with severe sepsis or septic shock. Multiple subsequent nonrandomized trials supported the concept of EGDT, and this became standard of care in sepsis resuscitation for more than a decade.

In order to determine which components of EGDT are appropriate to use in all or some patients, it is first necessary to understand who was enrolled in the initial EGDT study and the treatment protocol. Patients were enrolled in the emergency department if they had suspicion of infection, SIRS criteria, and either a systolic blood pressure less than 90 mm Hg or a blood lactate of greater than 4 mmol/L. After cultures were obtained and antibiotics were initiated, patients in the EGDT arm had mandatory placement of a central venous catheter with the capacity for continuous central venous oxygen saturation ($ScvO_2$) monitoring as well as an arterial line. In the first 6 hours, patients received a 500-mL bolus of crystalloid every 30 minutes until the patient achieved a

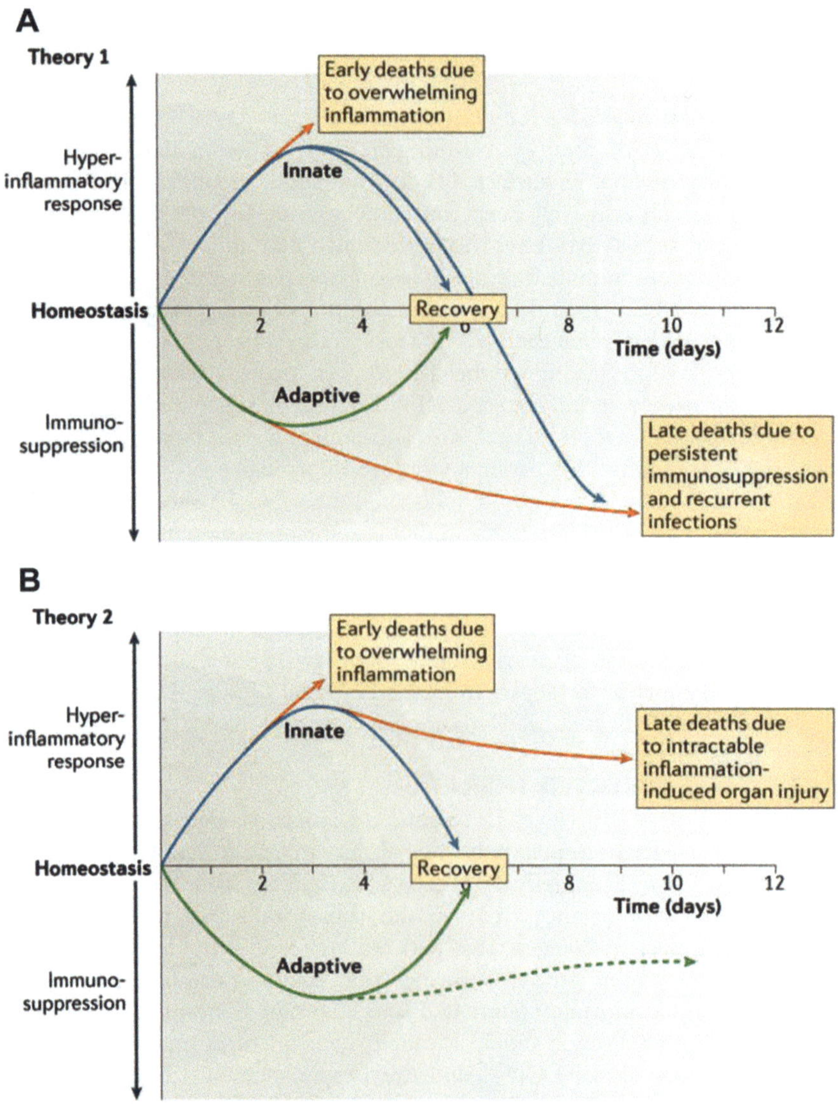

Fig. 2. Competing theories of the host immune response in sepsis. (*A*, Theory 1): Recent studies show that activation of both proinflammatory and anti-inflammatory immune responses occurs promptly after sepsis onset. Cells of the innate immune system including monocytes and neutrophils release large amounts of pro-inflammatory cytokines that drive inflammation (*blue line*, days 1–3). The intensity of the initial inflammatory response varies in individual patients, depending on multiple factors, including pathogen load and virulence, patient comorbidities, and host genetic factors. Early deaths in sepsis (*top red line*, day 3) are typically due to a hyperinflammatory "cytokine storm" response with fever, refractory shock, acidosis, and hypercatabolism. An example of this scenario would be a young patient dying of toxic shock syndrome or meningococcemia. Most patients have restoration of innate and adaptive immunity and survive the infection (recovery, day 6). If sepsis persists, failure of

central venous pressure (CVP) of 8 to 12 mm Hg (or 12–15 mm Hg if intubated). If a patient had a mean arterial blood pressure of less than 65 mm Hg despite reaching goal CVP, they were started on vasopressors. If the patient had a $ScvO_2$ less than 70% despite reaching both CVP and blood pressure goals, they were transfused with packed red blood cells to obtain a hematocrit of 30%. If all elements of EGDT were performed and a patient still had a $ScvO_2$ less than 70%, they were started on a dobutamine drip. The protocol had to be completed within 6 hours. Of note, as compared with the usual care group, patients randomized to EGDT received more total intravenous fluids, more red cell transfusions, and more inotropic support.

EFFICACY OF EARLY GOAL-DIRECTED THERAPY

Although the results of the original EGDT were remarkably impressive, the study was performed in only a single academic medical center. As such, it was unclear how generalizable the results were outside of this specialized setting. Furthermore, even if the results could be replicated, it was not clear whether all elements of EGDT were actually required for its success in light of subsequent trials demonstrating lack of efficacy for isolated portions of the protocol (discussed later). To address this, 3 international, multicenter randomized controlled trials were conducted to evaluate the effectiveness of EGDT, all published in 2014 and 2015. Each found no benefit to EGDT.

The protocol-based care for early septic shock (ProCESS) study was based in the emergency departments of 31 hospitals in the United States [20]. The trial enrolled patients into 3 different treatment arms: protocol-based EGDT as per Rivers and colleagues, protocol-based standard therapy that did not require inotropes or blood transfusions, and a usual care group. The primary endpoint was 60-day mortality. A total of 1341 patients were enrolled, with an initial $ScvO_2$ of 71% (compared with 49% in the original EGDT study). Volume of intravenous fluid administration, vasopressor use, inotrope use, and packed red cell transfusion differed significantly among the groups with the usual care arm having significant less use of intravenous fluids, vasopressors, inotropes, and blood transfusion as compared with EGDT. Notably, 60-day

critical elements of both innate and adaptive immune system occurs such that patients enter a profound immunosuppressive state (*blue and red lines*, after day 6). Deaths are due to an inability of the patient to clear infections and development of secondary infections. (*B*, Theory 2): A competing theory of sepsis agrees that there is an early activation of innate immunity and suppression of adaptive immunity. This theory holds that deaths in sepsis are due to persistent activation of the innate immunity with resultant intractable inflammation and organ injury. According to this theory, late deaths in sepsis are due to persistent underlying innate immune-driven inflammation. (*From* Hotchkiss RS, Monneret G, Payen D. Sepsis-induced immunosuppression: from cellular dysfunctions to immunotherapy. Nat Rev Immunol 2013;13(12):862–74; with permission.)

mortality ranged from 18.2% to 21.0% in the 3 groups, and no differences were noted in 90-day mortality, 1-year mortality, or need for organ support.

The ARISE (Australasian Resuscitation In Sepsis Evaluation) trial was the second study published evaluating the effectiveness of EGDT [21]. A total of 1600 patients were enrolled from the emergency departments of 51 centers primarily in Australia and New Zealand. The trial entered patients in 2 different treatment arms: protocol-based EGDT or usual care. The primary endpoint was 90-day mortality. Similarly to the ProCESS study, the patients in the EGDT group on average received a higher volume of intravenous fluid resuscitation, more vasopressors, more inotrope infusions, and more packed red cell transfusions. However, there was no difference in mortality with rates of death ranging from 18.6% to 18.8%.

Finally, the ProMISe (Protocolised Management in Sepsis) trial was the final study published as part of an international evaluation of EGDT [22]. A total of 1260 patients were enrolled in 56 hospitals in England, and the primary endpoint was all-cause mortality at 90 days in patients receiving either EGDT or usual care. The patients in the EGDT group on average received a higher volume of intravenous fluid resuscitation, more vasopressors, and more packed red cell transfusions, and notably, this was associated with worse organ failure scores, more cardiovascular support, and longer ICU stays. There was no difference in mortality with rates of death ranging from 29.2% to 29.5%, and quality of life was similar in both groups.

WHY DID EARLY GOAL-DIRECTED THERAPY FAIL?

The reasons these 3 landmark trials failed to show a benefit of EGDT can simplistically be broken down into (a) changes in sepsis management over time and (b) lack of efficacy of specific elements of EGDT when followed in every septic patient.

Changes in sepsis management over time

It is clear that what represents "usual care" has changed significantly in the 15 years between the original study of Rivers and colleagues and the 3 large randomized controlled trials of EGDT. Recognition of sepsis has gone up significantly. The reasons for this are multifactorial. Professional awareness efforts such as the Surviving Sepsis Campaign have clearly changed public consciousness with comprehensive guidelines, and evidence in the peer review literature that following sepsis bundles is associated with improved outcome; this has been coupled with numerous high-profile randomized controlled studies in high-impact journals on sepsis. Next, awareness in the public sector by groups such as the Rory Staunton Foundation and events such as World Sepsis Day have brightened the spotlight on a disease in which there has historically been a marked disconnect between burden of disease and public (and professional) awareness. Next, increased regulatory interest with sepsis quality measures and public reporting has also increased awareness. In addition, there are data that the incidence of sepsis is increasing. It is unclear how much of this is due to a true change in disease burden versus increasing recognition of the disease and increased billing in some countries due to favorable reimbursement for sepsis management, but it is reasonable to think increased familiarity with the disease would be associated with improved knowledge based on the part of health care providers. This thinking is consistent with a recent observational study that demonstrated sepsis-related mortality has decreased approximately 1.3% per year from 2000 to 2012 [23]. All of these manifest themselves in what now constitutes usual care. In the first 6 hours of the ProCESS trial, patients in the usual care arm received 2.3 L of fluid; 57.9% had a central venous catheter placed; 44.1% required vasopressors, and 76.1% received intravenous antibiotics (which increased to 96.9% thereafter). In other words, patients in the usual care arm were generally treated consistent with the Surviving Sepsis Campaign bundles.

Efficacy of individual elements of early goal-directed therapy

Central venous pressure

A key component to EGDT revolves around the mandatory placement of a central venous catheter for trending of CVP to target fluid resuscitation as well as following $ScvO_2$ to manipulate oxygen delivery. As an invasive procedure, the placement of a central venous catheter is associated with some risks, including pneumothorax, thrombosis, and central line–associated bloodstream infection. These risks and associated patient discomfort would be acceptable if the information obtained was vital to patient outcome. However, although it is appropriate to place a central venous catheter in a patient with septic shock to administer vasopressors, the data do not support placement in 100% of septic patients; this relates to the utility of CVP in guiding management. There is no debate that adequate fluid resuscitation is a cornerstone of sepsis management. Unfortunately, there is no gold standard for monitoring what constitutes adequate fluid resuscitation. Although a comprehensive overview of available options are outside the scope of this review, it is notable that many publications have demonstrated the limitations of CVP as a surrogate for intravascular volume [24]. Although trending CVP may be helpful in some patients, an isolated CVP is a poor static marker of circulating blood volume. Depending on the patient's underlying physiology, a low CVP may be associated with volume overload, whereas a high CVP may be associated with volume depletion. Instead, CVP is a more precise monitor of the compliance of the right ventricle rather than volume status.

Mean arterial pressure

The original EGDT trial targeted a mean arterial pressure of greater than 65 mm Hg, a goal also adopted by the Surviving Sepsis Campaign bundles and national quality indicators. There is a relative paucity of literature suggesting what the target blood pressure goal should be in sepsis. To address this, the SEPSISPAM (Sepsis and Mean Arterial Pressure) trial evaluated outcomes in patients randomized to undergo resuscitation with a mean arterial target of either 65 to 70 mm Hg or 80 to 85 mmgHg [25]. A total of 776 patients were enrolled, and there was no difference in outcome with 28-day mortality ranging from 34.0% to 36.6%. In addition, the incidence of newly diagnosed atrial fibrillation was higher in patients with higher mean arterial blood pressure, whereas patients with chronic hypertension required less renal replacement therapy if a higher mean arterial blood pressure was targeted.

Central venous oxygen saturation

Theoretically, $ScvO_2$ represents the balance between oxygen delivery and oxygen utilization in the tissues. Because of microcirculatory shunting and alterations in mitochondrial function in sepsis, $ScvO_2$ is typically elevated. Conceptually, when $ScvO_2$ is low (ie, <70%), this could be due to inadequate oxygen delivery from either low hematocrit or cardiac output. However, it is not clear how accurately $ScvO_2$ acts as a surrogate for mixed venous oxygen saturation (much like CVP is frequently not an appropriate approximation for end-diastolic left ventricular volume). Furthermore, $ScvO_2$ is most accurate as a predictor of mortality in patients with sepsis when it is high ($ScvO_2$ >90%), likely due to ineffective oxygen utilization in the tissues [26]. Notably, mortality was not different in septic shock in a study of 300 patients when they were randomized to a target of $ScvO_2$ of 70% versus a lactate clearance of at least 10%, suggesting a less invasive strategy is equally efficacious [27].

Transfusion

The rationale behind transfusing packed red blood cells in EGDT made physiologic sense: transfusion could theoretically increase oxygen delivery. However, because of the pathology of sepsis and disruption of the microcirculation and ineffective aerobic metabolism in the face of appropriate oxygen delivery, augmenting available oxygen by increasing hematocrit may not actually improve oxygen utilization in the tissues. There is now a robust literature suggesting that transfusing to a hemoglobin of 10 mg/dL is not helpful and may even be potentially harmful in the ICU. The TRICC (Transfusion Requirements in the Critical Care) trial evaluated a liberal versus restrictive transfusion goal in critically ill patients and found that those patients in the liberally transfused group (10 g/dL) had higher hospital mortality and significantly more cardiopulmonary complications than the restrictive transfusion group [28]. Subsequent trials found no benefit to transfusing patients undergoing cardiac surgery or having gastrointestinal bleeds. Importantly, the TRISS (Transfusion Requirements In Septic Shock) trial also compared lower vs higher hemoglobin threshold in septic shock in 998 patients and found no difference in 90-day mortality between the 2 treatment groups [29]. The absence of efficacy in transfusion in septic shock is consistent with the results of the ProCESS trial, which did not demonstrate a benefit in the EGDT arm that included transfusion compared with the protocol-based standard therapy that did not include transfusion.

PERSONALIZED CARE: TODAY

It is clear from the results of the 3 large-scale EGDT trials that the original Rivers protocol for EGDT does not improve outcomes if initiated on all septic patients in the emergency department. Mandatory central venous catheter placement does not improve outcomes nor does mandating continuous $ScvO_2$ monitoring, transfusing to a hematocrit greater than 30% or starting dobutamine if $ScvO_2$ is less than 70%. A protocol that supports these interventions on every patient cannot be supported based on existing literature.

However, it would be a grave mistake to interpret these studies as demonstrating that there are no global principles that are relevant to the management of septic patients. A close look at what constitutes usual care in the studies demonstrates several underlying principles that are imperative for the treatment of any newly diagnosed septic patients.

First, early treatment is critical. No different from the "golden hour" in trauma or myocardial infarction, the sooner a patient is recognized as septic and treatment is initiated, the better the outcome will be. Early antibiotic administration saves lives because it has been demonstrated that mortality increases by 7.6% for every hour antibiotics are delayed in septic shock [30]. Fluid resuscitation is also critical. An appropriate starting point is giving 30 mL/kg of crystalloid as recommended in sepsis bundles. Finally, vasopressors must be initiated if a patient is not responsive to volume resuscitation, and lactate levels should be followed to determine if therapy results in successful clearance of lactate.

After these core principles, care must be individualized. Although a patient needs as much fluid as is required for them to be fully volume resuscitated, the amount of fluid required to get to this point can vary significantly from patient to patient. Unfortunately, there are negative consequences to both underresuscitation and overresuscitation [31], so an accurate assessment of patient volume status is critical. Current bundles and public reporting require either focused physical examination, including vital signs, cardiopulmonary, capillary refill, pulse, and skin findings, or 2 of the following: (a) CVP, (b) $ScvO_2$, (c) bedside cardiovascular ultrasound, or (d) dynamic assessment of fluid responsiveness with passive leg raise or fluid challenge. Other options that are used by many practitioners include stroke volume variation, plethysmography variability index, and arterial pulse pressure variation. Ultimately, each of these techniques has a combination of advantages and disadvantages, and the optimal method of assessing volume status for each patient needs to be individualized based on the skill set of the provider, the tools available to the provider, as well as patient-specific characteristics (such as if they are intubated, their cardiac rhythm, and if adequate echocardiographic views can be obtained).

Furthermore, the goal mean arterial pressure in a septic patient is generally 65 mm Hg. However, in a patient with chronic hypertension, a higher blood pressure might be required to assure appropriate tissue perfusion. Alternatively, in a patient with chronic low blood pressure, a lower mean arterial blood pressure may be acceptable as long as the patient is showing signs of adequate tissue perfusion (normal mental status, urine output, lactate).

In addition, while continuous $ScvO_2$ measurement is not associated with improved outcomes, this does not mean the test has no value. A markedly depressed $ScvO_2$ is suggestive of inadequate tissue perfusion, even if the patient is at the goal mean arterial blood pressure. Obtaining an abnormal value might lead to additional diagnostic tests (echocardiogram, ruling out a pulmonary embolism, for example) or additional therapeutic interventions (volume, inotropes, depending on the clinical circumstance).

PERSONALIZED CARE: THE FUTURE

The patient's response to an invading micro-organism depends on both host and pathogen factors. Unfortunately, little can be done today at the bedside to assay the host response to sepsis outside of basic bedside assays of organ failure, such as the SOFA score, and simple blood tests. There are no biomarkers able to quantify and evaluate patients' response easily to allow for more personalized care. However, it is possible that omics approaches–genomics, transcriptomics, proteomics, metabolomics, microbiomics–will identify "signatures" for sepsis that could help guide treatment. This approach is currently being used in cancer, and although there are additional complexities seen in sepsis, the concept has significant promise. An early glimpse of a potential future lies in genetic studies in pediatric septic patients. Based on the varying expression of a group of biomarkers, 168 patients were subdivided into 2 broad endotypes of septic shock, characterized by either excessive inflammation or immune suppression. This model had an area under the curve of 0.83, with a sensitivity of 93% for predicting a complicated course [32]. A similar study examining the capacity of 100 subclass-defining genes was able to predict a 2.7-fold increase in mortality [33]. Notably, steroid usage in this patient group was independently associated with a 4.1-fold increase in mortality, suggesting the possibility that in the future, interrogating the host response to an infection on an individual basis could potentially determine whether an intervention should be given.

SUMMARY

The exciting results initially seen with EGDT have not been borne out in subsequent larger trials. However, an improvement in usual care over the past 15 years has led to markedly improved outcomes from sepsis. Core elements of sepsis management that are appropriate for all patients include rapid antibiotic administration after drawing cultures, fluid resuscitation, administration of vasopressors (if indicated), and assaying blood lactate levels to determine the success of treatment. However, patients also require individualized management when attempting to meet goals that are more difficult to protocolize, such as assessing volume resuscitation. The promise of genetic-based personalized medicine guiding administration of specific therapeutic agents holds substantial promise for the future.

References

[1] Kompanje EJ, Jansen TC, van der Hoven B, et al. The first demonstration of lactic acid in human blood in shock by Johann Joseph Scherer (1814-1869) in January 1843. Intensive Care Med 2007;33(11):1967–71.

[2] American College of Chest Physicians/Society of Critical Care Medicine Consensus Conference: definitions for sepsis and organ failure and guidelines for the use of innovative therapies in sepsis. Crit Care Med 1992;20(6):864–74.
[3] Levy MM, Fink MP, Marshall JC, et al. 2001 SCCM/ESICM/ACCP/ATS/SIS International Sepsis Definitions Conference. Crit Care Med 2003;31(4):1250–6.
[4] Singer M, Deutschman CS, Seymour CW, et al. The Third International Consensus definitions for sepsis and septic shock (sepsis-3). JAMA 2016;315(8):801–10.
[5] Shankar-Hari M, Phillips GS, Levy ML, et al. Developing a new definition and assessing new clinical criteria for septic shock: for the Third International Consensus definitions for sepsis and septic shock (sepsis-3). JAMA 2016;315(8):775–87.
[6] Seymour CW, Liu VX, Iwashyna TJ, et al. Assessment of clinical criteria for sepsis: for the Third International Consensus definitions for sepsis and septic shock (sepsis-3). JAMA 2016;315(8):762–74.
[7] Angus DC, Seymour CW, Coopersmith CM, et al. A framework for the development and interpretation of different sepsis definitions and clinical criteria. Crit Care Med 2016;44(3):e113–21.
[8] Seymour CW, Coopersmith CM, Deutschman CS, et al. Application of a framework to assess the usefulness of alternative sepsis criteria. Crit Care Med 2016;44(3):e122–30.
[9] Gaieski DF, Edwards JM, Kallan MJ, et al. Benchmarking the incidence and mortality of severe sepsis in the United States. Crit Care Med 2013;41(5):1167–74.
[10] Lagu T, Rothberg MB, Shieh MS, et al. Hospitalizations, costs, and outcomes of severe sepsis in the United States 2003 to 2007. Crit Care Med 2012;40(3):754–61.
[11] Zimmerman JE, Kramer AA, Knaus WA. Changes in hospital mortality for United States intensive care unit admissions from 1988 to 2012. Crit Care 2013;17(2):R81.
[12] Hotchkiss RS, Monneret G, Payen D. Sepsis-induced immunosuppression: from cellular dysfunctions to immunotherapy. Nat Rev Immunol 2013;13(12):862–74.
[13] Limaye AP, Kirby KA, Rubenfeld GD, et al. Cytomegalovirus reactivation in critically ill immunocompetent patients. JAMA 2008;300(4):413–22.
[14] Martin GS, Mannino DM, Moss M. The effect of age on the development and outcome of adult sepsis. Crit Care Med 2006;34(1):15–21.
[15] McConnell KW, McDunn JE, Clark AT, et al. Streptococcus pneumoniae and Pseudomonas aeruginosa pneumonia induce distinct host responses. Crit Care Med 2010;38(1):223–41.
[16] Danai PA, Moss M, Mannino DM, et al. The epidemiology of sepsis in patients with malignancy. Chest 2006;129(6):1432–40.
[17] Dellinger RP, Levy MM, Rhodes A, et al. Surviving sepsis campaign: international guidelines for management of severe sepsis and septic shock: 2012. Crit Care Med 2013;41(2):580–637.
[18] Levy MM, Rhodes A, Phillips GS, et al. Surviving sepsis campaign: association between performance metrics and outcomes in a 7.5-year study. Crit Care Med 2015;43(1):3–12.
[19] Rivers E, Nguyen B, Havstad S, et al. Early goal-directed therapy in the treatment of severe sepsis and septic shock. N Engl J Med 2001;345(19):1368–77.
[20] Yealy DM, Kellum JA, Huang DT, et al. A randomized trial of protocol-based care for early septic shock. N Engl J Med 2014;370(18):1683–93.
[21] Peake SL, Delaney A, Bailey M, et al. Goal-directed resuscitation for patients with early septic shock. N Engl J Med 2014;371(16):1496–506.
[22] Mouncey PR, Osborn TM, Power GS, et al. Trial of early, goal-directed resuscitation for septic shock. N Engl J Med 2015;372(14):1301–11.
[23] Kaukonen KM, Bailey M, Suzuki S, et al. Mortality related to severe sepsis and septic shock among critically ill patients in Australia and New Zealand, 2000-2012. JAMA 2014;311(13):1308–16.
[24] Marik PE, Baram M, Vahid B. Does central venous pressure predict fluid responsiveness? A systematic review of the literature and the tale of seven mares. Chest 2008;134(1):172–8.

[25] Asfar P, Meziani F, Hamel JF, et al. High versus low blood-pressure target in patients with septic shock. N Engl J Med 2014;370(17):1583–93.
[26] Pope JV, Jones AE, Gaieski DF, et al. Multicenter study of central venous oxygen saturation (ScvO(2)) as a predictor of mortality in patients with sepsis. Ann Emerg Med 2010;55(1): 40–6.
[27] Jones AE, Shapiro NI, Trzeciak S, et al. Lactate clearance vs central venous oxygen saturation as goals of early sepsis therapy: a randomized clinical trial. JAMA 2010;303(8): 739–46.
[28] Hebert PC, Wells G, Blajchman MA, et al. A multicenter, randomized, controlled clinical trial of transfusion requirements in critical care. Transfusion Requirements in Critical Care Investigators, Canadian Critical Care Trials Group. N Engl J Med 1999;340(6):409–17.
[29] Holst LB, Haase N, Wetterslev J, et al. Lower versus higher hemoglobin threshold for transfusion in septic shock. N Engl J Med 2014;371(15):1381–91.
[30] Kumar A, Roberts D, Wood KE, et al. Duration of hypotension before initiation of effective antimicrobial therapy is the critical determinant of survival in human septic shock. Crit Care Med 2006;34(6):1589–96.
[31] Raimundo M, Crichton S, Martin JR, et al. Increased fluid administration after early acute kidney injury is associated with less renal recovery. Shock 2015;44(5):431–7.
[32] Wong HR, Cvijanovich NZ, Anas N, et al. Prospective testing and redesign of a temporal biomarker based risk model for patients with septic shock: implications for septic shock biology. EBioMedicine 2015;2(12):2087–93.
[33] Wong HR, Cvijanovich NZ, Anas N, et al. Developing a clinically feasible personalized medicine approach to pediatric septic shock. Am J Respir Crit Care Med 2015;191(3): 309–15.

Advances in Surgery 50 (2016) 235–256

ADVANCES IN SURGERY

Current Status of Carotid Stenting Versus Endarterectomy

Ali F. AbuRahma, MD[a,b,*], Albeir Y. Mousa, MD[b]

[a]Vascular Laboratory, Vascular Surgery Fellowship and Residency Programs, Vascular & Endovascular Surgery, Vascular Center of Excellence, 3110 MacCorkle Avenue, Southeast, Charleston, WV 25304, USA; [b]Department of Surgery, West Virginia University, 3110 MacCorkle Avenue, Southeast, Charleston, WV 25304, USA

Keywords

• Embolic protection • Carotid angioplasty/stenting (CAS)
• Carotid endarterectomy (CEA) • Filter • Reversal flow • Stent • Diffusion

Key points

- For symptomatic de novo carotid stenosis in good risk patients, carotid endarterectomy (CEA) remains the standard of care.
- The use of carotid artery stenting (CAS) should be selective at this stage and must be done by experienced operators/centers.
- CAS may also be preferable in most patients with post-CEA restenosis.

Stroke is the third most common cause of mortality worldwide. About 20% to 30% of strokes have been attributed to atherosclerotic disease of the extracranial carotid artery. According to the North American Symptomatic Carotid Endarterectomy Trial [1], more than 70% of stenosis is associated with a stroke risk of 26% in symptomatic patients at 2 years. Although it is not the only etiology, extracranial carotid atherosclerosis is the most common surgically treatable condition for prevention of ischemic stroke. Multiple randomized controlled studies over the last 2 decades for both symptomatic and asymptomatic carotid stenosis have shown the efficacy of carotid endarterectomy (CEA) in reducing the risk of stroke over medical therapy alone [2,3].

Disclosure: The authors have nothing to disclose.

*Corresponding author. Vascular Laboratory, Vascular Surgery Fellowship and Residency Programs, Vascular & Endovascular Surgery, Vascular Center of Excellence, Charleston, WV. *E-mail address:* ali.aburahma@camc.org

0065-3411/16/$ – see front matter
http://dx.doi.org/10.1016/j.yasu.2016.04.004

Since its early inception in 1980 by Kerber and colleagues [4], carotid artery transluminal angioplasty has evolved into an acceptable alternative to CEA in a select group of patients. Both options for treating carotid artery stenosis have been subjected to extensive comparison over the last 2 decades with multiple randomized trials, mainly regarding efficacy, safety, and durability. Although these trials carry significant weight, they may not represent, in great part, the real-world experience. The Carotid Revascularization Endarterectomy versus Stenting Trial (CREST) investigators [5] have shown that these 2 procedures (CEA and carotid artery stenting [CAS]) are somewhat comparable. This multicenter, well-designed, prospective, randomized, controlled study examined the primary endpoints of stroke, myocardial infarction (MI), and death in 2502 patients. Evaluation was initiated in the preoperative period and extended to 4 years after randomization. Although there were no differences in the composite endpoints as defined by periprocedural (within 30 days) death, stroke, or MI between CEA and CAS; strokes were more frequent after CAS (4.1% vs 2.3%; $P = .01$). All respected authorities agree that the lower risk of MI and cranial nerve injury with CAS compared with CEA is counterbalanced by an increased risk of ipsilateral stroke events.

REVIEW OF RANDOMIZED CONTROLLED CAROTID TRIALS (CAROTID ARTERY STENTING VS CAROTID ENDARTERECTOMY)

The Carotid and Vertebral Artery Transluminal Angioplasty Study

This multicenter randomized carotid trial included 504 patients (90% symptomatic) with carotid stenosis (carotid angioplasty [n = 251] or CEA [n = 253]), with a median follow-up of 5 years [6] in an intention-to-treat analysis. Within 30 days of treatment, there were more minor strokes that lasted less than 7 days in the endovascular group (8 [3.2%] vs 1 [0.4%]), but the number of other strokes in any territory or death was the same (25 [10%] vs 25 [9.9%]). By comparing endovascular treatment with CEA after the 30-day posttreatment period, the 8-year incidence and hazard ratio (HR) at the end of follow-up for ipsilateral nonperioperative stroke was 11.3% versus 8.6% (HR, 1.2; 95% CI, 0.59–2.54); for ipsilateral nonperioperative stroke or transient ischemic attack it was 19.3% versus 17.2% (HR, 1.3; 95% CI, 0.78–2.14); and for any nonperioperative stroke was 21.1% versus 15.4% (HR, 1.7; 95% CI, 0.99–2.80). The primary endpoint of 70% or greater restenosis was higher in the angioplasty group (HR, 3.17; $P < .0001$). It should be noted that carotid stents were used only in 26% of the angioplasty group. Patients who received stents had a significantly lower incidence of restenosis than patients who underwent angioplasty alone (HR, 0.43; $P = .04$).

The Stenting and Angioplasty with Protection in Patients at High Risk for Endarterectomy Trial

This noninferiority trial included 334 patients and was the first randomized carotid trial to use mandatory cerebral protection devices [7]. High-risk surgical patients were randomly assigned to CEA (n = 167) or CAS (n = 167) and 70% of patients were 80% or greater asymptomatic and 30% were 50% or greater symptomatic. The 30-day combined perioperative major adverse events (MAE; stroke, MI, and death) rate was 4.8% for CAS versus 9.8% for CEA (P = .09). The combined MAE rate at 1 year was 12.2% for CAS versus 20.1% for CEA (P = .004) for noninferiority of CAS for patients at high risk for CEA. The MAE rate was 16.8% for CAS versus 16.5% for CEA in symptomatic patients (P = .95) and 9.9% for CAS versus 21.5% for CEA in asymptomatic patients (P = .02). The significant difference was mainly secondary to non-Q wave MI with CEA.

The Endarterectomy Versus Angioplasty in Patients with Symptomatic Severe Carotid Stenosis Trial

This multicenter French noninferiority randomized carotid trial compared CAS with CEA only in symptomatic carotid patients with at least 60% stenosis [8,9]. This study randomized 527 patients and excluded high-risk patients with unstable angina, uncontrolled diabetes mellitus, hypertension, or previous CEA. The study reported an incidence of any stroke or death at 30 days of 9.6% for CAS versus 3.9% for CEA and at 6 months, the stroke/death rate was 6.1% for CEA versus 11.7% for CAS (P = .02; relative risk [RR], 2.5). This study was stopped prematurely owing to excessive deaths in the CAS group. It should be noted that in the CAS group, the risk of stroke/death was significantly lower when embolic protection devices were used (18/227 [7.9%] vs 5/20 [25%]; P = .03). Notably, cranial nerve injuries were more common after CEA, but major local complications were more common with CAS. In long-term data at 5 years, the cumulative probability of primary endpoint was 11% for CAS versus 6.3% for CEA (HR, 2; P = .03). There was no difference reported beyond the procedural period with regard to severe carotid stenosis or occlusion, death, MI, or revascularization procedure [10].

The main criticisms of the Endarterectomy Versus Angioplasty in Patients With Symptomatic Severe Carotid Stenosis (EVA-3S) trial include heterogeneity of operator experience and the types of stents and cerebral protection devices that were used. Although the surgeons participating in this study were required to perform at least 25 CEAs within 1 year before trial entry, interventionalists were certified after performing only one-half of that number of CAS procedures. However, a subgroup analysis failed to show any statistical significance between operations based on the level of experience. In the early days of the trial, cerebral protection devices for patients assigned to CAS were optional and the 30-day stroke/death was significantly lower in patients who received cerebral protection devices (7.9% vs 25%).

The Stent-supported Percutaneous Angioplasty of the Carotid Artery Versus Endarterectomy Trial

The Stent-supported Percutaneous Angioplasty of the Carotid Artery Versus Endarterectomy (SPACE) Trial was another multicenter European noninferiority trial designed to compare CAS with CEA in symptomatic patients.

Patients were randomized to CAS (n = 605) or CEA (n = 595) [11]. The 30-day stroke and death rate was 6.8% for CAS versus 6.3% for CEA (*P* = .09). A postmarket analysis showed that an older age in the CAS group, but not CEA, was significantly associated with higher stroke and death. There were no differences in the stroke/death rates between the 2 groups up to 2 years (9.5% vs 8.8% in intention-to-treat and 9.4% vs 7.8% per protocol). Notably, recurrent carotid stenosis of greater than 70% was more significant in CAS than CEA (10.7% vs 4.6%).

The main criticisms of the SPACE trial were that the use of cerebral protection devices was optional and the steering committee decided to terminate the study after the interim analysis on the basis of both futility and financial concern, because it was revealed that 2500 patients would be needed to power the study adequately [11,12]. In most endpoints, there was a favorable trend toward the surgical arm, although none were statistically significant.

The Carotid and Vertebral Artery Transluminal Angioplasty Study 2 (also called International Carotid Stenting Study)

The Carotid and Vertebral Artery Transluminal Angioplasty Study 2 (also Called ICSS) enrolled 1713 patients and excluded high-risk patients. At least 50 CEAs were required for operators and 50 stenting (≥10 of these were CAS) for interventionalists [13]. The interim analysis at 120 days showed stroke, MI, or death for CAS was 8.5% versus 5.2% for CEA (HR, 1.7; *P* = .006). This study used restenosis as its primary endpoint. CAS also had an increased stroke rate (7.7% vs 4.1%), higher stroke/death rate (8.5% vs 4.7%), and greater all-cause death rate (2.3% vs 0.8%). There was no difference between CAS and CEA with regard to disabling stroke or death (4% vs 3.2%). A subanalysis based on MRI showed new ischemic brain lesions on the fusion-weighted MRI, which was significantly increased for CAS versus CEA (50% vs 17%; odds ratio [OR], 5.2). At a mean follow-up of 4 years, there were more strokes in the CAS group than the CEA group (119 vs 72): the 5-year cumulative risk of all strokes was 15.2% versus 9.4% (HR, 1.7; *P*<.001; mainly nondisabling strokes); a 5-year risk of fatal/disabling stroke was not different (6.4% vs 6.5%) [13].

Carotid Revascularization Endarterectomy Versus Stenting Trial

The Carotid Revascularization Endarterectomy Versus Stenting Trial (CREST) was a National Institutes of Health–sponsored trial with a primary endpoint of 30-day stoke, MI, death, or any ipsilateral stroke during a 4-year follow-up. Patients were randomized from 117 centers in the United States and Canada (2502 symptomatic and asymptomatic). This trial required a rigorous credentialing of surgeons in that they should have performed at least 12 CEAs in the previous year, with stroke or death rates of less than 5% and less than 3% for symptomatic and asymptomatic patients, respectively. The interventionalists were certified after satisfactory evaluation of their past CAS experience and if that was acceptable, then completion of CREST training program was followed by participation in hands-on training with ACCULINK and

ACCUNET carotid systems, and a lead-in phase of up to 20 cases, that is, the best of the best were selected. The endpoint of this study for CAS versus CEA: any periprocedure stroke or postprocedure stroke (4.1% vs 2.3%; $P = .01$), major stroke (0.9% vs 0.6%; $P = .52$), minor stroke (3.2% vs 1.7%; $P = .01$), MI (1.1% vs 2.3%; $P = .01$), death (0.7% vs 0.3%; $P = .18$), perioperative primary study endpoint (5.2% vs 4.5%; $P = .38$), primary endpoint to 4 years (7.2% vs 6.8%; $P = .51$), and cranial nerve palsy (0% vs 5%; Table 1). When the endpoints were analyzed according to preoperative indications, any perioperative stroke for asymptomatic patients (2.5% for CAS vs 1.4% for CEA; $P = .07$), and for asymptomatic patients (5.5% vs 3.2; $P = .25$); meanwhile, the primary study endpoints were 3.5% versus 3.6% ($P = .56$) for asymptomatic and 6.7% versus 5.4% ($P = .69$) for symptomatic patients (Table 2). In the 1-year analysis, the quality of life (Short Form-36 questionnaire) was diminished significantly for patients who had a stroke, even a minor stroke (−15.8 points), compared with those who had an MI or cranial nerve palsy (−4.5 points). The 2-year analysis showed that for symptomatic patients, the stroke and death was significantly higher in CAS versus CEA (6% vs 3.2%; HR, 1.9). The 4-year rate of death alone was very similar for CAS (11.3%) and CEA (12.6%; $P = .45$). During CREST enrollment (2000–2008), concurrent registry studies demonstrated a steady decrease in the risk of adverse outcome with CAS. This may reflect better patient selection based on an improved understanding of patients who are at high risk for CAS–a tortuous or highly calcified arch, great vessel, or carotid bifurcation; that is, better results may be secondary to, not only more experience, but also better patient selection.

It should be noted that the primary objective of carotid interventions is stroke prevention and this is 1 situation where the heart should not rule the head [14]. Although it is appropriate to consider all of the 3 primary endpoints, it is totally inappropriate to consider them to be of equal importance.

Table 1
CREST trial results: endpoints according to treatment with CAS or CEA

Endpoint	CAS (n = 1262)	CEA (n = 1240)	*P* value
Any periprocedure stroke or postprocedure ipsilateral stroke (%)	4.1 ± 0.6	2.3 ± 0.4	.01
Major stroke (%)	0.9 ± 0.3	0.6 ± 0.2	.52
Minor stroke (%)	3.2 ± 0.5	1.7 ± 0.4	.01
Myocardial infarction (%)	1.1 ± 0.3	2.3 ± 0.4	.01
Death (%)	0.7 ± 0.2	0.3 ± 0.2	.18
Primary study endpoint* perioperative (%)	5.2 ± 0.6	4.5 ± 0.6	.38
Primary endpoint* to 4 y (%)	7.2 ± 0.8	6.8 ± 0.8	.51
Cranial nerve palsy	0	5%	—

Abbreviations: CAS, carotid artery stenting; CEA, carotid endarterectomy; CREST, Carotid Revascularization Endarterectomy versus Stenting Trial.

Data from Brott TG, Hobson RW 2nd, Howard G, et al; CREST Investigators. Stenting versus endarterectomy for treatment of carotid-artery stenosis. N Engl J Med 2010;363:16.

Table 2
CREST results: asymptomatic and symptomatic patients

Endpoint	CAS	CEA	*P* value
Any periprocedural stroke or postprocedural ipsilateral stroke (%)			
Asymptomatic	2.5 ± 0.6	1.4 ± 0.5	.07
Symptomatic	5.5 ± 0.9	3.2 ± 0.7	.25
Primary study endpoint* (%)			
Asymptomatic	3.5 ± 0.8	3.6 ± 0.8	.56
Symptomatic	6.7 ± 1.0	5.4 ± 0.9	.69

Abbreviations: CAS, carotid artery stenting; CEA, carotid endarterectomy; CREST, Carotid Revascularization Endarterectomy versus Stenting Trial.

Data from Brott TG, Hobson RW 2nd, Howard G, et al; CREST Investigators. Stenting versus endarterectomy for treatment of carotid-artery stenosis. N Engl J Med 2010;363:11–23.

Table 3 summarizes various randomized controlled trials comparing CAS versus CEA [5–8,11,15–20].

Metaanalysis of Clinical Trials: Carotid Artery Stenting Versus Carotid Endarterectomy

Table 4 summarizes these metaanalyses [21–35].

A metaanalysis of 7 trials (2973 patients) [23] noted that CAS carries a higher 30-day risk of stroke or death than CEA (8.2% vs 6.2%; $P = .04$; OR, 1.35), but when nondisabling strokes were excluded, the difference was not significant. However, CEA had a significantly higher risk of cranial nerve palsy (4.7% vs 0.2%; $P < .0001$; OR, 0.17) and MI (2.3% vs 0.9%; $P = .03$; OR, 0.37) than CAS.

In a metaanalysis of 10 trials using an intention-to-treat approach, Brahmanandam and colleagues [27] noted that CAS patients had a higher risk of 30-day stroke/death than CEA patients (RR, 1.30; 95% CI, 1.01–1.67). A sensitivity analysis of only the randomized controlled trials (8 trials) produced similar results. A subset analysis of trials that only enrolled symptomatic patients showed a higher risk of 30-day stroke/death (RR, 1.63; 95% CI, 1.18–2.25) in CAS patients.

A metaanalysis of 9 trials (3138 patients) by Jeng and colleagues [26] found that when a random effects model was used, there was no difference between CAS and CEA in 30-day event rates for any stroke (OR for CAS, 1.46; 95% CI, 0.91–2.36), death or any stroke (OR, 1.37; 95% CI, 0.9–2.1), or death, any stroke, or MI (OR, 1.02; 95% CI, 0.49–2.11). Also, there was no difference in the rates of death/any stroke at 6 months (OR, 1.50; 95% CI, 0.69–3.23) or 1 year (OR, 1.25; 95% CI, 0.59–2.63). However, when a fixed effects model was used, the 30-day event rate for death/any stroke was significantly greater after CAS than CEA (OR, 1.37; 95% CI, 1.04–1.81), and the risk of cranial nerve injury was much lower in CAS patients (OR, 0.12; 95% CI, 0.05–0.29).

Table 3
Summary of various randomized controlled studies: CEA versus CAS

Trial (year)	Inclusion criteria	No. of patients		Stroke		Death		Myocardial infarction		Stroke or death		Death or disabling stroke			
		CEA	CAS	CEA	CAS	CEA	CAS	CEA	CAS	CEA	CAS	CEA	CAS	EPD%	Follow-up (months)
Wallstent [15], 2001	>60% symptomatic stenosis	112	107	NR	NR	NR	NR	NR	NR	5	13	NR	NR	0	12
Kentucky-A [16], 2001	>70% symptomatic stenosis	51	53	0	0	1	0	1	0	1	0	1	0	0	48
EVA-3S et al [8], 2006	>60% symptomatic stenosis	262	265	9	24	3	2	2	1	10	25	4	9	92	6
SAPPHIRE [7,17], 2008	>50% symptomatic or >80% asymptomatic stenosis and high surgical risk	167	167	5	6	4	2	10	4	8	7	NR	NR	96	36
SPACE [11,18], 2008	≥70% symptomatic stenosis	589	607	37	44	5	6	NR	NR	39	45	23	31	27	1
CAVATAS [6,19], 2009	>50% symptomatic or asymptomatic stenosis	253	251	21	18	4	7	3	0	25	25	15	16	0	36
ICSS [20], 2010	>50% symptomatic stenosis	857	853	35	65	7	19	4	3	40	72	27	34	72	3
CREST [5], 2010	≥50% on angiography, ≥70% on US, CTA, MRA symptomatic stenosis or ≥60% on angiography, ≥70% on US, 80% on CTA or MRA asymptomatic stenosis	1240	1262	29	52	4	9	28	14	29	55	NR	NR	96	30

Abbreviations: CAS, carotid artery stenting; CAVATAS, Carotid and Vertebral Artery Transluminal Angioplasty Study; CEA, carotid endarterectomy; CREST, Carotid Revascularization Endarterectomy versus Stenting Trial; CTA, computed tomography angiography; EPD, embolic protection device; EVA-3S, Endarterectomy Versus Angioplasty in Patients With Symptomatic Severe Carotid Stenosis; ICSS, Carotid and Vertebral Artery Transluminal Angioplasty Study 2; MRA, MR angiography; SAPPHIRE, Stenting and Angioplasty With Protection in Patients at High Risk for Endarterectomy; SPACE, Stent-supported Percutaneous Angioplasty of the Carotid Artery Versus Endarterectomy Trial; US, ultrasonography.

Adapted from Gahremanpour A, Perin EC, Silva G. Carotid artery stenting versus endarterectomy: a systematic review. Tex Heart Inst J 2012;39(4):474–87.

Table 4
Metaanalysis of carotid trials comparing CEA and CAS

Authors, year	No. patients/ studies	CAS outcome vs CEA
Quereshi et al [21], 2005	1154/5	Rate of stroke/death was not different (RR, 1.3; $P = .4$).
Ederle et al [22], 2007	3227/12	Higher 30-d rate of stroke/death for CAS with fixed-effects model (OR, 1.4; $P = .02$) but not with random-effects model (OR, 1.4; $P = .12$). No difference in risk of disabling stroke/ death with fixed-effects model (OR, 1.2; $P = .31$) or with random-effects model (OR, 1.2; $P = .39$).
Wiesmann et al [23], 2008	2973/7	Higher 30-d rate of stroke/death (OR, 1.35; $P = .04$). Rate of disabling stroke/death not different.
Murad et al [24], 2008	3182/10	Nonsignificant reduction in rate of death (RR, 0.61; $P > .05$) and nonsignificant increases in risk of any stroke (RR, 1.3; $P > .05$) and disabling stroke (RR, 1.06; $P > .05$).
Ringleb et al [25], 2008	2985/8	Higher 30-d rate of stroke/death (OR, 1.3; $P = .03$). Rate for disabling stroke/death not significantly different (OR, 1.3; $P = .12$).
Jeng et al [26], 2008	3138/9	Random-effects showed no significant difference in rate of any stroke, death or any stroke, or MI at 30 d, 6 mo, or 1 y. Fixed-effects model associated CAS with higher 30-d rate of any stroke or death (OR, 1.37; $P < .05$).
Brahmanandam et al [27], 2008	3580/10	Higher 30-d rate of stroke/death (OR, 1.3; $P < .05$).
Gurm et al [28], 2008	2122/5	No significant difference for 30-d rate of any stroke/disabling stroke or death.
Liu et al [29], 2009	2942/8	Similar risk of stroke/death at 30 d (OR, 0.69; $P = .1$) and 1 y (OR, 0.8; $P = .72$).
Roffi et al [30], 2009	4648/10	Higher 30-d rate of stroke/death for CAS (OR, 1.6; $P < .05$).
Bonati et al [31], 2010	3433/3[a]	Significantly higher 3-mo risk of stroke/ death (RR, 1.5; $P = .0006$). With age <70 y RR was 1.00; with age ≥70 y. RR was 2.04 ($P = .0014$).
Meier et al [32], 2010	4796/11	Lower risk of stroke/death for CEA (OR, 0.67; $P = .025$) secondary to lower stroke rate; no difference for risk of death alone (OR, 1.14; $P = .727$) or for death/disabling stroke (OR, 0.74; $P = .9$). Risk of stroke/death no different up to 4-y follow-up (HR, 0.9; $P = .314$).

(*continued on next page*)

Table 4
continued

Authors, year	No. patients/ studies	CAS outcome vs CEA
Economopoulos et al [33], 2011	7477/13	Higher stroke rate in both periprocedural period and long-term follow-up (OR, 1.37), particularly for patients older than 68 y (OR, 1.7).
Bangalore et al [34], 2011	7477/13	Greater relative risk of periprocedural stroke/ death (20%) and less RR of MI (15%).
Yavin et al [35], 2011	6973/12	Significantly higher periprocedural stroke risk (OR, 1.72) and lower MI (OR, 0.47). Death rates were similar (OR, 1.1).

Abbreviations: CAS, carotid artery stenting; CEA, carotid endarterectomy; HR, hazard ratio; MI, myocardial infarction; OR, odds ratio; RR, risk ratio.

[a]Endarterectomy Versus Angioplasty in Patients With Symptomatic Severe Carotid Stenosis, Stent-supported Percutaneous Angioplasty of the Carotid Artery Versus Endarterectomy Trial, and Carotid and Vertebral Artery Transluminal Angioplasty Study 2.

Adapted from Gahremanpour A, Perin EC, Silva G. Carotid artery stenting versus endarterectomy: a systematic review. Tex Heart Inst J 2012;39(4):474–87.

In another metaanalysis of 10 randomized clinical trials, Murad and colleagues [24] associated CAS with a nonsignificant reduction in the risk of death (RR, 0.6; 95% CI, 0.27–1.37), nonfatal MI (RR, 0.43; 95% CI, 0.17–1.11), and a nonsignificant increase in any stroke (RR, 1.29; 95% CI, 0.73–2.26), and major/disabling stroke (RR, 1.06; 95% CI, 0.73–2.26). Meanwhile, Ringleb and colleagues [25], in a metaanalysis of 8 randomized controlled trials (2985 patients), of whom 89% were symptomatic, noted that the risk of stroke/death within 30 days was greater after CAS, compared with CEA (OR, 1.38; 95% CI, 1.04–1.83; $P = .024$). However, the odds of disabling stroke/death were not significant.

In another recent metaanalysis of 11 trials (4796 patients), Meier and colleagues [32] found that CEA was associated with significantly less risk of periprocedural death/stroke (OR, 0.67; 95% CI, 0.47–0.95; $P = .025$), mainly because of a lesser risk of stroke (OR, 0.65; 95% CI, 0.43–1.00; $P = .049$). Furthermore, the risk of death and the composite endpoint of death/disabling stroke did not differ significantly, whereas CEA was associated with a significantly higher risk of periprocedural MI (OR, 2.69; 95% CI, 1.06–6.79; $P = .036$) and cranial nerve injury (OR, 10.2; 95% CI, 4.0–26.1; $P < .001$).

CAROTID ARTERY STENTING RESULTS IN THE REAL WORLD

Despite the controversial debate regarding the exact role of CAS as compared with CEA, its use in clinical practice has exploded all over the world. However, the favorable results of CAS in some of the carotid stenting trials have not been reflected in the real-world experience, as noted in the following discussion.

Outcomes After Carotid Artery Stenting in Medicare Beneficiaries, 2005 to 2009 (Carotid Artery Stenting Linked to High Real-world Mortality)

In a large retrospective cohort study of the Centers for Medicare and Medicaid Services CAS Database (2005–2009) [36], the perioperative mortality was more than twice the rate in this patient population than those reported earlier in CREST and SAPPHIRE. In that study, 22,000 patients were evaluated with a mean age of 76 years. The majority of patients were men, one-half were symptomatic, 91% were at high surgical risk, and the mean follow-up was 2 years. It is worth noting that 80% of the physicians in that study did not meet the minimal CAS volume requirement and/or the minimal complication rate of the SAPPHIRE trial, and more than 90% of the physicians did not meet the requirements of the CREST trial. The unadjusted 30-day risks were 1.7% for mortality, 3.3% for stroke, and 2.5% for MI. Overall, the mortality rate was 42% for patients 80 years or older and 37% in patients who were at high surgical risk. The overall mortality rate for symptomatic patients who were at high surgical risk was 37%. In asymptomatic patients, the mortality rate after CAS exceeded one-third of those patients who were at least 50 years old. Of special interest, only a few patients had providers with proficiency levels similar to those required in CAS clinical trials. Most of these CAS patients were done by cardiologists (53%). The mean number of past year CAS procedures was only 13.9 for physicians and 30 for hospitals. This study concluded that a major concern must be raised regarding generalizing the results of randomized clinical trials in real-world practice.

Comparison of Trends and Outcomes of Carotid Artery Stenting and Carotid Endarterectomy in the United States (2001–2010)

Kim and colleagues [37] reported on a cross-sectional study for CAS (n = 124,265) and CEA patients (n = 1,260,647) over a 10-year period from the Nationwide Inpatient Sample Database. A multivariate propensity score-matched analysis showed that CAS was associated with an increased risk of stroke (OR, 1.4), increased risk of death (OR, 1.7), and MAE (increased risk of death, stroke, and MI [OR, 1.3]). In asymptomatic patients, there were no significant differences in MAEs (OR, 1.1); however, there were significant differences for symptomatic patients ($P<.0001$ between CAS and CEA), with significant improvement in CAS outcomes over the course of 10 years. In the symptomatic cohort, the unadjusted rate of death, MI, stroke, and MAE were all increased significantly for CAS versus CEA groups (5.1% vs 1.9% for death, 3.1% vs 1.6% for MI, 8.6% vs 6.1% for stroke, and 15.2% vs 8.4% for MAE [$P<.001$ for all outcomes]).

The unadjusted and adjusted association between CAS and in-hospital outcomes with CEA as a reference is summarized in Table 5. The effect of clinical

Table 5
Unadjusted and adjusted association between CAS and in-hospital outcomes (CEA as reference)

Outcome	Unadjusted OR (95% CI)	*P* value	Model no. 1* adjusted OR (95% CI)	*P* value	Model no. 2† adjusted OR with PS (95% CI)	*P* value	Model no. 3‡ adjusted OR, PS matched model (95% CI)	*P* value
Death	2.16 (1.91–2.45)	<.001	1.60 (1.38–1.85)	<.001	1.62 (1.40–1.88)	<.001	1.69 (1.40–2.04)	<.001
Stroke	1.82 (1.64–2.00)	<.001	1.32 (1.18–1.49)	<.001	1.24 (1.10–1.40)	<.001	1.43 (1.23–1.66)	<.001
MI	1.27 (1.13–1.43)	<.001	0.92 (0.82–1.05)	.21	0.89 (0.82–1.05)	.08	0.89 (0.75–1.06)	.18
Death/stroke	1.94 (1.79–2.10)	<.001	1.41 (1.29–1.55)	<.001	1.37 (1.23–1.51)	<.001	1.51 (1.33–1.70)	<.001
MAEs	1.69 (1.57–1.81)	<.001	1.22(1.13–1.32)	<.001	1.17(1.08–1.28)	<.001	1.25 (1.13–1.39)	<.001

Abbreviations: CAS, carotid artery stenting; CEA, carotid endarterectomy; MI, myocardial infarction; OR, odds ratio; PS, propensity score.

*Model No. 1 was adjusted for statistically significant predictor variables that had significant univariate association with outcomes (*P* <.05) from among symptoms status, angina, chronic ischemic heart disease, renal dialysis, effect of radiation, prior coronary artery bypass grafting, prior percutaneous coronary intervention, age, gender, race, hospital bed size, hospital teaching status, region, payer, anemia, collagen vascular disease, congestive heart failure, chronic pulmonary disease, diabetes mellitus, coagulopathy, hypertension, liver disease, neurological disorders, obesity, peripheral vascular disorders, renal failure, and valvular disease.

†Model No. 2 included as covariates the propensity score for use of CAS and was adjusted for variables listed for Model no. 1.

‡Model No. 3 was adjusted using further propensity score-matched cohorts as well as covariates listed for Model no. 1.

From Kim LK, Yang DC, Swaminathan RV, et al. Comparison of trends and outcomes of carotid artery stenting and endarterectomy in the United States, 2001 to 2010. Circ Cardiovasc Interv 2014;7:692–700; with permission.

indication on the association of CAS with death, stroke, MI, and MAE is presented in Table 6.

Comparative Effectiveness of Carotid Revascularization Treatment: Evidence from a National Hospital Discharge Database

Another comparative effectiveness study [38] evaluated carotid revascularization using the National Hospital Discharge Database from 2006 to 2011, where 33 clinical covariables associated with carotid revascularization were subjected to a 1:1 propensity score matching. This study included 24,004 asymptomatic patients (12,002 CEA and 12,002 CAS) and 3506 symptomatic patients (1753 CEA and 1753 CAS) and reported an increased primary composite endpoint (stroke, MI, or death) for CAS compared with CEA, in both asymptomatic (OR, 1.4; $P \leq .0001$) and symptomatic patients (OR, 2.3; $P < .0001$), regardless of age or sex. Interestingly, similar findings were noted using the modified composite endpoints (stroke/death) for both asymptomatic (OR, 1.5; $P < .0001$) and symptomatic patients (OR, 3; $P < .0001$). The risk of acute MI was not significant between the 2 groups, regardless of the clinical presentation. This study concluded the CAS is associated with an increased risk of MAEs and unfavorable discharges, compared with CEA for all ages and clinical presentations [38].

Table 6
Effect of clinical indication on association of CAS with death, stroke, MI, and MAEs

Outcome	Clinical indication	Unadjusted OR (95% CI)	*P* Value	Adjusted[a] OR (95% CI)	*P* value
Death	Asymptomatic	1.54 (1.28–1.86)	<.0001	1.36 (1.09–1.70)	.007
	Symptomatic	2.59 (2.19–3.06)	<.0001	2.00 (1.64–2.45)	<.001
					<.001[b]
Stroke	Asymptomatic	1.74 (1.55–1.96)	<.0001	1.37 (1.17–1.59)	<.001
	Symptomatic	1.79 (1.50–2.14)	<.0001	1.16 (0.93–1.44)	.19
					<.001[b]
MI	Asymptomatic	1.10 (0.95–1.28)	.20	0.79 (0.67–0.94)	.007
	Symptomatic	1.55 (1.27–1.89)	<.001	1.12 (0.89–1.42)	.14
					<.001[b]
Death/stroke	Asymptomatic	1.65 (1.49–1.83)	<.001	1.33 (1.17–1.52)	<.001
	Symptomatic	2.23 (1.97–2.54)	<.001	1.59 (1.36–1.86)	<.001
					<.001[b]
MAEs	Asymptomatic	1.42 (1.30–1.55)	<.001	1.08 (0.97–1.20)	.16
	Symptomatic	2.06 (1.84–2.30)	<.001	1.47 (128–1.68)	<.001
					<.001[b]

Adjusted odds ratio and CI values were listed if interaction *P* values were less than .05.

Abbreviations: CAS, carotid artery stenting; MAEs, major adverse events; OR, odds ratio.

[a]Propensity score-adjusted multivariable Cox regression analysis.

[b]Interaction *P* value.

From Kim LK, Yang DC, Swaminathan RV, et al. Comparison of trends and outcomes of carotid artery stenting and endarterectomy in the United States, 2001 to 2010. Circ Cardiovasc Interv 2014;7:692–700; with permission.

Systematic Review and Metaanalysis of Carotid Artery Stenting Versus Endarterectomy for Carotid Stenosis: a Chronologic and Worldwide Study

In an extensive comparative analysis to examine real practice outcomes between CAS and CEA, Zhang and colleagues [39] reported on 35 comparative studies encompassing 27,525 patients. The risk ratios of stroke/death for CAS compared with CEA within 30 days of treatment were 1.51 (95% CI, 1.32–1.74; $P < .001$) for the entire cohort, 1.50 (95% CI, 1.14–1.98; $P = .004$) from 2011 to 2015, 1.61 (95% CI, 1.35–1.91; $P < .001$) from 2006 to 2010, 1.59 (95% CI, 1.27–1.99; $P < .001$) in North America, 1.50 (95% CI, 1.24–1.81; $P < .001$) in Europe, 1.63 (95% CI, 1.31–2.02; $P < .001$) for randomized, and 1.44 (95% CI, 1.20–1.73; $P < .001$) for nonrandomized comparative studies. This study reported an associated decreased risk of transient ischemic attacks with CEA at 30 days (RR, 2.07; 95% CI, 1.50–2.85; $P < .001$) and restenosis at 1 year (RR, 1.97; 95% CI, 1.28–3.05; $P = .002$). Data from follow-up showed that the risk ratios of stroke or death were 0.74 (95% CI, 0.55–0.99; $P = .04$) at 1 year, 1.24 (95% CI, 1.04–1.46; $P = .01$) at 4 years, and 2.27 (95% CI, 1.39–3.71; $P = .001$) at 10 years. This study concluded that CEA is superior to CAS for freedom from stroke/death within 30 days, especially from 2006 to 2015, in North America and Europe. Meanwhile, superiority was also observed for restenosis at 1 year, transient ischemic attacks within 30 days, and stroke/death at the 4- and 10-year follow-up visits.

Repeat Carotid Endarterectomy Versus Carotid Artery Stenting for Patients with Restenosis After Carotid Endarterectomy: Systematic Review and Metaanalysis

Another metaanalysis [40] included 9 comparative studies and 41 noncomparative studies of 4399 patients. This report showed no beneficial differences in the 1-month perioperative mortality, stroke, and transient ischemic attack rates in the comparative studies ($P > .05$) and the noncomparative studies ($P > .05$). Patients undergoing redo CEA suffered more cranial nerve injuries than those undergoing CAS ($P < .05$), but most of these cases recovered within 3 months. Patients treated with redo CEA exhibited similar MI rates to those treated with CAS in the comparative studies ($P = .53$), but the rate was higher in the noncomparative studies ($P < .01$). However, a nonsignificant difference was noted in the freedom from stroke at 36 months in the comparative studies ($P = .47$) and at 12 months in the noncomparative studies ($P = .89$). The risk of restenosis was greater in CAS patients than in the redo CEA patients ($P < .05$ for comparative and noncomparative studies). This study concluded that both redo CEA and CAS are safe and feasible options after CEA. Although the incidences of cranial nerve injuries and MI were increased in the redo CEA group, most of the cranial nerve injury cases were reversible. Patients treated with CAS were more likely to develop restenosis than those treated with redo CEA over long-term follow-up.

Society for Vascular Surgery Carotid Vascular Registry: Carotid Artery Stenting Versus Carotid Endarterectomy Outcome Comparison

The 30-day outcomes in symptomatic patients (n = 1151) are summarized in Table 7. As noted, the combined death, stroke, and MI rate was twice as high for CAS as for CEA (7.1% vs 3.8%; *P* = .014). Similar observations were noted in other endpoints, including death and stroke. The 30-day outcomes of asymptomatic patients (n = 1667) are summarized in Table 8 [41].

Other Negative Predictors for Carotid Artery Stenting

Recently, several studies have indicated that increasing age, female gender, and lesser operator experience have a negative impact on the results of CAS. Others have shown that CAS has a higher hospital cost, in comparison with CEA.

Effect of Age on Carotid Artery Stenting Results

Multiple studies have shown that age has a negative impact on CAS outcomes. Bonati and colleagues [42] reported the results of a study showing that age modifies the relative risk of CAS versus CEA for symptomatic carotid stenosis from a pooled analysis of EVA-3S, SPACE and ICSS trials. Individual data from all 3433 patients randomized and analyzed in these trials were pooled and the primary outcome event was stroke or death. The primary outcome event for CAS was 8.9% versus 5.8% for CEA (risk ratio of 1.53; *P* = .0006). Age was the only subgroup variable that significantly modified treatment effect. In patients less than 70 years of age, the 120-day stroke or death risk was 5.8% for CAS versus 5.7% for CEA. In patients greater than 70 years of age, there was an estimated 2-fold increase in risk with CAS over CEA (12% vs 5.9%; relative risk, 2.04; *P* = .00053). They concluded that CEA was safer in the short-term than CAS because of the increasing risk of stroke/death associated with CAS in patients greater than 70 years old. They felt that CAS should be avoided in older patients, but that CAS may be as safe as CEA in younger patients [42]. Similar observations were noted in a 2012 Cochrane review of a metaanalysis of randomized trials, where the subset of patients 70 years of age or greater had a 2-fold increased risk of perioperative stroke/death with CAS, compared with CEA (OR, 2.2; 95% CI,

Table 7
SVS carotid vascular registry: CAS versus CEA outcome comparison for symptomatic patients

30-d outcome (n = 1151)	CAS (n = 645), %	CEA (n = 506), %	*P* value
Combined death/stroke/MI	7.1	3.8	.014
Death	2	0.8	.091
Stroke	5.3	2.4	.015
MI	0.9	0.6	.739
TIA	2.0	1.4	.499

Abbreviations: CAS, carotid artery stenting; CEA, carotid endarterectomy; MI, myocardial infarction; SVS, Society for Vascular Surgery; TIA, transient ischemic attack.

From Sidawy AN, Zwolak RM, White RA, et al. Risk-adjusted 30-day outcomes of carotid stenting and endarterectomy: results from the SVS vascular registry. J Vasc Surg 2009;49:71–9; with permission.

Table 8
SVS carotid vascular registry: CAS versus CEA outcome comparison for asymptomatic patients

30-d outcome (n = 1667)	CAS (n = 805), %	CEA (n = 862), %	*P* value
Combined death/stroke/MI	4.6	2.0	.003
Death	2.0	0.7	.030
Stroke	2.1	1.3	.252
MI	1.4	0.6	.131
TIA	1.2	0.5	.107

Abbreviations: CAS, carotid artery stenting; CEA, carotid endarterectomy; MI, myocardial infarction; SVS, Society for Vascular Surgery; TIA, transient ischemic attack.
From Sidawy AN, Zwolak RM, White RA, et al. Risk-adjusted 30-day outcomes of carotid stenting and endarterectomy: results from the SVS vascular registry. J Vasc Surg 2009;49:71–9; with permission.

1.47–3.29) [43]. Similar findings were noted in a 2010 metaanalysis [31] and in the CREST trial. In a 2013 metaanalysis of observational studies, Antoniou and colleagues [44] found that CAS was associated with an increased incidence of stroke in elderly patients.

Effect of Gender on Carotid Artery Stenting Results

A CREST subgroup analysis showed that CAS had 2.5 times more strokes in women than CEA (HR, 2.6; $P = .013$). Because of this finding, a CREST subgroup analysis and the Society for Vascular Surgery (SVS) Registry suggest that CAS should currently be avoided in females and should only be done when CEA is contraindicated [45–47].

Recently, an analysis of 20,000 CEA and CAS for 2007 through 2009 showed similar conclusions. In an analysis of 16,576 asymptomatic and 1744 symptomatic CEA, and 1943 asymptomatic and 350 symptomatic CAS in women, CAS was associated with a higher stroke and combined stroke and death rates compared with CEA in both symptomatic and asymptomatic patients. The risk of endpoint of stroke/mortality was 1.7% higher in symptomatic patients and 3.4% higher in asymptomatic female patients for CAS versus CEA [47].

Carotid Artery Stenting Is More Costly than Carotid Endarterectomy

Donovan and colleagues [48] analyzed hospital reimbursement for CAS and CEA and concluded that CAS is more costly than CEA and cannot be considered cost effective in most patients. The reason for this was felt to be the increased cost of CAS materials ($9396 vs $6673 for CEA). A policy of CAS centralization, leading to lower complication rates, may translate into a reduction of overall CAS costs. Patient selection may also improve CAS cost effectiveness by cutting perioperative complications [46].

Should the United States Centers for Medicare and Medicaid Services Extend Reimbursement Indications for Carotid Artery Stenting?

On January 25, 2012, the Centers for Medicare and Medicaid Services held a meeting to consider whether or not to expand reimbursement for CAS to include patients with asymptomatic disease and low/standard surgical risk symptomatic carotid disease. Various opinions were widely available regarding the justification of such expanded reimbursement; however, more than 40 worldwide authorities from multidisciplinary groups signed a letter to clarify this issue and objected to expanding these indications. These authorities came from various specialties, including vascular surgery, neurology (neurosciences), neurointerventional radiology, interventional radiology, and imaging departments. They highlighted their rationale behind why Centers for Medicare and Medicaid Services should not approve or change reimbursement for CAS, which is summarized in the following:

- For asymptomatic patients, CREST data showed the rate of perioperative stroke or death or later ipsilateral stroke up to 4 years was 4.5% for patients who had CAS versus 2.7% for CEA (67% higher; $P = .07$) and outcome measured reached statistical significance when symptomatic patients were added (6.4% vs 4.7%, 36% higher; $P = .03$).
- Supporters for routine CAS for asymptomatic patients tried to use a higher incidence of perioperative MI associated with CEA to justify a higher stroke/death risk with CAS. However, the groups felt this was invalid and distracting, because the main purpose of carotid intervention is prevention of stroke. Furthermore, a large proportion of patients who suffered perioperative MI associated with CAS, compared with CEA, died during follow-up.
- CAS has higher procedural costs than CEA. Because about 90% of CAS are for asymptomatic disease, this results in unnecessary risk and unjustified expenditures of at least $1 to $2 billion in health care expenditures each year. Extending approved indications for CAS will open floodgates for widespread CAS and expose patients to unnecessary risks and unjustifiable health care expenditures.
- CAS for symptomatic patients is also felt to be inappropriate because actual CREST data, and most other randomized trial data, metaanalyses, and registry data do not justify this presumed equivalence of CAS and CEA for symptomatic patients. CAS, overall, was associated with about double the 30-day, 120-day, 6-month, and/or 4-year risk of stroke/death compared with CEA, particularly in patients greater than 70 years of age. CAS is also associated with a much greater perioperative risk of brain damage detecting ischemic lesions than CEA and a higher incidence of carotid restenosis
- In summary, these authorities felt that the evidence does not support broadening reimbursement of CAS to routine management of patients with asymptomatic carotid disease or symptomatic carotid disease at low or standard risk from CEA, at least at the present time [49].

Guidelines of Various Specialties in Treating Carotid Artery Stenosis and the Differences in Their Recommendations for the Role of Carotid Artery Stenting

Five different specialty guidelines were published in 2011. These included the American College of Cardiology/American Heart Association (ACC/AHA) [50], the Society for Vascular Surgery [51], European Society of Cardiology

[52], Intercollegiate Committee of the RACP (ANZN, CSANZ, RACS, ANZSVS, RANZCR) [53], and the UK National Institute for Health and Clinical Excellence [54]. These guidelines vary in their recommendation in both the symptomatic and asymptomatic carotid artery stenosis.

For Symptomatic Carotid Artery Stenosis

The ACC/AHA guidelines recommended that CAS be used as an alternative to CEA in treating patients with symptomatic artery stenosis. They concluded that CAS is equivalent to CEA for these patients. However, in symptomatic patients, CEA was associated with a lesser stroke and death rate, compared with CAS in all randomized controlled trials to date. Therefore, CAS should not be accepted at the present time as an equivalent alternative to CEA in most patients with symptomatic carotid stenosis. It is feasible that the ACC/AHA guidelines in their interpretation of the CREST trial, which combined both symptomatic and asymptomatic patients that there was no difference in the estimated 4-year rate of primary endpoints (combined stroke, MI, and death) between CAS and CEA [55]. However, when each specific endpoint was analyzed, CAS was associated with nonsignificant (owing to small number), but a greater than 2-fold higher risk of periprocedural death (9 for CAS vs 4 deaths for CEA, respectively), a HR of 2.25, a significant P value of .01) and almost 2-fold increased risk of any perioperative stroke rate (52 vs 29 stroke for CAS vs CEA, respectively; HR, 1.79) and a highly significant greater than 2-fold increased risk of minor ipsilateral stroke (37 for CAS vs 17 for CEA, respectively; HR, 2.16; $P = .009$), compared with CEA. On the other hand, patients undergoing CAS, admittedly, suffered fewer MIs compared with those undergoing CEA (14 vs 28, HR, 0.50; $P = .03$).

The SVS and the Australian guidelines [51,53] specifically recommended CAS only for symptomatic patients who are at high risk for CEA, for example, scarred necks (status post previous endarterectomy), tracheal stoma, external beam radiotherapy, previous cranial nerve injury, and other medical comorbidities. Meanwhile, the European Society of Cardiology guidelines [52] provided a weak recommendation for CAS as an alternative CEA only in high surgical risk symptomatic patients or high-volume centers with documented stroke/death rates of less than 6%.

It should be noted that before publishing the ACC/AHA, the SVS Executive Committee raised the issue of rewriting the word "alternative" (for CAS vs CEA); however, the ACC/AHA guidelines committee felt it would be counterproductive because the document would have to be returned to all 16 sponsoring societies for altering that single word. Because of this decision, the SVS updated their guidelines [51] and clarified that issue accordingly.

For Asymptomatic Carotid Artery Stenosis

The ACC/AHA guidelines [50] felt that CAS may be considered as an option for asymptomatic carotid stenosis (class II-B, level I evidence B); in contrast, both the SVS [51] and the Australian [53] guidelines indicated that there is currently insufficient evidence to recommend CAS for asymptomatic stenosis. Similarly, the National Institute for Health and Clinical Excellence guidelines indicated that clinicians wishing to undertake CAS for asymptomatic carotid stenosis should insure that patients understand that the uncertainty about the procedure efficacy, the risk of complications, including stroke, and the reason for advising CAS rather than CEA or best medical treatment alone in their particular case [54]. The European Society of Cardiology guidelines gave class II-A recommendation for CEA and class II-B recommendation for CAS in asymptomatic patients [52]. They also emphasized that, for CAS to be performed for asymptomatic carotid stenosis, it should be done by providers in high-volume centers with documented stroke and death rates of less than 3%.

Recent Carotid Artery Stenting Data: Using the Enroute Transcarotid System (Investigation of Transcarotid CAS With Dynamic Flow Reversal in Subjects With Significant Extracranial Carotid Stenosis [ROADSTER Trial])

This prospective multicenter investigational device exemption (IDE) study designed to evaluate safety and effectiveness of the Enroute transcarotid neuroprotection system in a hybrid procedure (combined the best elements of CEA and CAS). The primary endpoint was combined stroke, death, and MI at 30 days. Direct access to the carotid artery, potentially reducing the risk of stroke by diverting debris away from the brain with surgery, inspired the mechanism to temporarily reverse blood flow was used. The study enrolled 208 symptomatic and asymptomatic patients who are high risk for CEA (26% were symptomatic), and 47% of patients were over 75 years of age. The 30-day stroke, death, and MI rates were 3.5% in intention-to-treat (n = 141) and 2.9% in per-protocol patients (n = 136). The stroke/death rate was 2.8% in intention-to-treat versus 2.2% in the per-protocol population. The rate of all stroke was 1.4% in the intention-to-treat and 0.7% in the per-protocol population. The investigators concluded that the stroke rates in high-surgical risk patients were the lowest to date for CAS and comparable with periprocedural rates in standard surgical risk patients for CEA [56].

Final Recommendation for the Role of Carotid Artery Stenting Versus Carotid Endarterecomy

1. The majority of patients with carotid stenosis who are candidates for intervention: CEA is preferred to CAS (grade I, level of evidence B) [51,55].
2. Data from CREST suggest that patients less than 70 year of age may do as well with CAS as CEA, but the data need further confirmation.
3. CEA is preferred over CAS in patients who are over 70 years of age (grade I, level of evidence A).
4. CAS is preferred over CEA in symptomatic patients with greater than 50% stenosis and prior ipsilateral CEA, tracheal stoma, external irradiation, prior cranial nerve injury, or high cervical lesion (grade 2, level of evidence B).

5. CAS is preferred over CEA in symptomatic patients with greater than 50% stenosis with severe and correctible coronary artery disease, congestive heart failure, and chronic obstruction pulmonary disease.
6. Presently, there are insufficient data to recommend CAS as the primary treatment for asymptomatic patients with 70% or greater stenosis, particularly those at low risk for CEA.
7. A similar recommendation can be made for asymptomatic patients with high surgical risk, at least at the present time.
8. Neurologically asymptomatic patients deemed at high-risk for CEA should be considered for primary medical treatment at this stage.

SUMMARY

For symptomatic de novo carotid stenosis in low-risk patients, CEA remains the standard of care. The use of CAS should be selective at this stage and must be done by experienced operators at experienced centers. CAS is better therapy for symptomatic patients who are at high surgical risk (anatomic/physiologic), for example, high cervical lesions (above C2) and previous irradiation for CEA. CAS may also be preferable in most patients with post-CEA restenosis. The value of CAS in high surgical risk asymptomatic patients is questionable at this stage. CAS with the flow reversal system may change these rules in the future.

References

[1] Inzitari D, Eliasziw M, Gates P, et al. The causes and risk of stroke in patients with asymptomatic internal-carotid-artery stenosis. North American Symptomatic Carotid Endarterectomy Trial Collaborators. N Engl J Med 2000;342(23):1693–700.

[2] North American Symptomatic Carotid Endaraterectomy Trial Collaborators. Beneficial effect of carotid endarterectomy in symptomatic patients with high-grade carotid stenosis. N Engl J Med 1991;325(7):445–53.

[3] Endarterectomy for asymptomatic carotid artery stenosis. Executive Committee for the Asymptomatic Carotid Atherosclerosis Study. JAMA 1995;273(18):1421–8.

[4] Kerber CW, Cromwell LD, Loehden OL. Catheter dilatation of proximal carotid stenosis during distal bifurcation endarterectomy. AJNR Am J Neuroradiol 1980;1(4):348–9.

[5] Brott TG, Hobson RW 2nd, Howard G, et al, CREST Investigators. Stenting versus Endarterectomy for Treatment of Carotid-Artery Stenosis. N Engl J Med 2010;363:11–23.

[6] Ederle J, Bonati LH, Dobson J, et al. Endovascular treatment with angioplasty or stenting versus endarterectomy in patients with carotid artery stenosis in the Carotid and Vertebral Artery Transluminal Angioplasty Study (CAVATAS): long-term follow-up of a randomised trial. Lancet Neurol 2009;8(10):898–907.

[7] Yadav JS, Wholey MH, Kuntz RE, et al. Protected carotid-artery stenting versus endarterectomy in high-risk patients. N Engl J Med 2004;351(15):1493–501.

[8] Mas JL, Chatellier G, Beyssen B, et al. Endarterectomy versus stenting in patients with symptomatic severe carotid stenosis. N Engl J Med 2006;355(16):1660–71.

[9] Mas JL, Chatellier G, Beyssen B, et al. Carotid angioplasty and stenting with and without cerebral protection: clinical alert from the Endarterectomy Versus Angioplasty in Patients With Symptomatic Severe Carotid Stenosis (EVA-3S) trial. Stroke 2004;35(1):e18–20.

[10] Mas JL, Arquizan C, Calvet D, et al. Long-term follow-up study of endarterectomy versus angioplasty in patients with symptomatic severe carotid stenosis trial. Stroke 2014;45(9):2750–6.

[11] SPACE Collaborative Group, Ringleb PA, Allenberg J, Bruckmann H, et al. 30 day results from the SPACE trial of stent-protected angioplasty versus carotid endarterectomy in symptomatic patients: a randomised non-inferiority trial. Lancet 2006;368(9543):1239–47.
[12] Hacke W, Brown MM, Mas JL. Carotid endarterectomy versus stenting: an international perspective [author reply]. Stroke 2006;37(2):344.
[13] Bonati LH, Dobson J, Featherstone RL, et al. Long-term outcomes after stenting versus endarterectomy for treatment of symptomatic carotid stenosis: the International Carotid Stenting Study (ICSS) randomised trial. Lancet 2015;385(9967):529–38.
[14] Naylor AR. Endarterectomy versus carotid stenting. Br J Surg 2012;99(2):149–51.
[15] Alberts MJ. Results of a multicenter prospective randomized trial of carotid artery stenting vs carotid endarterectomy [abstract]. Stroke 2001;32:325-d. Available at: http://stroke-meeting.ahajournals.org/cgi/content/abstract/32/325-3.
[16] Brooks WH, McClure RR, Jones MR, et al. Carotid angioplasty and stenting versus carotid endarterectomy: randomized trial in a community hospital. J Am Coll Cardiol 2001;38(6):1589–95.
[17] Gurm HS, Yadav JS, Fayad P, et al. Long-term results of carotid stenting versus endarterectomy in high-risk patients. N Engl J Med 2008;358(15):1572–9.
[18] Eckstein HH, Ringleb P, Allenberg JR, et al. Results of the Stent-Protected Angioplasty versus Carotid Endarterectomy (SPACE) study to treat symptomatic stenoses at 2 years: a multinational, prospective, randomised trial. Lancet Neurol 2008;7(10):893–902 [Erratum appears in Lancet Neurol 2009;8(2):135].
[19] Endovascular versus surgical treatment in patients with carotid stenosis in the Carotid and Vertebral Artery Transluminal Angioplasty Study (CAVATAS): a randomised trial. Lancet 2001;357:1729–37.
[20] International Carotid Stenting Study Investigators, Ederle J, Dobson J, Featherstone RL, et al. Carotid artery stenting compared with endarterectomy in patients with symptomatic carotid stenosis (International Carotid Stenting Study): an interim analysis of a randomised controlled trial. Lancet 2010;375:985–97.
[21] Qureshi AI, Kirmani JF, Divani AA, et al. Carotid angioplasty with or without stent placement versus carotid endarterectomy for treatment of carotid stenosis: a meta-analysis. Neurosurgery 2005;56:1171–81.
[22] Ederle J, Featherstone RL, Brown MM. Percutaneous transluminal angioplasty and stenting for carotid artery stenosis. Cochrane Database Syst Rev 2007;(4):CD000515.
[23] Wiesmann M, Schopf V, Jansen O, et al. Stent-protected angioplasty versus carotid endarterectomy in patients with carotid artery stenosis: meta-analysis of randomized trial data. Eur Radiol 2008;18:2956–66.
[24] Murad MH, Flynn DN, Elamin MG, et al. Endarterectomy vs stenting for carotid artery stenosis: a systematic review and meta-analysis. J Vasc Surg 2008;48:487–93.
[25] Ringleb PA, Chatellier G, Hacke W, et al. Safety of endovascular treatment of carotid artery stenosis compared with surgical treatment: a meta-analysis. J Vasc Surg 2008;47:350–5.
[26] Jeng JS, Liu HM, Tu YK. Carotid angioplasty with or without stenting versus carotid endarterectomy for carotid artery stenosis: a meta-analysis. J Neurol Sci 2008;270:40–7.
[27] Brahmanandam S, Ding EL, Conte MS, et al. Clinical results of carotid artery stenting compared with carotid endarterectomy. J Vasc Surg 2008;47:343–9.
[28] Gurm HS, Nallamothu BK, Yadav J. Safety of carotid artery stenting for symptomatic carotid artery disease: a meta-analysis. Eur Heart J 2008;29:113–9.
[29] Liu Z, Shi Z, Wang Y, et al. Carotid artery stenting versus carotid endarterectomy: systematic review and meta-analysis. World J Surg 2009;33:586–96.
[30] Roffi M, Mukherjee D, Clair DG. Carotid artery stenting vs. endarterectomy. Eur Heart J 2009;30:2693–704.
[31] Carotid Stenting Trialists' Collaboration, Bonati LH, Dobson J, Algra A, et al. Short-term outcome after stenting versus endarterectomy for symptomatic carotid stenosis: a preplanned meta-analysis of individual patient data. Lancet 2010;376(9746):1062–73.

[32] Meier P, Knapp G, Tamhane U, et al. Short term and intermediate term comparison of endarterectomy versus stenting for carotid artery stenosis: systematic review and meta-analysis of randomised controlled clinical trials. BMJ 2010;340:c467 [Erratum appears in BMJ 2010;340:c1798].
[33] Economopoulos KP, Sergentanis TN, Tsivgroulis G, et al. Carotid artery stenting versus carotid endarterectomy: a comprehensive meta-analysis of short-term and long-term outcomes. Stroke 2011;42:687–92.
[34] Bangalore S, Kumar S, Wetterslev J, et al. Carotid artery stenting vs carotid endarterectomy: meta-analysis and diversity-adjusted trial sequential analysis of randomized trials. Arch Neurol 2011;68:172–84.
[35] Yavin D, Roberts DJ, Tso M, et al. Carotid endarterectomy versus stenting: a meta-analysis of randomized trials. Can J Neurol Sci 2011;38:230–5.
[36] Jalbert JJ, Nguyen LL, Gerhard-Herman MD, et al. Outcomes after carotid artery stenting in Medicare beneficiaries, 2005 to 2009. JAMA Neurol 2015;72(3):276–86.
[37] Kim LK, Yang DC, Swaminathan RV, et al. Comparison of trends and outcomes of carotid artery stenting and endarterectomy in the United States, 2001 to 2010. Circ Cardiovasc Interv 2014;7:692–700.
[38] McDonald RJ, McDonald JS, Therneau TM, et al. Comparative effectiveness of carotid revascularization therapies: evidence from a National Hospital Discharge Database. Stroke 2014;45(11):3311–9.
[39] Zhang L, Zhao Z, Ouyang Y, et al. Systematic review and meta-analysis of carotid artery stenting versus endarterectomy for carotid stenosis: a chronological and worldwide study. Medicine (Baltimore) 2015;94(26):e1060.
[40] Tu J, Wang S, Huo Z, et al. Repeated carotid endarterectomy versus carotid artery stenting for patients with carotid restenosis after carotid endarterectomy: Systematic review and meta-analysis. Surgery 2015;157(6):1166–73.
[41] Sidawy AN, Zwolak RM, White RA, et al. Outcomes Committee for the Society for Vascular Surgery. Risk-adjusted 30-day outcomes of carotid stenting and endarterectomy: results from the SVS Vascular Registry. J Vasc Surg 2009;49(1):71–9.
[42] Bonati LH, Fraedrich G. Carotid Stenting Trialists C. Age modifies the relative risk of stenting versus endarterectomy for symptomatic carotid stenosis–a pooled analysis of EVA-3S, SPACE and ICSS. Eur J Vasc Endovasc Surg 2011;41(2):153–8.
[43] Bonati LH, Lyrer P, Ederle J, et al. Percutaneous transluminal balloon angioplasty and stenting for carotid artery stenosis. Cochrane Database Syst Rev 2012;(9):CD000515.
[44] Antoniou GA, Georgiadis GS, Georgakarakos EI, et al. Meta-analysis and meta-regression analysis of outcomes of carotid endarterectomy and stenting in the elderly. JAMA Surg 2013;148(12):1140–52.
[45] Howard VJ, Lutsep HL, Mackey A, et al, CREST Investigators. Influence of sex on outcomes of stenting versus endarterectomy: a subgroup analysis of the Carotid Revascularization Endarterectomy versus Stenting Trial (CREST). Lancet Neurol 2011;10(6):530–7.
[46] Paraskevas KI, Moore WS, Veith FJ. Commentary: carotid artery stenting: still not as cost-effective as carotid endarterectomy, but the contest continues. J Endovasc Ther 2014;21(2):303–5.
[47] Vouyouka AG, Egorova NN, Sosunov EA, et al. Analysis of Florida and New York state hospital discharges suggests that carotid stenting in symptomatic women is associated with significant increase in mortality and perioperative morbidity compared with carotid endarterectomy. J Vasc Surg 2012;56(2):334–42.
[48] Donovan MJ, Ramirez DE, Crenshaw GD, et al. Hospital reimbursement for carotid stenting and endarterectomy. J Endovasc Ther 2014;21(2):296–302.
[49] Veith FJ. CMS considers expanding reimbursement for carotid stenting. Vascular 2012;20:1–11.
[50] Brott TG, Halperin JL, Abbara S, et al. 2011 ASA/ACCF/AHA/AANN/AANS/ACR/ASNR/CNS/SAIP/SCAI/SIR/SNIS/SVM/SVS guidelines on the management of patients

with extracranial carotid and vertebral artery disease. A report of the American College of Cardiology Foundation/American Heart Association Task Force on Practice Guidelines, and the American Stroke Association, American Association of Neuroscience Nurses, American Association of Neurological Surgeons, American College of Radiology, American Society of Neuroradiology, Congress of Neurological Surgeons, Society of Atherosclerosis Imaging and Prevention, Society for Cardiovascular Angiography and Interventions, Society of Interventional Radiology, Society of NeuroInterventional Surgery, Society for Vascular Medicine, and Society for Vascular Surgery. Circulation 2011;124:e54–130.

[51] Ricotta JJ, AbuRahma A, Ascher E, et al, Society for Vascular Surgery. Updated Society for Vascular Surgery guidelines for management of extracranial carotid disease. J Vasc Surg 2011;54:e1–31.

[52] Authors/Task Force Members, Tendera M, Aboyans V, et al. ESC Guidelines on the diagnosis and treatment of peripheral artery diseases. Eur Heart J 2011;32:2851–906.

[53] Carotid Stenting Guidelines Committee: An Intercollegiate Committee of the RACP (ANZAN, CSANZ), RACS (ANZSVS) and RANZCR. Guidelines for patient selection and performance of carotid artery stenting. Intern Med J 2011;41:344–7.

[54] UK National Institute for Health and Clinical Excellence. Carotid artery stent placement for asymptomatic carotid artery stenosis. 2011. Available at: http://www.nice.org.uk/nicemedia/live/13026/54241/54241.pdf. Accessed October 17, 2001.

[55] Mohler ER III, Fairman RM. Management of symptomatic carotid atherosclerotic disease. UpToDate; 2014. Available at: www.uptodate.com.

[56] Kwolek CJ, Jaff MR, Leal JI, et al. Results of the ROADSTER multicenter trial of transcarotid stenting with dynamic flow reversal. J Vasc Surg 2015;62:1227–34.

FSC
www.fsc.org
MIX
Papier | Fördert
gute Waldnutzung
FSC® C083411

Kolibri 360 GmbH
Ferdinand-Jühlke-Straße 7
99095 Erfurt, Deutschland
produktsicherheit@kolibri360.de